# Ultrasonography in Gynecology and Early Pregnancy

*Editors*

LAWRENCE D. PLATT
CHRISTINA S. HAN

## OBSTETRICS AND GYNECOLOGY CLINICS OF NORTH AMERICA

www.obgyn.theclinics.com

*Consulting Editor*
WILLIAM F. RAYBURN

December 2019 • Volume 46 • Number 4

**ELSEVIER**

1600 John F. Kennedy Boulevard • Suite 1800 • Philadelphia, Pennsylvania, 19103-2899

http://www.theclinics.com

**OBSTETRICS AND GYNECOLOGY CLINICS OF NORTH AMERICA Volume 46, Number 4**
**December 2019 ISSN 0889-8545, ISBN-13: 978-0-323-70908-8**

Editor: Kerry Holland
Developmental Editor: Kristen Helm



*Obstetrics and Gynecology Clinics* (ISSN 0889-8545) is published quarterly by Elsevier Inc., 360 Park Avenue South, New York, NY 10010-1710. Months of issue are March, June, September, and December. Periodicals postage paid at New York, NY, and additional mailing offices. Subscription price per year is $322.00 (US individuals), $685.00 (US institutions), $100.00 (US students), $404.00 (Canadian individuals), $865.00 (Canadian institutions), $225.00 (Canadian students), $459.00 (international individuals), $865.00 (international institutions), and $225.00 (international students). To receive student/resident rate, orders must be accompanied by name of affiliated institution, date of term, and the signature of program/residency coordinator on institution letterhead. Orders will be billed at individual rate until proof of status is received. Foreign air speed delivery is included in all *Clinics* subscription prices. All prices are subject to change without notice. POSTMASTER: Send address changes to *Obstetrics and Gynecology Clinics*, Elsevier Health Sciences Division, Subscription Customer Service, 3251 Riverport Lane, Maryland Heights, MO 63043. **Customer Service: Telephone: 1-800-654-2452 (U.S. and Canada); 314-447-8871 (outside U.S. and Canada). Fax: 314-447-8029. E-mail: journalscustomerservice-usa@elsevier.com (for print support); journalsonlinesupport-usa@elsevier.com (for online support).**

*Reprints.* For copies of 100 or more of articles in this publication, please contact the Commercial Reprints Department, Elsevier Inc., 360 Park Avenue South, New York, New York 10010-1710. Tel.: 212-633-3874; Fax: 212-633-3820; E-mail: reprints@elsevier.com.

*Obstetrics and Gynecology Clinics of North America* is also published in Spanish by McGraw-Hill Interamericana Editores S.A., P.O. Box 5-237, 06500, Mexico; in Portuguese by Reichmann and Affonso Editores, Rio de Janeiro, Brazil; and in Greek by Paschalidis Medical Publications, Athens, Greece.

*Obstetrics and Gynecology Clinics of North America is covered in MEDLINE/PubMed (Index Medicus), Excerpta Medica, Current Concepts/Clinical Medicine, Science Citation Index, BIOSIS, CINAHL, and ISI/BIOMED.*

# Contributors

## CONSULTING EDITOR

**WILLIAM F. RAYBURN, MD, MBA**
Associate Dean, Continuing Medical Education and Professional Development, Distinguished Professor and Emeritus Chair, Obstetrics and Gynecology, University of New Mexico School of Medicine, Albuquerque, New Mexico, USA

## EDITORS

**LAWRENCE D. PLATT, MD**
Clinical Professor, Division of Maternal-Fetal Medicine, Department of Obstetrics and Gynecology, David Geffen School of Medicine, University of California, Los Angeles, Center for Fetal Medicine and Women's Ultrasound, Los Angeles, California, USA

**CHRISTINA S. HAN, MD**
Associate Clinical Professor, MFM Fellowship Program Director, David Geffen School of Medicine, University of California, Los Angeles, Center for Fetal Medicine and Women's Ultrasound, Los Angeles, California, USA

## AUTHORS

**YALDA AFSHAR, MD, PhD**
Assistant Professor, Division of Maternal-Fetal Medicine, Department of Obstetrics and Gynecology, University of California, Los Angeles, Los Angeles, California, USA

**BERYL R. BENACERRAF, MD**
Clinical Professor of OB/GYN and Radiology, Harvard Medical School, Brigham & Women's Hospital, Brookline, Massachusetts, USA

**BRYANN BROMLEY, MD**
Department of Obstetrics and Gynecology, Massachusetts General Hospital, Harvard Medical School, Boston, Massachusetts, USA; Diagnostic Ultrasound Associates, Brookline, Massachusetts, USA

**GIUSEPPE CALÌ, MD**
Department of Obstetrics and Gynaecology, Arnas Civico Hospital, Palermo, Italy

**STUART CAMPBELL, DSc(Lon), FRCPE, FROG**
Director of Ultrasound, Create Fertility, London, United Kingdom

**JOSHUA A. COPEL, MD**
Professor of Obstetrics, Gynecology, and Reproductive Sciences and Pediatrics, Yale School of Medicine, New Haven, Connecticut, USA

**FRANCESCO D'ANTONIO, MD**
Fetal Medicine Unit, Department of Obstetrics and Gynecology, University of Foggia, Foggia, Italy

**VERED H. EISENBERG, MD, MHA**
Department of Obstetrics and Gynecology, Medical Assistant to the Associate Director General of the Sheba Medical Center, Sheba Medical Center, Tel Hashomer, Israel; Sackler Faculty of Medicine, Tel Aviv University, Tel Aviv, Israel

**ADAM T. EVANS, MD**
Resident, Department of Obstetrics and Gynecology, University of Rochester Medical Center, Rochester, New York, USA

**WOUTER FROYMAN, MD**
Department of Development and Regeneration, KU Leuven, Department of Obstetrics and Gynecology, University Hospitals Leuven, Leuven, Belgium

**PHYLLIS GLANC, MD, FRCPC**
Professor, University of Toronto, Radiologist, Sunnybrook Health Sciences Centre, Toronto, Ontario, Canada

**STEVEN R. GOLDSTEIN, MD, FACOG**
New York University School of Medicine, New York, New York, USA

**KALESHA HACK, MD, FRCPC**
Clinician Teacher, University of Toronto, Radiologist, Sunnybrook Health Sciences Centre, Toronto, Ontario, Canada

**CHRISTINA S. HAN, MD**
Associate Clinical Professor, MFM Fellowship Program Director, David Geffen School of Medicine, University of California, Los Angeles, Center for Fetal Medicine and Women's Ultrasound, Los Angeles, California, USA

**ANDREA KAELIN AGTEN, MD**
Nottingham University Hospitals NHS, Nottingham, United Kingdom

**HADAS ALLOUCHE KAM, MD**
Department of Obstetrics and Gynecology, Hadassah Mount Scopus – Hebrew University Medical Center Jerusalem, Jerusalem, Israel

**ASHRAF KHAFAGA, MBBCh**
Icahn School of Medicine at Mount Sinai, New York, New York, USA

**MARTINA LEOMBRONI, MD**
Fondazione Policlinico Universitario Agostino Gemelli, IRCCS, Dipartimento Scienze della Salute della Donna, del Bambino e di Sanità Pubblica, Rome, Italy

**MAHAN MATHUR, MD**
Associate Professor of Radiology and Biomedical Imaging, Section of Body Imaging, Yale School of Medicine, New Haven, Connecticut, USA

**JENNY Y. MEI, MD**
Resident Physician, Department of Obstetrics and Gynecology, University of California, Los Angeles, Los Angeles, California, USA

**ANA MONTEAGUDO, MD**
Department of Obstetrics, Gynecology, and Reproductive Science, Icahn School of Medicine at Mount Sinai, New York, New York, USA

**FRANCESCA MORO, MD, PhD**
Fondazione Policlinico Universitario Agostino Gemelli, IRCCS, Dipartimento Scienze della Salute della Donna, del Bambino e di Sanità Pubblica, Rome, Italy

**LAWRENCE D. PLATT, MD**
Clinical Professor, Division of Maternal-Fetal Medicine, Department of Obstetrics and Gynecology, David Geffen School of Medicine, University of California, Los Angeles, Center for Fetal Medicine and Women's Ultrasound, Los Angeles, California, USA

**EMILY W. SCIBETTA, MD**
Department of Obstetrics and Gynecology, Harbor-UCLA Medical Center, Torrance, California, USA

**LESLIE M. SCOUTT, MD**
Professor of Radiology and Biomedical Imaging, Section of Ultrasound, Yale School of Medicine, New Haven, Connecticut, USA

**JAMES M. SHWAYDER, MD, JD**
President and CEO, Shwayder Consulting, LLC, Venice, Florida, USA

**HINDI STOHL, MD, JD**
Assistant Professor, Department of Obstetrics and Gynecology, Director of Perinatology and Obstetric Quality, Harbor-UCLA Medical Center, Torrance, California, USA

**KAM SZLACHETKA, RDMS, RDCS, RVT**
Chief Sonographer, Department of Obstetrics and Gynecology, University of Rochester Medical Center, Rochester, New York, USA

**ANTONIA CARLA TESTA, MD, PhD**
Fondazione Policlinico Universitario Agostino Gemelli, IRCCS, Dipartimento Scienze della Salute della Donna, del Bambino e di Sanità Pubblica, Università Cattolica del Sacro Cuore, Istituto di Ginecologia ed Ostetricia, Roma, Italy

**LORALEI L. THORNBURG, MD**
James R. Woods, Jr. Professor, Department of Obstetrics and Gynecology, University of Rochester Medical Center, Rochester, New York, USA

**DIRK TIMMERMAN, MD, PhD**
Department of Development and Regeneration, KU Leuven, Department of Obstetrics and Gynecology, University Hospitals Leuven, Leuven, Belgium

**ILAN E. TIMOR-TRITSCH, MD**
Department of Obstetrics and Gynecology, NYU School of Medicine, NYU Langone Health, New York, New York, USA

**SIMCHA YAGEL, MD**
Department of Obstetrics and Gynecology, Head of the Division of Obstetrics and Gynecology, Hadassah – Hebrew University Medical Centers, Director, Obstetrics and Gynecology Ultrasound Unit, Head of Center for Human Placenta Research, Jerusalem, Israel

# Contents

# OBSTETRICS AND GYNECOLOGY CLINICS

**FORTHCOMING ISSUES**

***March 2020***
**The Human Placenta in Health and Disease**
D. Michael Nelson and Leslie Myatt, *Editors*

***June 2020***
**Telemedicine and Connected Health in Obstetrics and Gynecology**
Curtis L. Lowery, Jr., *Editor*

***September 2020***
**New Postpartum Visit: Beginning of Lifelong Health**
Haywood Brown, *Editor*

**RECENT ISSUES**

***September 2019***
**Women's Preventive Health Care**
Jeanne Conry and Maureen Phipps, *Editors*

***June 2019***
**Patient Safety in Obstetrics and Gynecology**
Paul A. Gluck, *Editor*

***March 2019***
**Gynecologic Cancer Care: Innovative Progress**
Carolyn Y. Muller, *Editor*

# Foreword

# A Practical and Contemporary Guide to Gynecologic Ultrasonography

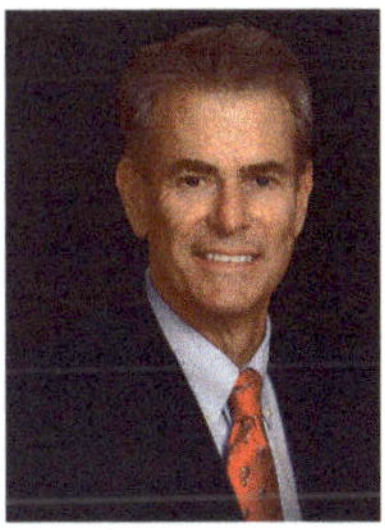

William F. Rayburn, MD
*Consulting Editor*

Being a maternal-fetal medicine specialist, I have devoted many years to fetal evaluation by direct sonographic visualization. Gynecologic ultrasound performance seemed to be less routine and more as an adjunct in confirming clinical suspicions. At last, we have an issue in *Obstetrics and Gynecology Clinics of North America* that addresses the many advances of ultrasonography in gynecology and early pregnancy. A repeat editorial overview by Dr Lawrence Platt with valuable input from the coeditor Dr Christina Han has led to the production of an excellent resource for any gynecologist.

This issue nicely covers the multiple indications for gynecologic ultrasound examination. Much needed discussions cover the following common clinical subjects: gynecologic and nongynecologic pelvic pain, natural or stimulated follicular development during interfertility therapy, intrauterine device localization, abnormal uterus and uterine bleeding, assessment of a pelvic and ovarian mass, pelvic floor dysfunction, endometriosis, and screening for malignancy. Diagnostic ultrasound examination has no direct harmful effects when used appropriately. Early pregnancy topics in this issue include viability, unknown or ectopic pregnancy, and evaluation of any prior cesarean scar. Coding and legal issues are nicely covered in the final article.

Sonography is an operator-dependent technology. Competence in gynecologic imaging can only be achieved by experience with many normal and abnormal examinations. The sonographer should know the indication for the examination and results of any other evaluations related to the patient's problem. This information is essential for focusing upon specific pelvic structures (ie, uterine size, shape, and orientation; endometrium, myometrium, and cervix; ovaries and adnexa; cul-de-sac), choosing a transabdominal or transvaginal technique or both, and deciding whether further evaluation is necessary. Impressions from real-time ultrasound examination can be enhanced, if

Obstet Gynecol Clin N Am 46 (2019) xiii–xiv
https://doi.org/10.1016/j.ogc.2019.08.004
0889-8545/19/© 2019 Published by Elsevier Inc.

necessary, by saline infusion sonohysterography, high-frequency transvaginal transducers, 3-dimensional sonography, or color Doppler velocimetry.

Transabdominal scanning is important for evaluating the upper pelvis and abdomen, such as with enlarged fibroids and ovaries extending above the pelvis. Transvaginal scanning may be insufficient, or pathology may be missed as the distance is increased from the area under investigation to the vagina. Translabial or transperineal ultrasound is being used increasingly to evaluate the pelvic floor of women with pelvic organ prolapse and urinary or anal incontinence. Pelvic floor sonography includes the evaluation of urethral diverticula, mesh location, residual urine volume, and rectal intussusception.

A written ultrasound report should be included in the patient's medical record and sent to the referring clinician in a timely manner. Consultative services to remote or resource-poor areas allow patient care to occur, which may not have happened otherwise. Significant imaging findings should be called and transmitted to the referring clinician to ensure and facilitate appropriate follow-up.

I appreciate Dr Platt and Dr Han for their efforts in assembling a group of well-known authors. A wealth of knowledge is covered in an easy-to-read format from published research spanning the past several years. Each article is well illustrated and comprehensive. The contributors provided their evidence-based interpretation of the current peer-review literature and, when appropriate, pushed the limits of technological advancements to educate the present and future generations of learners.

William F. Rayburn, MD
Continuing Medical Education and Professional Development
University of New Mexico School of Medicine
MSC 10 5580, 1 University of New Mexico
Albuquerque, NM 87131-0001, USA

*E-mail address:*
wrayburn@salud.unm.edu

# Preface

# Moving Ultrasound First in Women's Health

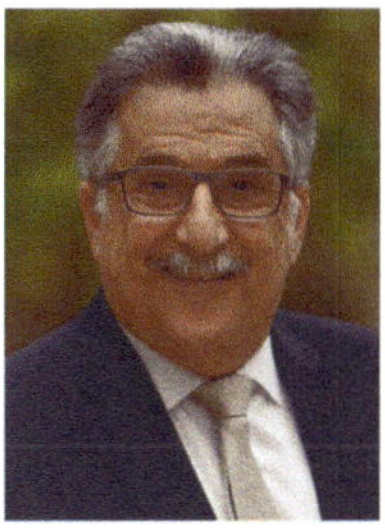

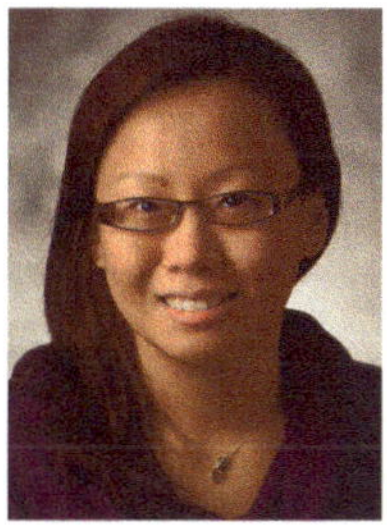

Lawrence D. Platt, MD Christina S. Han, MD
*Editors*

It is hard to believe that it was in 1984, and again in 1991, when one of us was a guest editor of the *Obstetrics and Gynecology Clinics of North America* on two issues focused on "Diagnostic Ultrasound." Within those 2 issues, there were only 3 articles that were dedicated to imaging in the nonpregnant woman. Thirty years later, we now have an entire issue focused on ultrasound in the gynecologic patient. Even with 17 articles allotted, we did not find sufficient room to fully cover the wealth of knowledge that has been accrued over the last few decades.

We are both honored to be part of this important contribution to the care of the gynecologic patient, and we are thankful for the input from so many world experts on the topic. These authors are each well known for being "frontline physicians," working daily to optimize patient care, conduct research, teach the next generation, and push the boundaries of technological advancements. What is deeply humbling is to know that some of these individuals were also contributors to the previously mentioned issues of *Obstetrics and Gynecology Clinics of North America*.

Within this issue, we aimed to cover all essential areas of sonographic imaging in gynecology. We followed the reproductive journey of the female patient by discussing normal and pathologic imaging of the pelvic organs, infertility and intrauterine contraceptives, and pregnancies of unknown locations. You will find articles on common pathologic conditions, such as endometriosis, abnormal uterine bleeding, pelvic floor dysfunction, and pelvic pain. We drew from the expertise of the "modern father" of ultrasound to provide 2 outstanding articles on the workup of the infertile patient. We included the groundbreaking work by the International Ovarian Tumor Analysis group, which provides "simple rules" for a systematic approach to evaluating ovarian masses. With the dramatic rise in cesarean rates over the past few decades, an important and new addition is a thorough discussion on evaluation of cesarean scar pregnancies, drawn from the world's leading experts.

Obstet Gynecol Clin N Am 46 (2019) xv–xvi
https://doi.org/10.1016/j.ogc.2019.08.003
0889-8545/19/© 2019 Published by Elsevier Inc.

Throughout this issue, we also focused on optimizing ultrasound imaging using technologies, such as high-frequency transvaginal transducers, color Doppler, and 3-dimensional ultrasound rendering. These technological advances have made the diagnosis of many pathologies, such as IUD localization and pregnancies of unknown locations, easier and safer. Last, as we all practice in the real world, we close with a practical article on coding and legal concerns in gynecologic imaging.

This issue would not be possible without the outstanding contributors who have made our job feel easy with their brilliant, comprehensive, beautifully illustrated, and easy-to-read articles. Working with the professional editors at Elsevier, especially Kristen Helm, could not have been a more efficient and streamlined process. We hope all of these combined efforts will prove beneficial to the current and future practitioners in women's health.

Lawrence D. Platt, MD
Center for Fetal Medicine and
Women's Ultrasound
Department of Obstetrics and Gynecology at
David Geffen School of Medicine at UCLA
6310 South San Vicente Boulevard
Suite 520
Los Angeles, CA 90048, USA

Christina S. Han, MD
Center for Fetal Medicine and
Women's Ultrasound
Department of Obstetrics and Gynecology at
David Geffen School of Medicine at UCLA
6310 South San Vicente Boulevard
Suite 520
Los Angeles, CA 90048, USA

*E-mail addresses:*
ldplatt@gmail.com (L.D. Platt)
chrishanmd@gmail.com (C.S. Han)

# Normal Pelvic Anatomy

James M. Shwayder, MD, JD*

**KEYWORDS**

- Pelvic ultrasonography • Doppler sonography • 3D sonography
- Sonohysterography

**KEY POINTS**

- Ultrasonography is the preferred imaging modality for gynecologic disorders.
- The vaginal and abdominal imaging approaches are complementary.
- Timing of the ultrasonographic study is critical in predicting the findings in reproductive women.
- Determining if organs move during an ultrasonographic examination is critical in predicting pelvic adhesions.

**Video content accompanies this article at http://www.obgyn.theclinics.com.**

Gynecologic ultrasonography has emerged as the preferred imaging technique in women.[1] It provides the ability to promptly evaluate patients and correlate one's clinical findings. The proximity of the pelvic anatomy via the vaginal approach allows the use of higher-frequency transducers, offering enhanced image resolution. There are circumstances in which pathology extends out of the pelvis or the pelvic anatomy is incompletely visualized, necessitating an abdominal imaging approach.[2] Thus, one must not confine the ultrasonographic assessment of the pelvis to one approach, recognizing that both approaches are complementary.

In premenopausal women, not on ovarian suppression, timing of the study critically affects the findings at ultrasonography.[3,4] Imaging a patient early in the menstrual cycle is considered ideal, as the endometrium is usually thin, less than 5 mm thick, and ovarian follicles are in a resting state, $\leq$10 mm in diameter (**Figs. 1** and **2**). At midcycle, at or near ovulation, the endometrium is approximately 10 mm thick and a dominant follicle approaches 20 to 24 mm in diameter (**Figs. 3** and **4**). Finally, in the luteal phase, the endometrium is 15 to 18 mm thick, with a corpus luteum in an ovary[4] (**Figs. 5** and **6**). A basic history, including the patient's pregnancy history, her last menstrual period, any hormone use or suppression, and any previous pelvic surgery, can help predict

Disclosure: J.M. Shwayder is a consultant for GE Ultrasound and Siemens Ultrasound.
Shwayder Consulting, LLC, Venice, FL, USA
* 13413 Orino Street, Venice, FL 34293.
*E-mail address:* jshwayder@hotmail.com

Obstet Gynecol Clin N Am 46 (2019) 563–580
https://doi.org/10.1016/j.ogc.2019.06.001

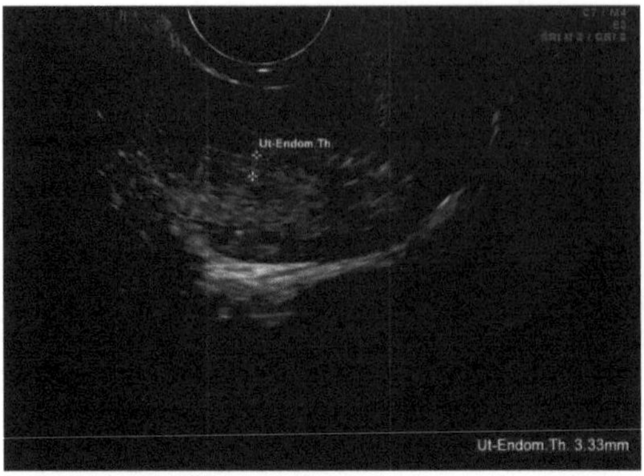


**Fig. 1.** Thin endometrium in the early proliferative phase of the menstrual cycle.

ultrasonographic findings and highlight those that are not consistent with the patient's menstrual cycle.

## VAGINAL VERSUS ABDOMINAL STUDIES

Vaginal ultrasonography is ideal for evaluation of the normal pelvis, as most target organs are in close proximity to the vagina, regardless of body habitus. This allows complete evaluation in many patients via the vaginal route only. In addition, vaginal ultrasonography is ideally performed with an empty bladder, which is also desired for a typical pelvic examination. The higher frequencies in vaginal transducers allows enhanced detailed imaging, but limits penetration to 10 to 12 cm. Thus, all relevant anatomy may not be adequately visualized using a vaginal sonographic approach, for example, nonvisualization of both ovaries, adnexal or ovarian masses rising out of the pelvis, or when the uterus is enlarged (**Figs. 7** and **8**). An abdominal approach may also be required with a uterus oriented in the midsagittal plane. Finally, ureteric obstruction due to endometriosis warrants evaluation of the kidneys for obstructive changes, for example, hydronephrosis. As opposed to previous practice, abdominal ultrasonography does not always require a distended bladder to visualize pertinent pelvic anatomy, although some patients, for example, pediatric or adolescent patients, often require a distended bladder for optimal visualization.

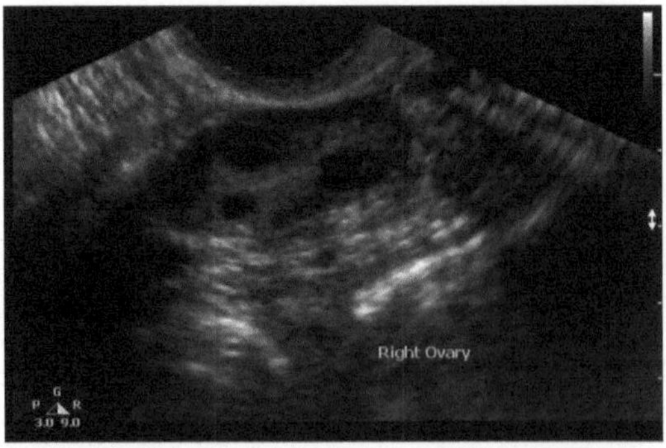


**Fig. 2.** Resting follicles in the early follicular phase of the menstrual cycle.

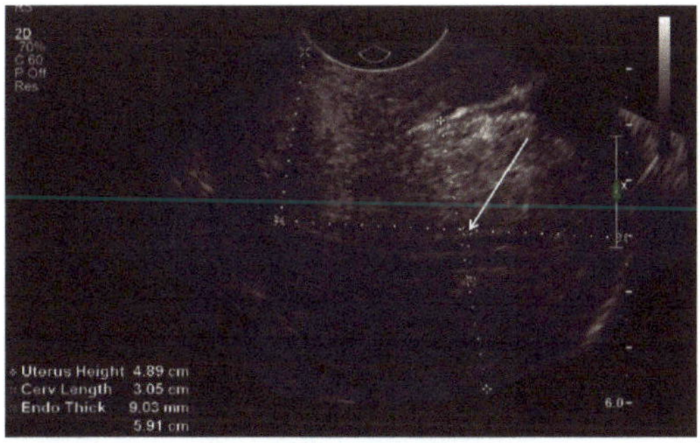


**Fig. 3.** Midcycle endometrium with trilaminar appearance (*arrow*).

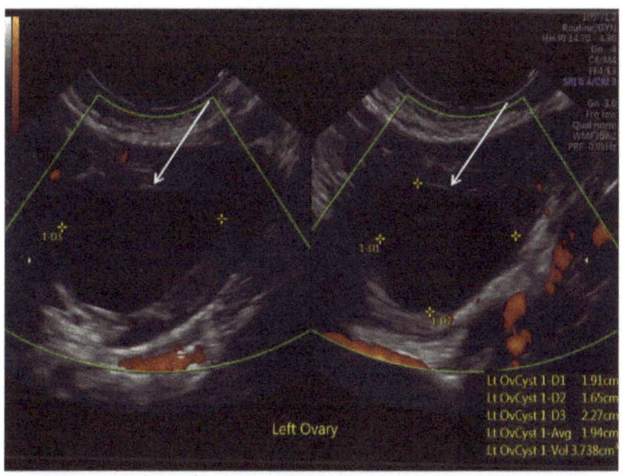


**Fig. 4.** Preovulatory follicle (*arrow*) at midcycle.

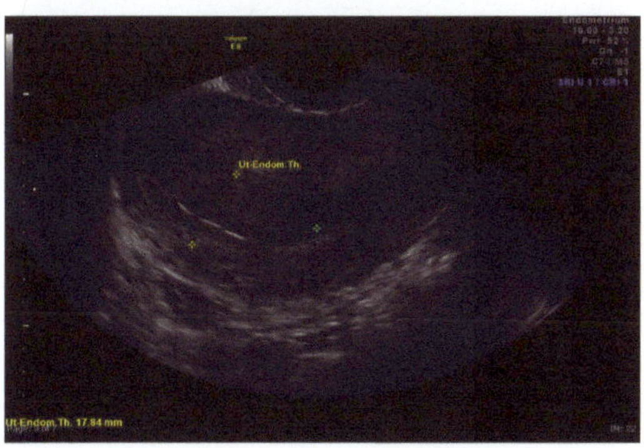


**Fig. 5.** Thickened endometrium is the secretory (luteal) phase.

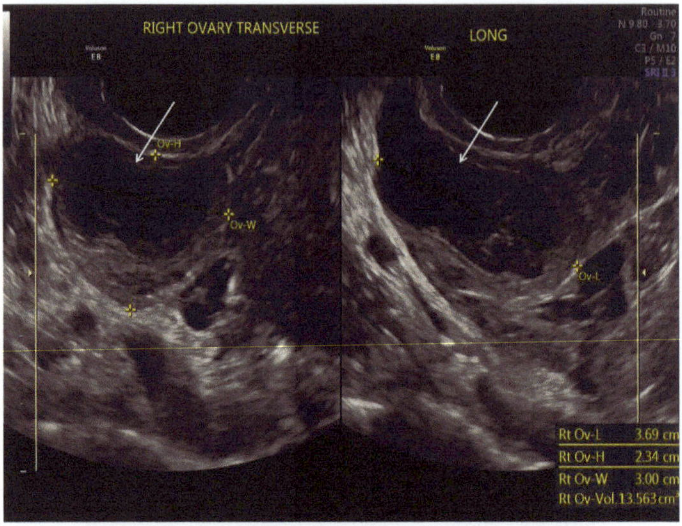


**Fig. 6.** Corpus luteum (*arrow*) during the luteal phase of the menstrual cycle.

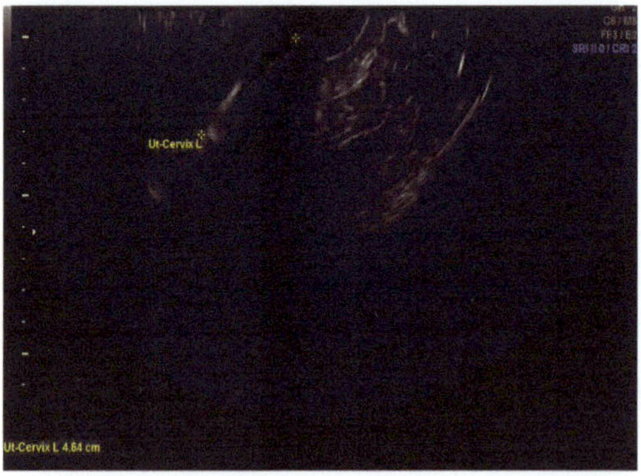


**Fig. 7.** Large fibroid uterus on vaginal ultrasound showing lack of adequate visualization of the uterus.

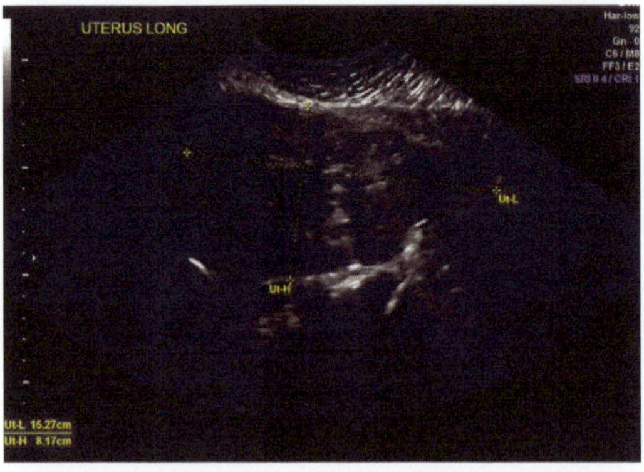


**Fig. 8.** Enlarged fibroid uterus with adequate visualization on abdominal ultrasonography.

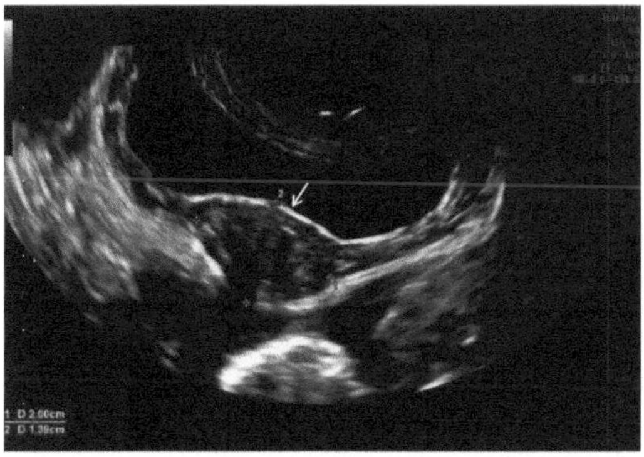

**Fig. 9.** Mass in the wall of bladder (*arrow*) consistent with an invasive endometrioma.

## SCANNING PROTOCOL

A scanning protocol should be established such that studies are consistent and complete. This consistent approach to pelvic ultrasonography optimizes detection of significant abnormalities. One such approach follows the following sequence:

- Vagina (on entry on transvaginal imaging)
- Bladder
- Uterus and cervix
- Endometrium
- Right ovary and adnexa
- Left ovary and adnexa
- Cul-de-sac and uterosacral ligaments
- Rectum
- Kidneys and ureters

The pertinent ultrasonographic findings and techniques are described in the following sections.

## BLADDER

Sweep from the patient's right to left, scanning the bladder wall and mucosa. The mucosa should be smooth, although an irregular contour can occasionally be seen when the bladder is not distended. Masses, such as with an invasive endometrioma, can be identified during bladder evaluation (**Fig. 9**). The wall of the bladder is usually

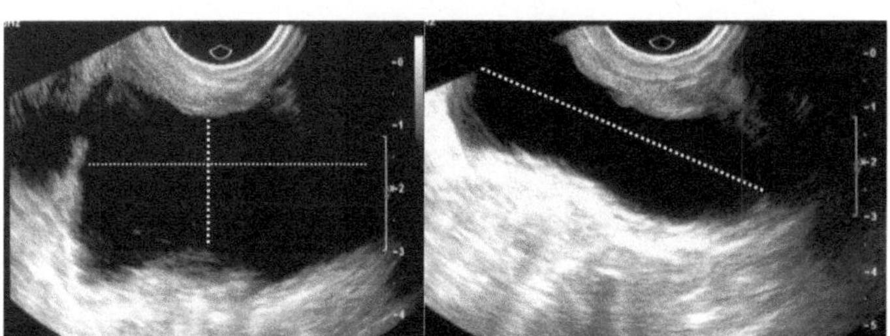

**Fig. 10.** Measuring the postvoid residual (PVR) in 3 dimensions using 2 orthogonal planes. In this example the PVR = (6.3 × 2.3 × 5.8) × 0.5233 = 43.9 mL.

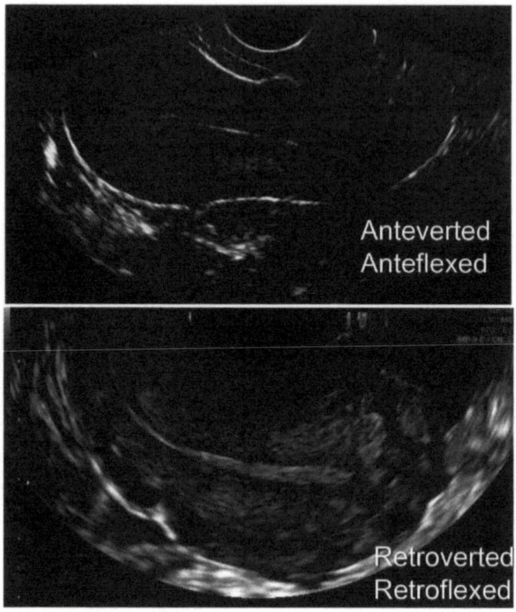


Fig. 11. Orientation of the uterus demonstrating an anteverted, anteflexed uterus and a retroverted, retroflexed uterus.

homogeneous and less than 5 mm thick. A thickness greater than 5 mm can be seen with chronic cystitis. A postvoid residual can be obtained by measuring in 2 orthogonal planes and calculating volume using 3 dimensions (**Fig. 10**). Echogenic debris may also be seen in the bladder lumen during imaging, and may represent a urinary tract infection.

## UTERUS, INCLUDING CERVIX

Sweep from the patient's right to left, evaluating the orientation, contour, and size of the uterus, the characteristics of the myometrium, findings such as fibroids or adenomyosis,[5] and the morphology of the cervix, such as Nabothian cysts. Both version and flexion are noted in the orientation (**Fig. 11**). Version describes the relationship of the body of the uterus to the vagina, with the cervix to the right of the image with an anteverted uterus. Flexion describes the relationship of the body of the uterus to the cervix.

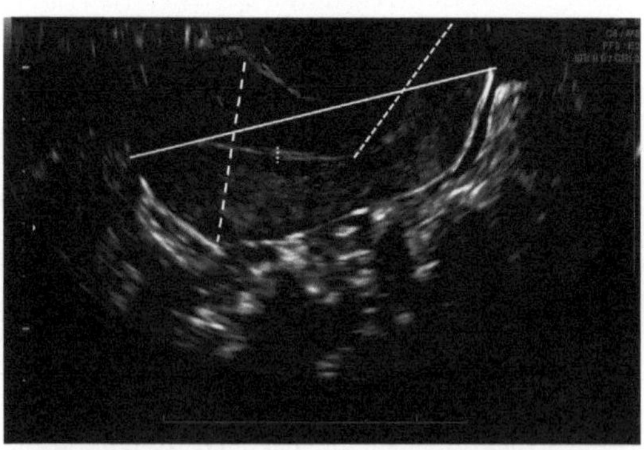

Fig. 12. Sagittal view. Measurements of the uterus in the longitudinal view.

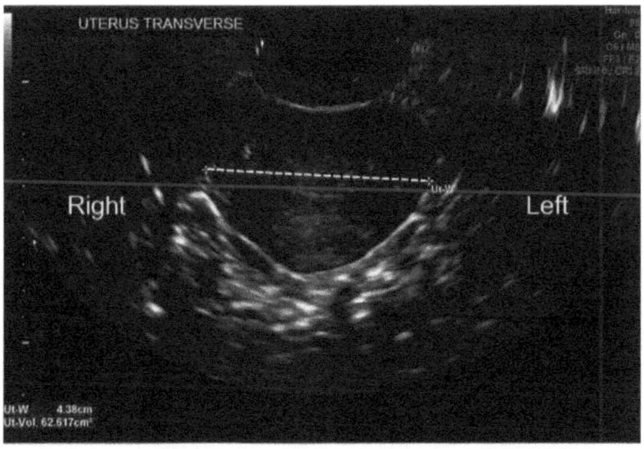


**Fig. 13.** Transverse view. Measurements of the uterus (width) in the transverse view.

The midsagittal plane of the uterus is then evaluated (**Fig. 12**):

- This allows measurement of the length and height of the uterus.
- The cervical length can be determined by measuring from the internal os to the external os.
- The thickness of the myometrium anteriorly and posteriorly can be measured. Significant discrepancies can be found with adenomyosis.[6]
- The myometrial echogenicity is assessed, noting homogeneity or heterogeneity (as seen with adenomyosis).
- The endometrial thickness is measured at the thickest anterior-posterior dimension in this midsagittal view.

Sweep the uterus in a transverse view, rotating the transducer 90° counterclockwise, such that the right side of the uterus is viewed on the left side of the ultrasound monitor. Rotating the transducer in the counterclockwise manner maintains the same orientation of the pelvic anatomy and the image on the video monitor. The sweep traces from the cervix to the uterine fundus and returns to the maximum width of the uterus. The uterine width is measured at this level (**Fig. 13**).

### *Uterine Volume*

When calculating the uterine volume, one only measures the length of the uterine body, excluding the cervix (**Fig. 14**). The volume is calculated using this uterine length, the uterine height and width. The equation is $[L \times H \times W] \times 0.5233$.

### *Uterine Motion*

The uterine sliding sign is demonstrated by visualizing the uterus in the midsagittal plane and gently advancing the transducer 1 to 2 cm. Normal mobility is demonstrated

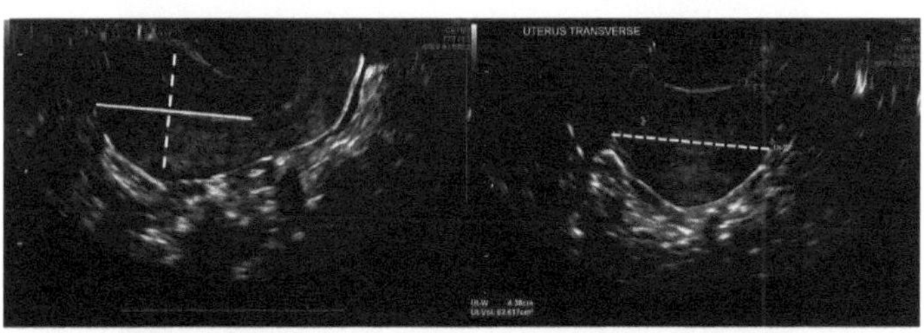


**Fig. 14.** Measurements used to calculate the uterine volume. The length measurement does NOT include the cervical length.

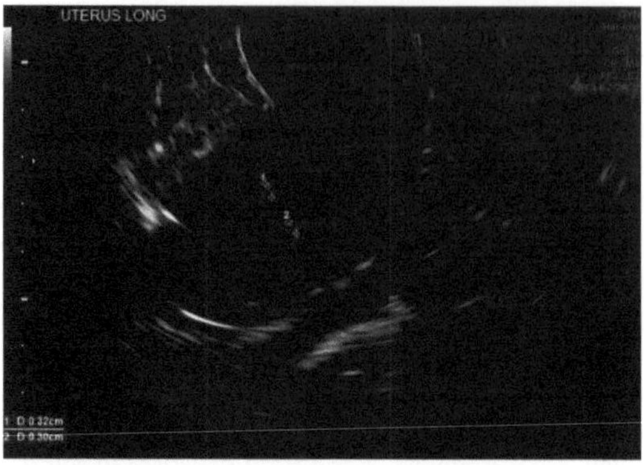


Fig. 15. Measuring the endometrium when fluid is present.

when the bowel moves along the posterior cervix, posterior uterine body, and over the uterine fundus (Video 1). The lack of mobility is considered a *negative uterine sliding sign* (Video 2) and is associated with obliteration of the cul-de-sac in 93% of cases.[7,8]

## ENDOMETRIUM

The endometrium should be measured in the anterior-posterior measurement at the widest point, including both layers of the endometrium. In cases where fluid is visualized in the endometrium then each layer is measured individually and added together (**Fig. 15**). Evaluate the echogenicity of the endometrium, for example, homogeneous, heterogeneous, or trilaminar. Note any cystic spaces, irregularities, or possible masses. Cystic spaces raise concern for an endometrial polyp (**Fig. 16**). In such cases, color power angiography can be placed over the endometrium, using a pulse repetition frequency (PRF) of 0.3 kHz. The presence of Doppler flow within the endometrium (**Fig. 17**) suggests the presence of an endometrial polyp, which can be confirmed with further study, such as sonohysterography (**Fig. 18**).

## RIGHT OVARY AND ADNEXA

There are several technical approaches to identifying the ovaries. Each is replicated on both the right and left side until adequate visualization is obtained. The approach follows in a sequential manner until the ovary is visualized:

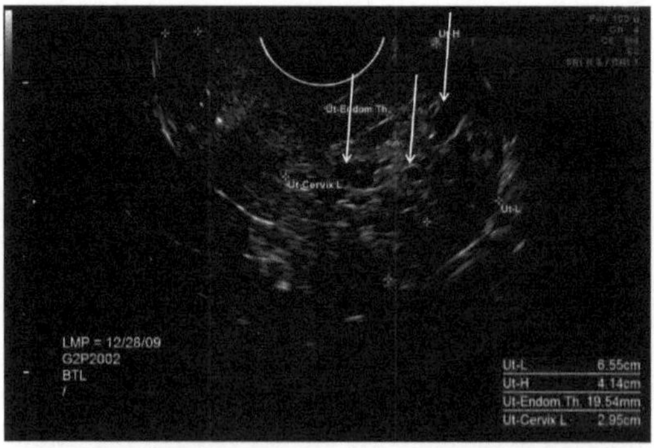


Fig. 16. Cystic spaces in the endometrium (*arrows*) suggesting an endometrial polyp.

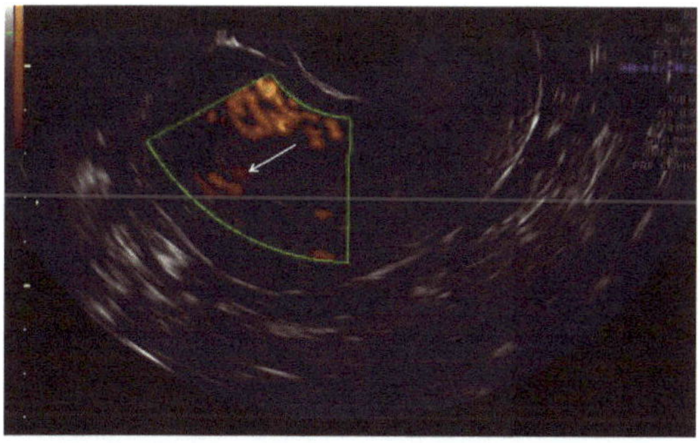

Fig. 17. Doppler flow demonstrated with color power angiography (*arrow*), consistent with an endometrial polyp.

- Sweep laterally in a sagittal plane.
- Sweep the adnexa from the cervix to the fundus with the transducer in a transverse plane.
- Start at the fundus in the transverse plane and follow the utero-ovarian ligament (or approximate location of the ligament) out laterally, then sweeping from the fundus to the cervix.
- Apply gentle abdominal pressure to displace the bowel and bring the ovary into the imaging field and repeat the above procedures.
- On the patient's right side, rotate the transducer counterclockwise, such that the top of the transducer is at the 7 o'clock position and rotate it clockwise, identifying the internal iliac vessels, and move the transducer medially. On the patient's left side, rotate the transducer clockwise, such that the top of the transducer is at the 5 o'clock position and rotate it counterclockwise, identifying the internal iliac vessels, and move the transducer medially. Of note, when evaluating the left adnexa in this manner, the iliac vessel image will appear as if it is on the right side of the patient.
- If the ovary is not identified with a vaginal approach, one should scan the patient abdominally (see abdominal protocol), which may lead to ovarian identification or visualization of an enlarged ovary that is out of the pelvis.
- Once identified, the ovary is visualized in 2 orthogonal planes with appropriate measurements obtained (**Fig. 19**). A split screen image is used that allows visualization of both planes. The first image is frozen; the transducer is rotated 90°

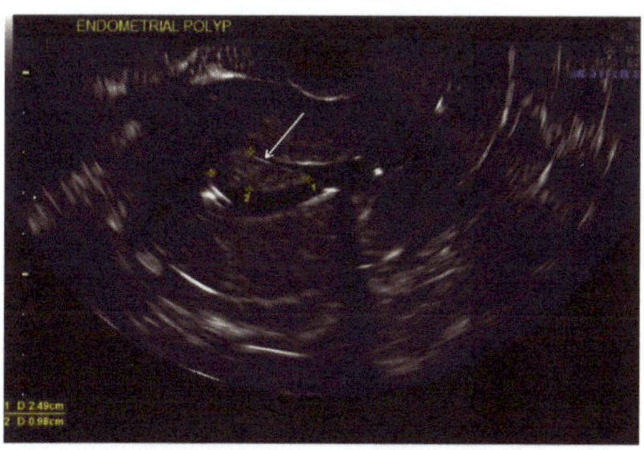


**Fig. 18.** Endometrial polyp (*arrow*) from **Fig. 17** on sonohysterography.

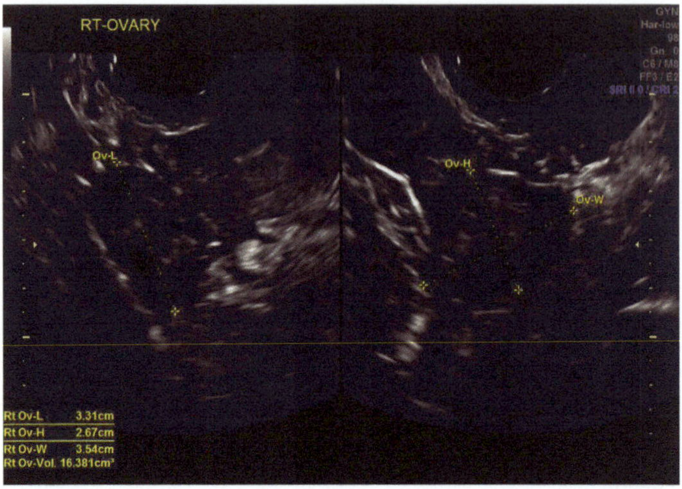


**Fig. 19.** Right ovary, using split screen images, measured in 2 orthogonal planes.

toward the pelvic sidewall, which keeps the ovary relatively fixed against the sidewall.

- *Mobility of the ovary* is demonstrated with the ovarian sliding sign[9] (Video 3). In 1 study of patients with previous abdominal surgery, the lack of ovarian mobility (Video 4) was associated with significant adhesions in 96.3% of patients.
- The adnexa is further interrogated to identify the fallopian tube, which is usually not visualized unless there is fluid in the cul-de-sac (**Fig. 20**) or the tube is dilated, for example, a hydrosalpinx (**Figs. 21** and **22**).

## LEFT OVARY AND ADNEXA

The approach to identifying the left ovary is the same as described for the right ovary, with 1 difference being the rotational sweep in the left adnexa. On the left side, the transducer is rotated clockwise, such that the top of the transducer is at the 5 o'clock position to start the rotational sweep. Transducer rotation occurs in the counterclockwise manner, until the transducer is in the sagittal orientation. Otherwise, the technical steps replicate those on the right side.

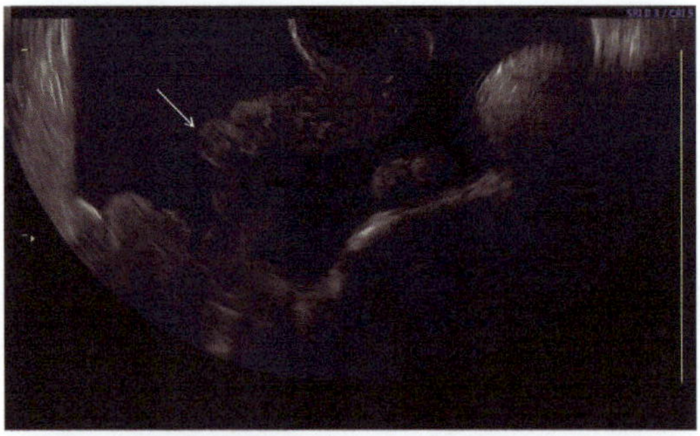

**Fig. 20.** Large amount of fluid, associated with malignant ascites, allows visualization of the fallopian tube (*arrow*).

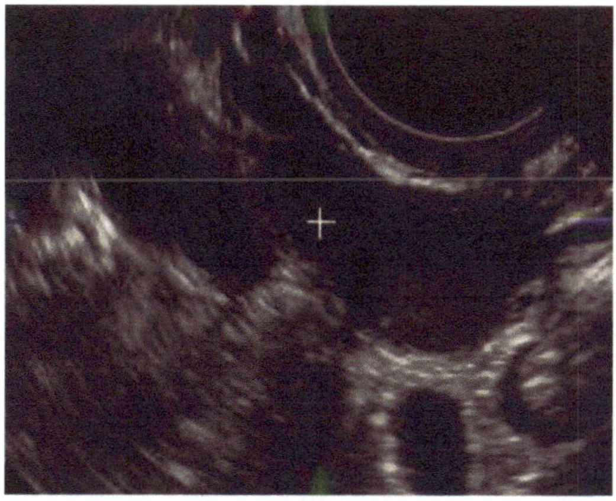

**Fig. 21.** Hydrosalpinx on 2D with cystic areas lining up in the adnexa.

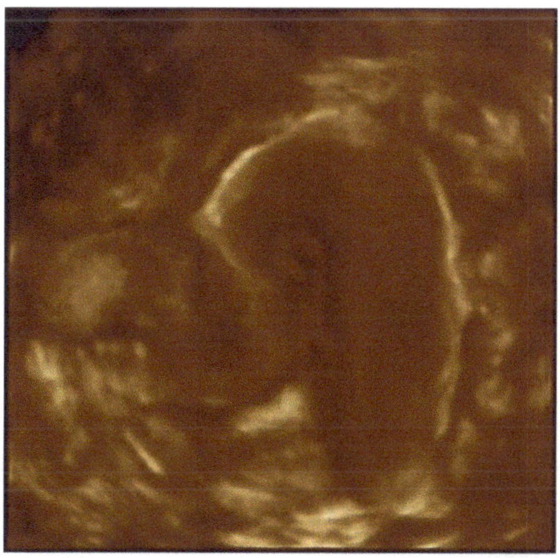

**Fig. 22.** Hydrosalpinx on 3D rendered view with a serpiginous tubular structure of a hydrosalpinx.

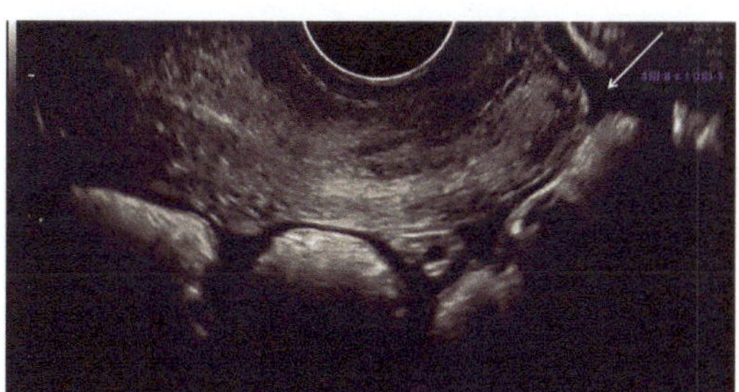

**Fig. 23.** Small amount of clear fluid (*arrow*) in the cul-de-sac, which is normal.

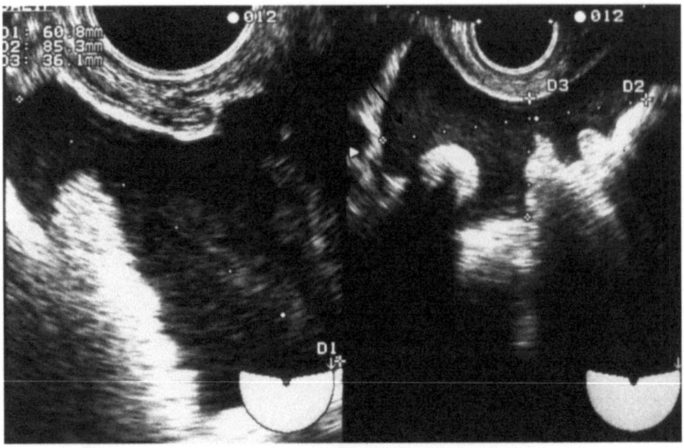


Fig. 24. Blood in the cul-de-sac with a ruptured ectopic pregnancy.

## CUL-DE-SAC AND UTEROSACRAL LIGAMENTS

The cul-de-sac may have a small amount of fluid present, the amount varying during the menstrual cycle.[10] One study found that 40% of patients have fluid in the cul-de-sac, with up to a third of patients having fluid present from midcycle to menses. The fluid may range from clear (**Fig. 23**) to having low-level echoes, associated with blood (**Fig. 24**) or ascites (see **Fig. 20**). The uterosacral ligaments are usually not visualized unless there is an abnormal pathologic condition, for example, implants of endometriosis.[11] Again, mobility of the uterus (see Uterus, above) is critical in evaluating the presence or absence of cul-de-sac adhesions or obliteration.

## RECTUM

The rectum is not routinely interrogated with a normal pelvic ultrasonography. However, in cases of deep infiltrating endometriosis (DIE), bowel wall thickening, masses, or distortion may indicate significant bowel involvement with endometriosis (**Fig. 25**). The rectum is carefully evaluated in cases of pelvic floor dysfunction, as seen with tears in the internal or external sphincter (**Figs. 26** and **27**).

## KIDNEYS AND URETERS

The kidneys and ureters are not routinely visualized with a normal pelvic ultrasonography. However, with suspected ureteric compression or obstruction, for example, with DIE, one would be prudent to evaluate the kidney for any signs of retrograde obstruction (**Fig. 28**).

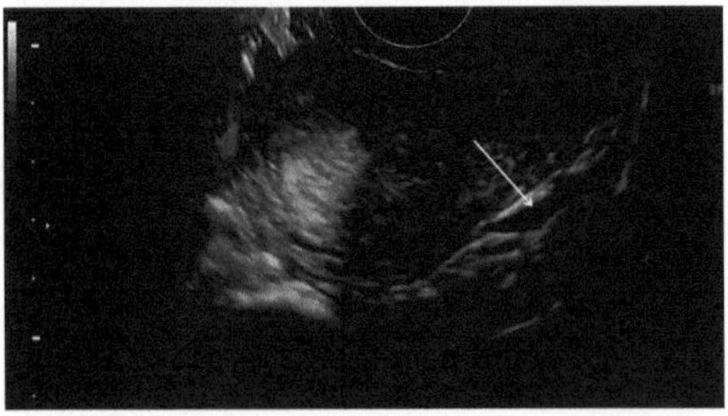

Fig. 25. Thickened bowel wall in area of deep infiltrating endometriosis (*arrow*).

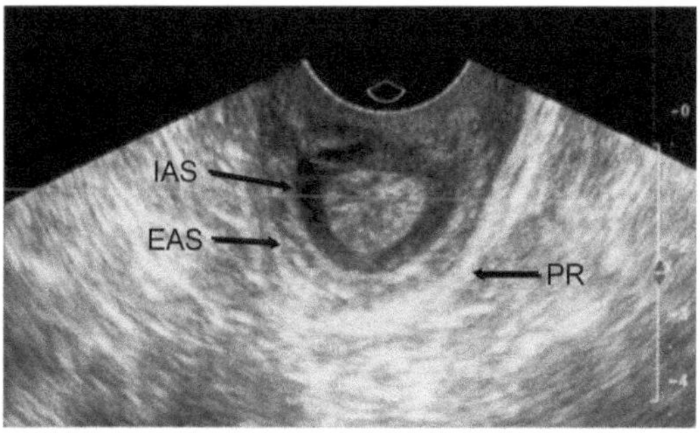


**Fig. 26.** Normal rectal sphincter demonstrating the internal anal sphincter (IAS), the external anal sphincter (EAS), and the puborectalis muscle (PR).

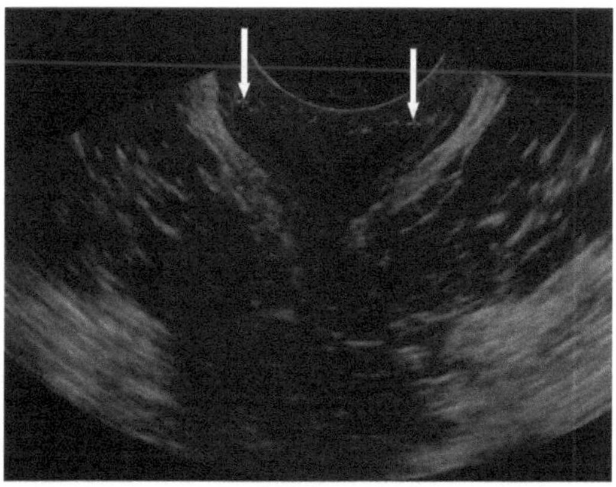

**Fig. 27.** Abnormal rectal sphincter with significant disruption of the normal continuity of the sphincter (*arrows*).

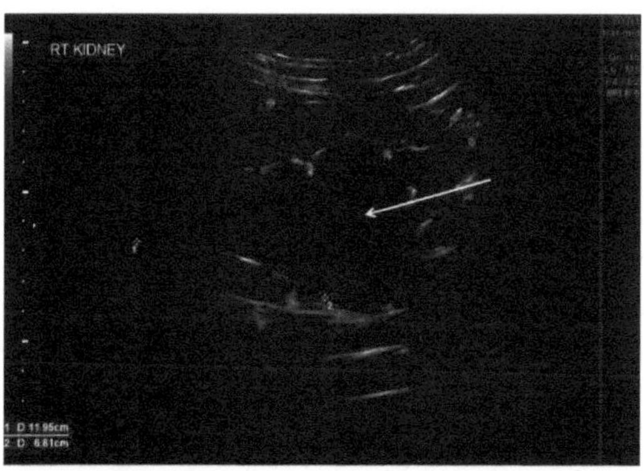


**Fig. 28.** Significant hydronephrosis (*arrow*) in a patient with partial obstruction of the right ureter due to deep infiltrating endometriosis.

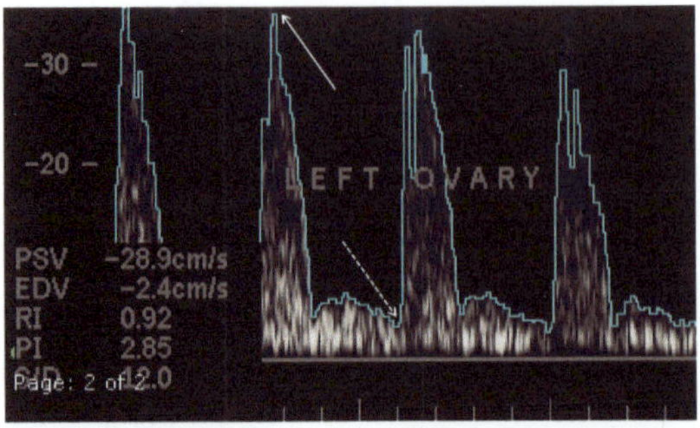


**Fig. 29.** Color Doppler with normal flow spectral analysis showing the peak systolic velocity (PSV) (*solid arrow*) and the end diastolic velocity (EDV) (*dotted arrow*).

## *Additional Studies*

### *Doppler sonography*

It is common to augment 2-dimensional (2D) ultrasonographic studies with Doppler studies and 3D ultrasonography. This is particularly helpful in determining if a mass is cystic (lacking central vascular flow) or solid (central Doppler flow identified). Doppler is applied using 2 primary methods: color Doppler flow and power Doppler. Color Doppler flow identifies vascular flow toward and away from the transducer. There is some angle-dependency with color Doppler flow, as well as some interference from background noise, particularly in low-velocity states. Color Doppler measures the frequency shift (eg, velocity) between 2 different points in a vessel. It is expressed as a spectral analysis, with the Resistance Index (RI), the ratio of the peak systolic velocity (PSV) minus the end diastolic velocity (EDV) divided by the PSV, and the Pulsatility Index (PI), the ratio of the PSV minus EDV divided by the mean of the PSV and EDV. The RI is always a lower number than the PI. Normal resistance to flow is demonstrated with an RI >0.5 and a PI >1.0 (**Fig. 29**). Low-resistance flow, signified by an RI <0.5 and a PI <1.0 (**Fig. 30**), is found with neovascularization, such as in early pregnancy, with a corpus luteum, and in malignancy. Unfortunately, there is significant overlap with some malignancies showing normal-resistance flow parameters, and some normal findings, for example, a corpus luteum, showing low-resistance flow parameters.

Increasingly, studies are demonstrating that vessel distribution may be more indicative of malignant transformation.[12] As such, power Doppler sonography has emerged

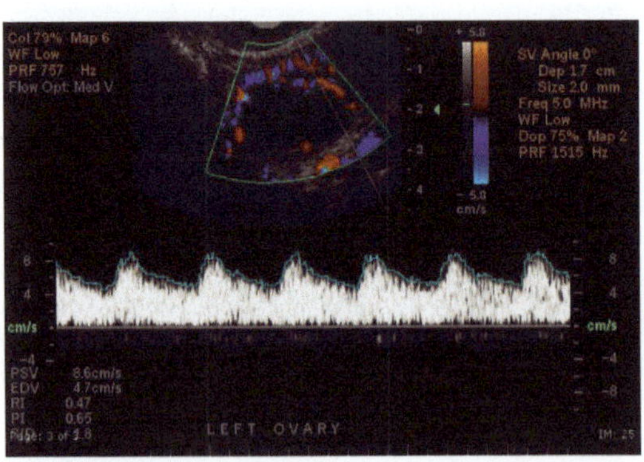


**Fig. 30.** Color Doppler with abnormal spectral analysis showing a low Resistance Index (RI <0.5) and a low Pulsatility Index (PI <1.0).

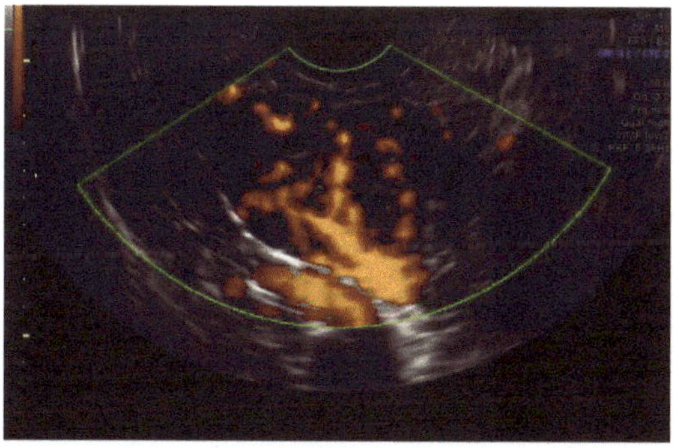

Fig. 31. Power Doppler sonography in a postmenopausal patient with a granulosa cell tumor. Note the relatively abundant vascular flow within the mass (IOTA 3).

as a preferred alternative in sonographic evaluation of pelvic vasculature. Power Doppler demonstrates the amplitude of the Doppler signal, rather than velocity, and is more sensitive than color Doppler, particularly in low-velocity states. By convention, power Doppler is adjusted to a PRF of 0.3 kHz for evaluation of the adnexa and other pelvic organs.[13] A more recent development is Spectral Doppler, which is directionally dependent power Doppler sonography. This allows visualization of the amplitude of Doppler flow, as well as calculating the velocity of flow, particularly helpful in low-velocity flow states. The International Ovarian Tumor Analysis (IOTA) group has standardized the description of the flow,[13] by assigning a "vascularity score" as follows:

1. No flow
2. Minimal flow
3. Moderate flow
4. Strong flow throughout

A vascularity score of 3 or 4 increases concern for malignancy (**Fig. 31**). The IOTA method is covered in Wouter Froyman and Dirk Timmerman's article, "Methods of Assessing Ovarian Masses: IOTA Approach," in this issue.

***Three-dimensional sonography***

The ability to capture 2D images and manipulate them to demonstrate 3D planes has dramatically improved the ultrasonographic assessment of various gynecologic findings. An in-depth discussion of 3D is beyond the scope of this article. A basic understanding of several modalities is important. The 3D image can be obtained in the longitudinal (sagittal) plane or the transverse plane (which may be better for some uterine anomalies, eg, a bicornuate uterus or uterine didelphys). The image representing the plane of acquisition is always displayed in the upper left corner. The perpendicular orthogonal plane is the upper right corner. The coronal view is in the lower left corner. The rendered view is in the lower right corner (**Fig. 32**). Abuhamad and colleagues described a method (the "Z-technique") of rapidly and easily manipulating the images to obtain the best coronal view of the uterus.[14] Rotating the C-plane image 90° allows visualization of the coronal view of a normal uterus in its correct orientation (**Fig. 33**). An in-depth discussion of 3D and its ability to diagnose several pelvic abnormalities is covered in Beryl R. Benacerraf's article, "Three-Dimensional Volume Imaging in Gynecology," in this issue.

Sonohysterography is a technique of inserting fluid into the uterus during 2D or 3D sonography, enhancing the ability to assess the endometrium and evaluate the presence of any intracavitary focal lesions, for example, endometrial polyps, submucous myomas, focal hyperplasia, or cancer. A normal uterus will have uniform and

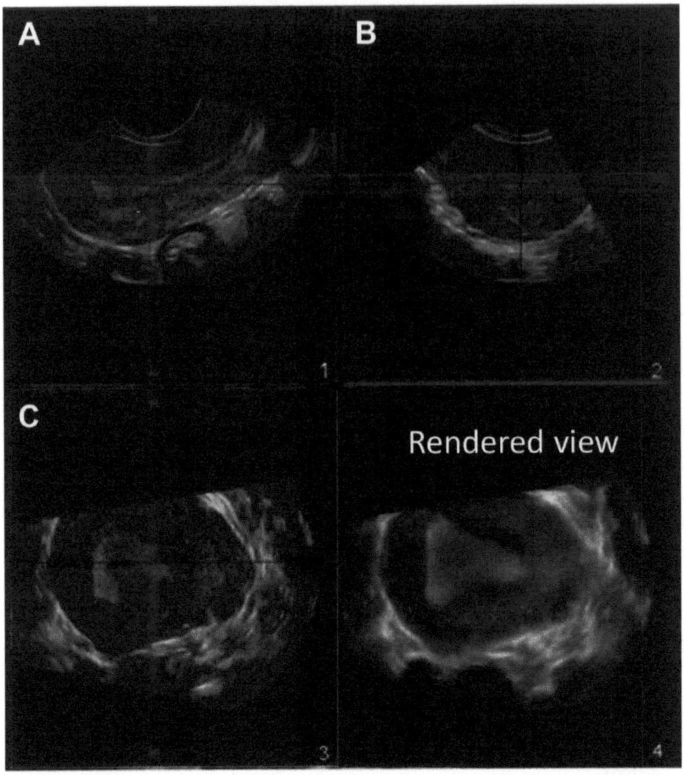


Fig. 32. Uterine image captured in 3D demonstrating (*A*) the acquisition plane, (*B*) the perpendicular orthogonal plane, and (*C*) the coronal view and the rendered view.

symmetric endometrial echoes, with no focal lesions in the cavity (**Fig. 34**). This is covered in more detail in Beryl R. Benacerraf's article, "Three-Dimensional Volume Imaging in Gynecology," in this issue.

Sonosalpingography, so-called hystero-contrast-sonography or HyCoSy, is a technique to demonstrate tubal patency at the time of pelvic sonography.[14] The technique

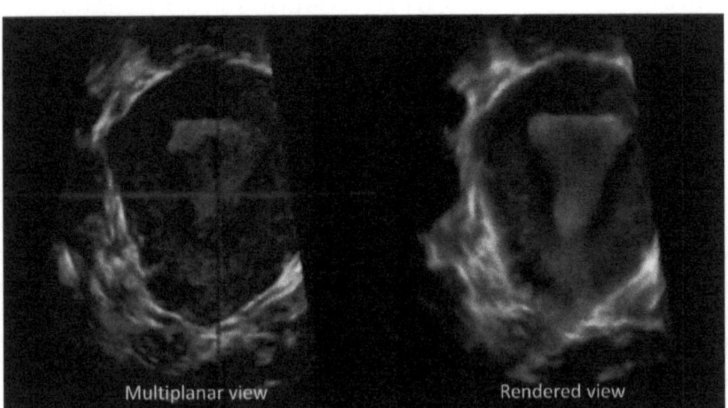


Fig. 33. Rotation of the coronal view allows correct anatomic orientation of a normal uterus for the coronal multiplaner view and rendered view.

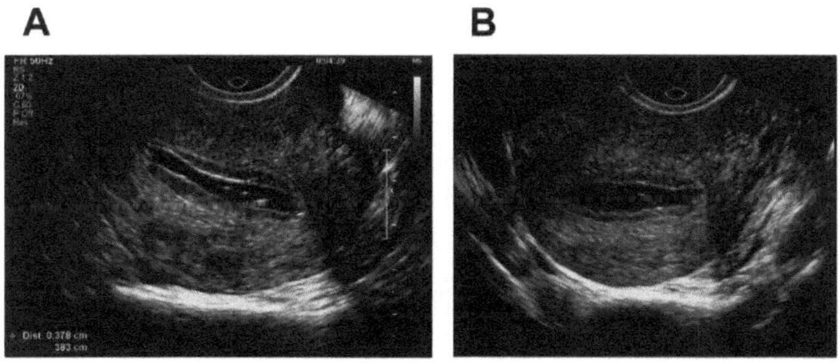

**Fig. 34.** Fluid inserted into the uterine cavity during sonohysterography demonstrates endometrial echoes that are uniform and symmetric with no focal lesions present. (*A*) Longitudinal view and (*B*) transverse view.

involves injecting a contrast agent, either fluid or foam, into the uterus, allowing flow of the contrast into and out of the fallopian tube, and documenting such flow with ultrasonography. This is covered in more detail in Beryl R. Benacerraf's article, "Three-Dimensional Volume Imaging in Gynecology," in this issue.

Pelvic floor ultrasonography is an emerging application using both 2D and 3D ultrasonography. It involves multiple approaches including the abdominal approach, a vaginal approach, a transperineal approach, and a transrectal approach. Application of ultrasonography to assessment of pelvic floor disorders is increasing exponentially. This application is discussed in detail in Hadas Allouche Kam and colleagues' article, "Ultrasound in Pelvic Floor Dysfunction," in this issue.

## SUPPLEMENTARY DATA

Supplementary data related to this article can be found online at https://doi.org/10.1016/j.ogc.2019.06.001.

## REFERENCES

1. Benacerraf B, Abuhamad AZ, Bromley B, et al. Consider ultrasound first for imaging the female pelvis. Am J Obstet Gynecol 2015;212(5):450–5.
2. Gollub E, Westhoff C, Timor-Tritsch I. Detection of ovaries by transvaginal sonography in postmenopausal women. Ultrasound Obstet Gynecol 1993;3(6):422–5.
3. Fleischer A, Kalemeris G, Entman S. Sonographic depiction of the endometrium during normal cycles. Ultrasound Med Biol 1986;12(4):271–7.
4. Santolaya-Forgas J. Physiology of the menstrual cycle by ultrasonography. J Ultrasound Med 1992;11(4):139–42.
5. Shwayder JM, Sakhel K. Imaging for uterine myomas and adenomyosis. J Minim Invasive Gynecol 2014;21(3):362–72.
6. Van den Bosch T, Dueholm M, Leone FP, et al. Terms, definitions and measurements to describe sonographic features of myometrium and uterine masses: a consensus opinion from the Morphological Uterus Sonographic Assessment (MUSA) group. Ultrasound Obstet Gynecol 2015;46(3):284–98.
7. Hudelist G, Fritzer N, Staettner S, et al. Uterine sliding sign: a simple sonographic predictor for presence of deep infiltrating endometriosis of the rectum. Ultrasound Obstet Gynecol 2013;41(6):692–5.

8. Reid S, Condous G. Transvaginal sonographic sliding sign: accurate prediction of Pouch of Douglas obiliteration. Ultrasound Obstet Gynecol 2013;41(6):605–7.
9. Ayachi A, Bouchahda R, Derouich S, et al. Accuracy of preoperative real-time dynamic transvaginal ultrasound sliding sign in prediction of pelvic adhesions in women with previous abdominopelvic surgery: prospective, multicenter, double-blind study. Ultrasound Obstet Gynecol 2018;51(2):253–8.
10. Davis J, Gosnik BB. Fluid in the female pelvis: cyclic patterns. J Ultrasound Med 1986;5:75–9.
11. Guerriero S, Condous G, Van den Bosch T, et al. Systematic approach to sonographic evaluation of the pelvis in women with suspected endometriosis, including terms, definitions and measurements: a consensus opinion form the International Deep Endometriosis Analysis (IDEA) group. Ultrasound Obstet Gynecol 2016;48:318–32.
12. Medeiros LR, Rosa DD, da Rosa MI, et al. Accuracy of ultrasonography with color Doppler in ovarian tumor: a systematic quantitative review. Int J Gynecol Cancer 2009;19(2):230–6.
13. Valentin L, Ameye L, Savelli L, et al. Adnexal masses difficult to classify as benign or malignant using subjective assessment of gray-scale and Doppler ultrasound findings: logistic regression models do not help. Ultrasound Obstet Gynecol 2011;38(4):456–65.
14. Saunders RD, Shwayder JM, Nakajima ST. Current methods of tubal patency assessment. Fertil Steril 2011;95(7):2171–9.

# Gynecologic Ultrasound Evaluation of the Nongravid Woman with Pelvic Pain

Bryann Bromley, MD[a,b]

**KEYWORDS**

• Pelvic pain • Ultrasound • Uterus • Ovaries • Adnexa

**KEY POINTS**

- Pelvic pain is a common although nonspecific condition in women, which may be due to multiple etiologies (gynecologic, urologic, gastrointestinal, musculoskeletal, vascular, neurologic, and metabolic causes).
- Pelvic ultrasound is the first-line imaging modality to evaluate the female patient with pelvic pain and must be interactive, include a transvaginal assessment, and be tenderness guided.
- The use of 3-dimensional and power Doppler enhance the detection of pathologic conditions.
- A detailed history is crucial in helping the imager to focus on the correct clinical scenario to support any ultrasound findings.

**Video content accompanies this article at http://www.obgyn.theclinics.com.**

## INTRODUCTION

Pelvic pain is a common although nonspecific condition in women, which may be due to multiple etiologies, including gynecologic, urologic, gastrointestinal, musculoskeletal, vascular, and metabolic etiologies. The prevalence is difficult to ascertain but has been reported in 15% to 24% of women and accounts for 2% to 10% of outpatient gynecologic consultations and 20% of laparoscopies.[1,2] The pain itself may be debilitating and has been reported to have significant impact on quality of life, as well as economic repercussions.[2] If a gynecologic etiology is suspected, ultrasound examination is the optimal first choice imaging technique because it is an extension of the bimanual examination, readily available and affordable, and not associated with ionizing radiation.[3] This article focuses on gynecologic etiologies of pelvic pain in

No disclosures.

[a] Department of Obstetrics and Gynecology, Massachusetts General Hospital, Harvard Medical School, Boston, MA, USA; [b] Diagnostic Ultrasound Associates, One Brookline Place, Suite 506, Brookline, MA 02445, USA

Obstet Gynecol Clin N Am 46 (2019) 581–594
https://doi.org/10.1016/j.ogc.2019.06.002 obgyn.theclinics.com
0889-8545/19/

the nonpregnant patient, specifically those conditions that may be identified by pelvic ultrasound examination.

In evaluating the patient with pelvic pain, it is critical to take a detailed history, both general and reproductive. The differential diagnosis of pelvic pain is strongly guided by the exclusion of pregnancy and therefore a serum human chorionic gonadotropin should be obtained in patients of reproductive age. The gynecologic history should include menopausal status, last menstrual period, presence of irregular bleeding, any methods of contraception, prior pelvic surgery or procedures, history of infections, and medications, including hormone replacement therapy. The patient should be asked about the presence of vaginal discharge, dysmenorrhea, or dyspareunia. Associated symptoms such fevers, chills, and gastrointestinal changes should be noted. Inquiring further as to what factors provoke or alleviate the pain may be helpful in identifying associations between the gastrointestinal and urinary tract systems, as well as the potential association with conditions, such as deep infiltrating endometriosis. The patient should also be questioned as to chronic medical conditions involving bowel, bladder, musculoskeletal, and vascular conditions.

Acute pelvic pain is sudden in onset and lasts less than 3 months. It is often associated with other symptoms such as nausea, vomiting, and diarrhea or laboratory findings such as leukocytosis. Chronic pelvic pain is a noncyclic pain occurring for at least 6 months leading to disability or medical care.[4]

## ULTRASOUND TECHNIQUE

Ultrasound examination is the primary imaging modality for evaluating the patient with pelvic pain. The ultrasound evaluation of the patient is optimally accomplished by a transabdominal approach through a slightly distended bladder, followed by a transvaginal study with the bladder empty. These 2 methods of imaging are complimentary, each adding to the overall diagnostic quality of the examination. The transabdominal approach permits the visualization of a panoramic view of the pelvis so that normal structures and masses or fluid collections that are located higher in the pelvis may be visualized. The transvaginal approach enhances image resolution because a higher frequency transducer is used, resulting in finer detail of the anatomy but within a limited depth of penetration.[3] Importantly, the transvaginal ultrasound examination is an enhancement of the bimanual examination. Gentle manipulation of pelvic organs with the transducer aided by opposing pressure of a hand on the patient's abdomen can be used to demonstrate the mobility of the pelvic structures against the peritoneal surface and with reference to each other and pelvic masses (sliding organ sign).[5] The transvaginal ultrasound evaluation is guided by the patient's symptoms and should include the bladder, rectovaginal septum, and cul-de-sac. Attention should be focused in areas of increased pain. In patients who are unable to tolerate a transvaginal examination, a transrectal evaluation may be helpful.[6] In many circumstances, color Doppler imaging should be added to the evaluation to aid in diagnostic performance. The use of 3-dimensional (3D) reconstruction to demonstrate the coronal view of the uterus is particularly useful in determining the position of an intrauterine device (IUD), mapping out the position of fibroids, and evaluating the junctional zone in patients with adenomyosis. It may also help in distinguishing an adnexal mass as ovarian or tubal in origin. Attention to adjacent structures such as the bladder and cul-de-sac may lead to the identification of deep infiltrating endometriosis, bladder endometriosis, or nongynecologic conditions.

## ACUTE PELVIC PAIN

Gynecologic considerations include ovarian masses, which may be simple, hemorrhagic, or ruptured. Ovarian hyperstimulation may be a source of pain in a patient undergoing augmented ovulation. Ovarian or tubal torsion is a well-described cause of acute pelvic pain. Other potential gynecologic etiologies include pelvic inflammatory disease (PID), malpositioned or penetrating/perforating intrauterine contraceptive devices, and acutely degenerating fibroids. The details of the individual pathologies described can be found in the corresponding articles dedicated to their specific imaging characteristics within this issue.

## ADNEXAL ETIOLOGIES

Hemorrhagic cysts (HC) are a common cause of abrupt onset of midcycle pelvic pain, although they may also be seen in asymptomatic patients as well. HC occur during ovulation when the luteinized granulosa layer becomes vascularized and vessels within the wall cyst rupture.[7] The ultrasound appearance of the corpus luteum reflects hemorrhage and therefore depends on the time course since the bleeding began. In the initial phases, the blood is anechoic; however, when a clot forms, it becomes echogenic. This echogenicity decreases over time owing to hemolysis. HC range in size between 2.5 and 8.5 cm with an average of 3.0 to 3.5 cm.[7] They have a thin wall and posterior enhancement owing to the cystic nature. HC often have a fish net or reticular pattern characterized by wavy strands of fibrin. There is no internal color flow (**Fig. 1**). The cyst may evolve to have layered echoes, reflecting separated components of blood after formation of the clot (**Fig. 2**). Circumferential color flow is characteristic of a corpus luteum (**Fig. 3**). A transvaginal tenderness-guided examination in which the ultrasound transducer is used to manipulate cyst contents may demonstrate waves within the material located within the interior of the cyst (Video 1). During the acute phase, the HC may rupture and echogenic fluid (blood) may be seen in the dependent portions of the pelvis. This type of ultrasound appearance is nonspecific and can be due to other conditions such as infection or cellular debris. A fever or leukocytosis would not be expected with an HC and there should be no internal color

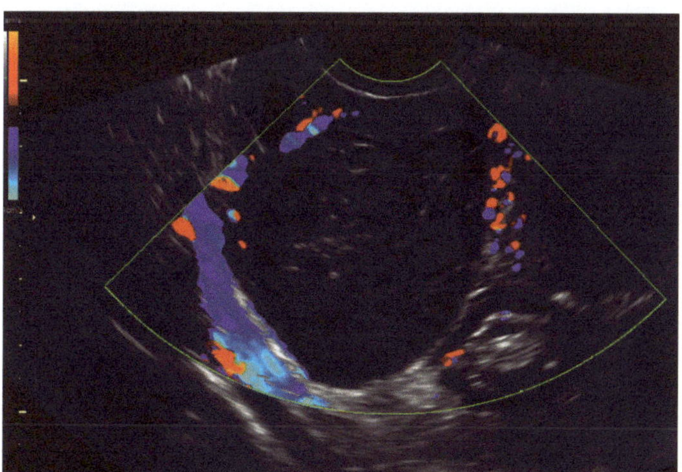

**Fig. 1.** Transvaginal examination of the ovary demonstrating reticular internal echoes characteristic of a HC. Note that there is no color flow to the interior of the cyst.

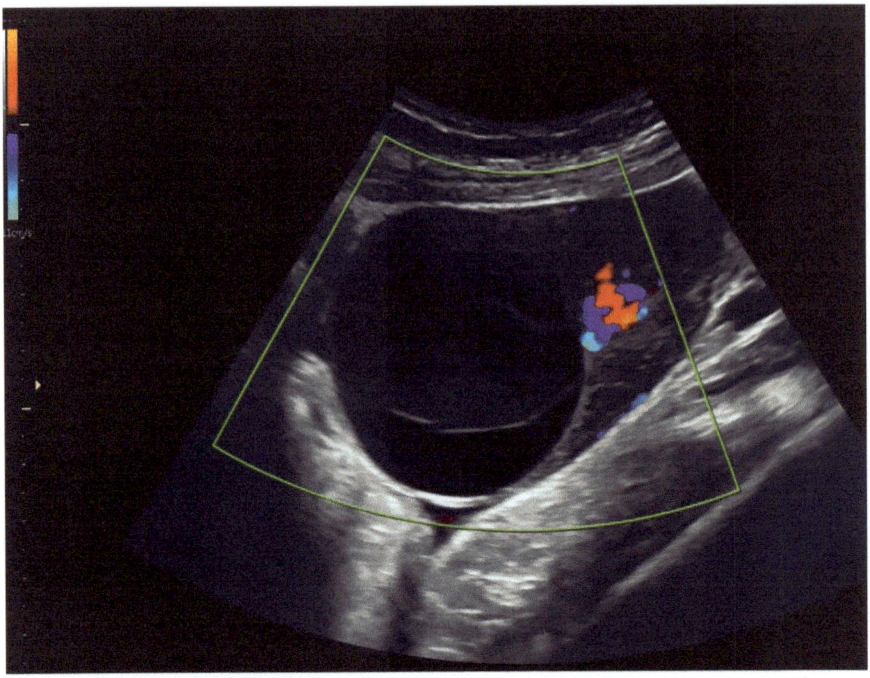

Fig. 2. Transvaginal examination of the ovary demonstrating a cyst with layered echoes and no internal color flow. Note the smooth border of the layering, characteristic of a clot, the and absence of internal color flow in this HC.

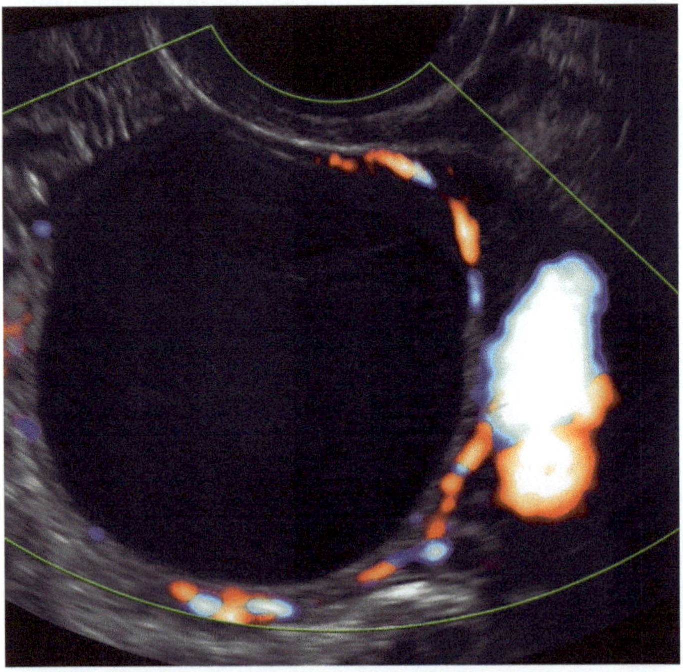

Fig. 3. Transvaginal examination of the ovary demonstrating a cyst with internal echoes. There is circumferential flow characteristic of a hemorrhagic corpus luteum. The patient also had a 5-week intrauterine gestation.

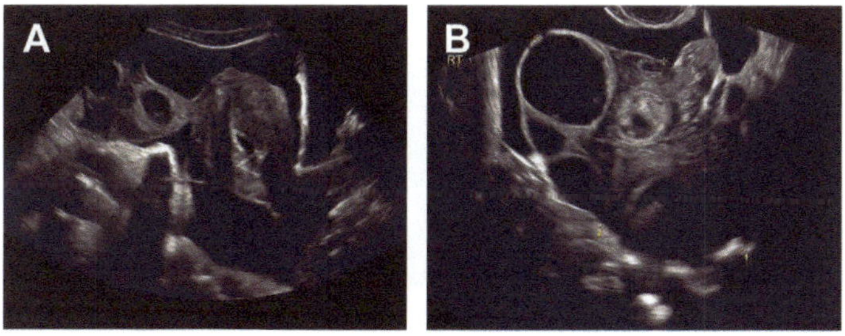


**Fig. 4.** (*A*) Transabdominal ultrasound demonstrating a uterus that is surrounded by free fluid extending into the upper abdomen of a patient with ovarian hyperstimulation syndrome. (*B*) Transvaginal view of the enlarged 12-cm ovary showing multiple follicles associated with hyperstimulation.

flow to the cyst. Owing to the physiologic nature of these cysts, they will usually resolve over 6 to 8 weeks.[7] They may occur with pregnancy and differentiation from an ectopic pregnancy may be challenging in some circumstances. A knowledge of the serum human chorionic gonadotropin status is important. Augmented ovulation with hyperstimulation may be an etiology of acute lower abdominal pain and can be associated with a significant amount of free fluid (**Fig. 4**).

## ENDOMETRIOSIS AND DEEP INFILTRATING ENDOMETRIOSIS

Endometriosis is an estrogen-dependent lesion, occurring in reproductive age women and refers to the presence of endometrial tissue (glands and stroma) outside the uterus. It is often associated with pelvic pain. Endometriosis may involve the ovaries (endometrioma) or may extend to adjacent organs resulting in implants in the bladder, bowel, and cul-de-sac as well as remote locations such as the diaphragm, pleural cavity, or abdominal wall. An endometrioma is fairly straightforward to identify by ultrasound examination. It is most commonly a unilocular cystic lesion with ground glass echogenicity (**Fig. 5**). It may contain up to 4 locules, but should not contain any solid components and should not have any color flow internally.[8] Deep infiltrating endometriosis occurs when endometrial glands and stroma infiltrate more than 5 mm into the subperitoneal tissue and occurs in 1% to 2% of patients with endometriosis[9,10] (**Fig. 6**). This condition is often associated with severe pain, which can be reproduced

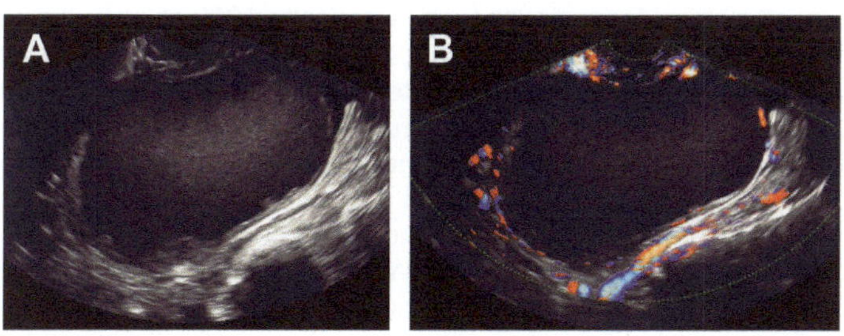


**Fig. 5.** (*A*) Transvaginal examination of the ovary demonstrating an 8-cm (not measured in this image) unilocular cyst with uniform low-level echoes and a slightly lobulated internal wall. Note the peripheral ovarian tissue. These features are characteristic of an endometrioma in a premenopausal patient. (*B*) Color flow Doppler imaging does not demonstrate any flow to the interior of the cyst.

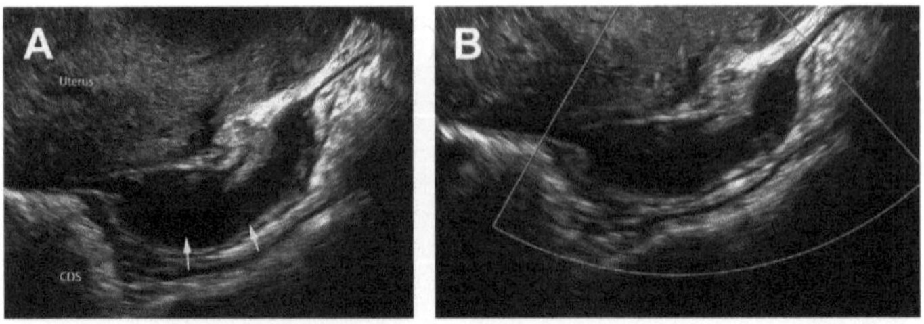


**Fig. 6.** (*A*) Transvaginal examination demonstrating the uterus and cul-de-sac that contains a comet-shaped lesion (*arrows*) characteristic of deep infiltrating endometriosis. This implant was extremely tender to pressure applied with the transvaginal transducer. (*B*) Color Doppler imaging demonstrating no color flow to the implant area.

by pushing on the area of the implant with the transvaginal transducer. Another clue to the extent of endometriosis can be obtained by using the transvaginal ultrasound transducer to gently manipulate and slide the pelvic organs against each other.[5] In cases of endometriosis, the organs may not move, suggesting adhesions. Another useful tip is to maintain a slight amount of fluid in the maternal bladder, which may help in identifying endometriotic implants in that location. The ability to perform an interactive ultrasound evaluation is an important and unique feature of ultrasound examination that distinguishes it from other remote imaging modalities and should be used in every gynecologic ultrasound examination (see Francesca Moro and colleagues' article, "Ultrasound Imaging in Endometriosis," in this issue).

## ADNEXAL TORSION

The ovary and/or fallopian tube may twist around the axis of the ovarian ligament and the infundibulopelvic ligament, resulting in torsion. Adnexal torsion involves both the ovary and fallopian tube in the majority of cases, although rarely the fallopian tube may torse alone.[11] The twisting of the pedicle results in venous stasis and altered lymphatic flow, leading to ovarian edema. If torsion persists, eventual loss of arterial flow leads to ischemia and necrosis. The mainstay of early treatment involves untwisting of the pedicle.

The clinical presentation of ovarian torsion overlaps with many other etiologies, both gynecologic and nongynecologic, making it an elusive diagnosis. Acute lower abdominal pelvic pain, often unilateral, is reported in the majority of patients with surgical confirmation of ovarian torsion, although historically 20% of patients with torsion were identified at elective surgery for other indications given the "lack of impressive symptoms."[12] The pain associated with torsion may be constant or intermittent because the vascular pedicle may twist and untwist over time. It is right sided approximately two-thirds of cases.[13] The patient may also experience nausea and vomiting, fever, and leukocytosis.[14] Although ovarian masses are predisposing factors, in one study, 46% of torsion occurred in the absence of demonstrated pathology.[14] Ovarian masses that are most commonly associated with torsion include simple cysts, corpora lutea, and dermoid cysts.[15] Owing to their adherent nature, endometriomas and malignancies are not usually associated with torsion. Adnexal torsion is most common in women of reproductive age; however, 15% of patients with torsion are premenarchal and 15% occur during or after menopause.[11]

The diagnosis of ovarian torsion may be elusive, with only 55% of women undergoing surgery for suspected adnexal torsion having this condition.[15] Ultrasound accuracy has been reported to range from 23% to 75% in different studies, which has been attributed to operator experience.[11] Additionally, the ultrasound findings may vary with the duration of the condition given the potential for intermittent vascular compromise.[16]

The most common ultrasound findings are indirect features such as ovarian enlargement (>4 cm) in a clinical setting suspicious for ovarian torsion[14,17] (**Fig. 7**A). Other indirect signs include ovarian edema and the presence of free fluid around the ovary or in the pouch of Douglas.[15,17] Direct features such as the visible twisting of the vascular pedicle can be demonstrated by evaluating the suspensory ligaments and demonstrating alternating concentric hyperechoic and hypoechoic circles known as the whirlpool sign (**Fig. 7**B).[18] The whirlpool sign may occur medial or lateral to the ovary.[19] The presence of the whirlpool sign has added value to the preoperative diagnosis of adnexal torsion, decreasing the false-positive rate.[20] Although venous and arterial flow abnormalities are described in cases of ovarian torsion, the sensitivity and specificity have been suboptimal.[21] In a recent study of 78 women undergoing laparoscopy for suspected ovarian torsion, abnormal ovarian flow had a sensitivity of 43.8% and specificity of 91.7%, with positive and negative predictive values of 78% and 71%, respecitvely.[22] Normal vascular supply does not exclude ovarian torsion, which may be related to the intermittent nature of torsion as well as the dual blood supply to the ovary via the ovarian branch of the uterine artery and the ovarian artery (**Fig. 7**C).

A recent study using the multiple ultrasound features (unilateral ovarian enlargement >4 cm, ovarian edema with hyperechogenic ovary and peripherally displaced follicles, free fluid in Pouch of Douglas, absence or reduced Doppler flow, a

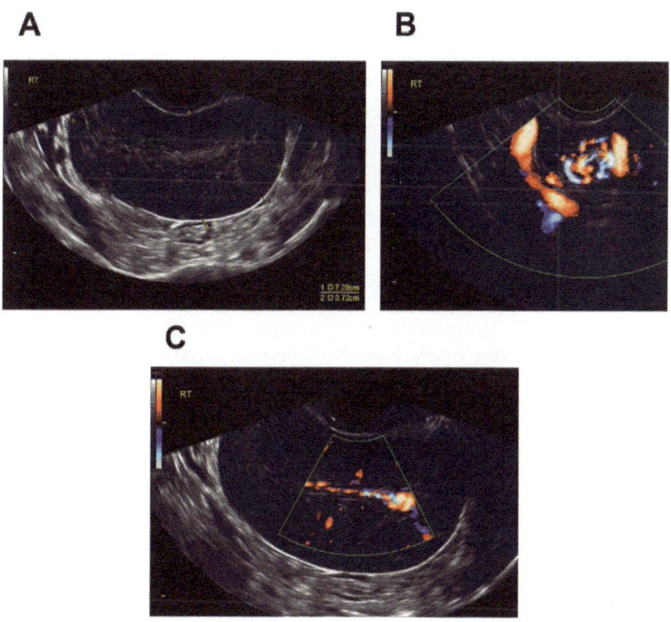


**Fig. 7.** (*A*) Transvaginal ultrasound showing a uniformly enlarged edematous ovary characteristic of ovarian torsion. (*B*) Color Doppler evaluation reveals the whirlpool sign, which is characteristic of rotated vessels. (*C*) The ovary maintains blood supply owing to the redundant nature of the vasculature.

whirlpool sign, and abnormal ovarian position) reported the presence of at least 2 findings resulted in a sensitivity of 0.84, a specificity of 0.77, a positive predictive value of 0.82, a negative predictive value of 0.79, and an overall accuracy of 0.81 for the detection of adnexal torsion.[11] The absence of ultrasound features does not rule out ovarian torsion when clinical symptoms are suggestive of this diagnosis.[17]

## UTERINE ETIOLOGIES

### *Leiomyoma*

Leiomyoma or uterine fibroids are a common benign tumor that can be associated with painful menses, painful intercourse, and acute pain from degeneration or torsion. Fibroids may outgrow their blood supply and undergo degeneration owing to venous or hemorrhagic infarction. Patients with degeneration may have a low-grade fever, uterine tenderness, elevated white blood cell count, and peritoneal signs. Pelvic ultrasound examination has a high sensitivity to detect uterine fibroids and fibroid degeneration is suspected in the setting of acute clinical pain when scanning over the fibroid. There is no typical appearance for degeneration, although they may appear cystic and edematous[23] (**Fig. 8**). The pain associated with the degeneration of uterine fibroids may be intense, but usually resolves over the course of several days to weeks. In some cases, especially if the fibroid is pedunculated or in the broad ligament, it may masquerade as an ovarian malignancy. It is incumbent on the imager to use their ultrasound skills to attempt to demonstrate a possible connection between the fibroid and the uterus and to identify a normal separate ovary.

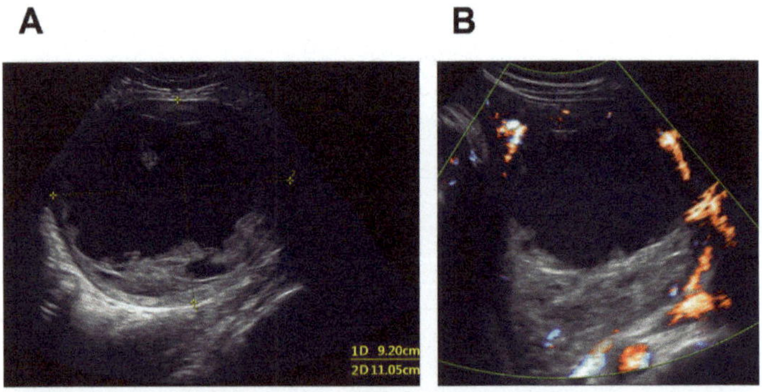


**Fig. 8.** (*A*) Transabdominal ultrasound showing a large pedunculated fibroid that has undergone cystic degeneration. The ovary was identified as separate from this mass and was normal in architecture. (*B*) Color Doppler demonstration reveals no internal color flow.

### *Hematometra Status Post Ablation or with a Mullerian Duct Anomaly*

Endometrial ablation is a procedure that surgically destroys the endometrium. On occasion, ablation of the entire endometrial lining may not be accomplished.[24] In a patient who has undergone endometrial ablation in which some endometrial tissue may have been retained, cyclic bleeding may occur. The blood can be trapped within pockets of the endometrium owing to synechiae and adhesions, resulting in significant pain.[25] Pain after endometrial ablation may also occur in the absence of an identifiable etiology on ultrasound examination.[26] Acute pelvic pain in a patient with a Müllerian duct anomaly and obstructed horn is a well-known clinical condition (**Fig. 9**).

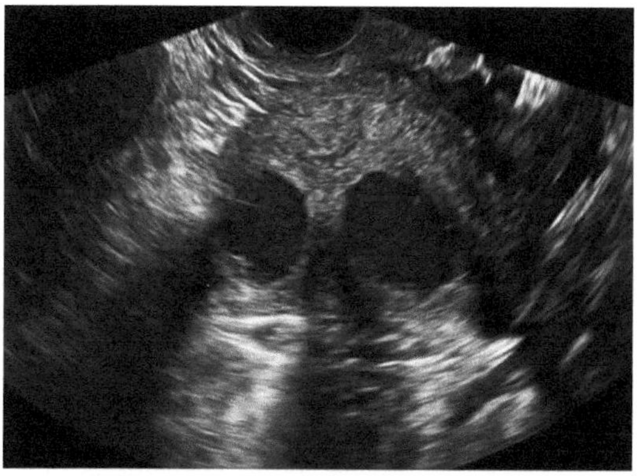

**Fig. 9.** Axial scan through the fundus of a septate uterus in a patient with pelvic pain after a septal resection. Note the hypoechoic collections with low level echoes on either side of the midline uterine septum, representing blood retained within the endometrial cavity (hematometra).

### *Adenomyosis*

Adenomyosis occurs when endometrial glands and stroma are present within the myometrium. The ectopic tissue is thought to induce hypertrophy and hyperplasia of the surrounding myometrium. The prevalence of the condition is difficult to ascertain because the definitive diagnosis is based on pathologic evaluation of the uterus and many women do not undergo hysterectomy. Adenomyosis is estimated to occur in 20% to 35% of women of reproductive age.[27,28] Some women with this condition are asymptomatic, although many have pelvic pain and menorrhagia. Adenomyosis and endometriosis often occur together within the same patient and are more common in later reproductive years and in multiparous women.[29,30] The disease process is heterogeneous and may be diffuse, focal, or associated with an adenomyoma.

The 2-dimensional ultrasound findings associated with adenomyosis include an enlarged globular uterus with heterogeneous myometrium, myometrial lucencies (**Fig. 10**A), asymmetry of the anterior and posterior myometrium (**Fig. 10**A, B), hypoechoic linear striations, and an indistinct endometrial-myometrial border[31] (**Fig. 10**C). Three-dimensional imaging will optimize evaluation of the junctional zone, which normally appears as a hypoechoic halo between the endometrium and myometrium, and which may be indistinct or interrupted in the presence of adenomyosis (**Fig. 10**D, E). Color and power Doppler ultrasound imaging can be used to differentiate glands from vascular structures and to differentiate leiomyoma from adenomyoma based on color flow. Characteristically, the capsule of a leiomyoma contains vascular flow as opposed to diffuse vascularity, which may be seen in an adenomyoma.[28]

Adenomyosis can be an elusive entity, with a recent study of highly heterogeneous studies reporting a pooled sensitivity of transvaginal ultrasound examination for the detection of adenomyosis (all subtypes) of between 0.72 and 0.82, a pooled specificity of 0.85 to 0.81, and a pooled positive likelihood ratio of 4.67 to 3.7.[32] Recent expert consensus groups have proposed uniform terms, definitions, and measurements with respect to uterine findings.[33] A correlation between the number of ultrasound findings and the degree of pelvic pain has been reported.[34]

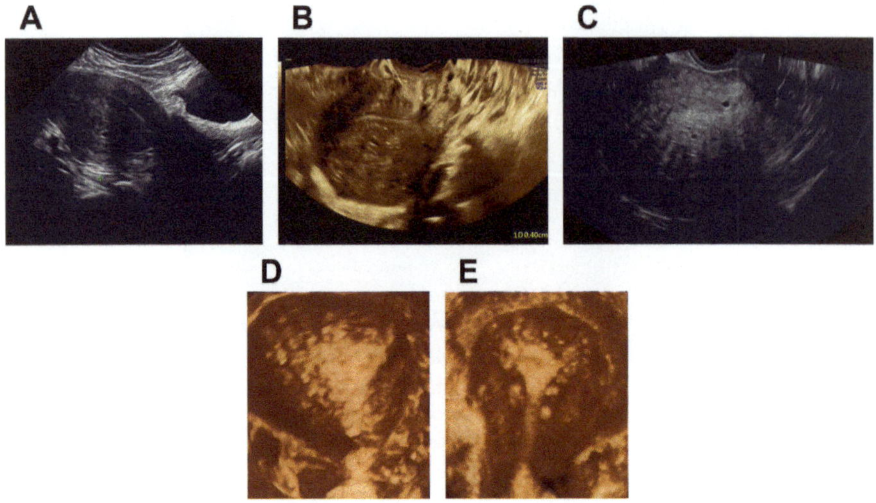


Fig. 10. (*A*) Transabdominal sagittal image of an asymmetrically thickened uterus. Note the anterior myometrium is much thinner than the posterior myometrium. The posterior myometrium is heterogeneous and contains a hypoechoic echolucent space consistent with an endometrial gland embedded in the myometrium. These ultrasound findings are typical of adenomyosis. (*B*) Transvaginal sagittal scan of a uterus demonstrating an asymmetrically thickened globular uterus. The anterior myometrium is thinner than the posterior myometrium. The posterior myometrium is mottled. In this case, the endometrium is well seen (+ calipers), which is not always the situation with adenomyosis. (*C*) Transvaginal sagittal scan of a globular uterus with adenomyosis. In this case, the endometrium cannot be distinguished and there are glandular lucencies and hypoechoic linear striations. (*D*) Three-dimensional coronal view of the uterus showing an irregular junctional zone related to extensive adenomyosis. (*E*) Three-dimensional coronal view of the uterus showing an irregular junctional zone and pockets of endometrial glands extending into the myometrium characteristic of adenomyosis.

### *Intrauterine Contraceptive Devices*

Intrauterine contraceptive devices are commonly used method of contraception, being used in approximately 10% of contraceptive users in the United States.[35] They are safe and generally well-tolerated by most women; however, side effects and complications may occur. Discontinuation of IUD use in the first 6 months after placement is approximately 7% and the most common reason is cramping.[36] A malpositioned IUD can occur in up to 10% of patients and is more common in those with a retroflexed uterus, uterine anomaly, or fibroids.[37,38] A malpositioned IUD is displaced into the lower uterine segment or cervix, is embedded in the myometrium, or penetrates the serosa, being either partially or completely extruded from the uterine cavity (**Fig. 11**). It is more commonly associated with pain and bleeding than a normally positioned IUD. The placement of the IUD shaft and especially the arms is optimally demonstrated using the 3D coronal view of the uterus.[39] Malposition of the IUD may be associated with higher pregnancy rates, although much of this occurrence can be attributed to a lack of initiation of an alternative contraceptive method after IUD removal (see Adam T. Evans and colleagues' article, "Ultrasound Assessment of the Intrauterine Device," in this issue).[37,40]

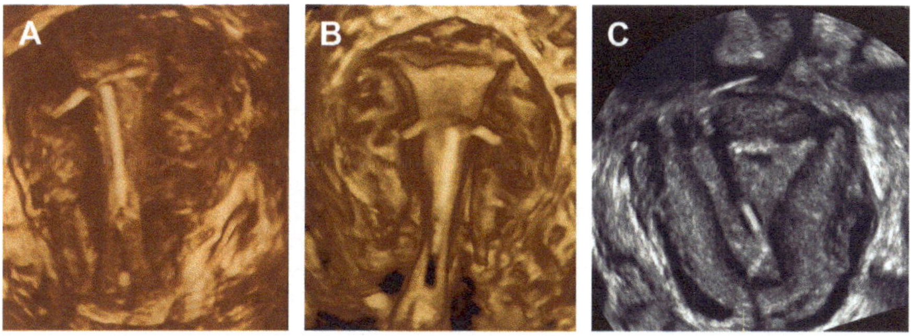


Fig. 11. (*A*) Three-dimensional coronal view of the uterus showing an IUD in the endometrial cavity; however, the right arm is embedded into the myometrium. (*B*) Three-dimensional coronal view of the uterus demonstrating an IUD in the lower part of the endometrial cavity. Both arms of the IUD are embedded in the myometrium. (*C*) Three-dimensional coronal view of the uterus demonstrating an intrauterine contraceptive device that is perforating through the serosa of the uterus, extending out the right cornua.

### *Pelvic Inflammatory Disease*

PID is an acute or subclinical infection of the uterus, fallopian tubes, and ovaries. PID is a spectrum with numerous potential pathogenic etiologies. The patient usually presents with abdominal pain, which may be associated with fever, chills, vaginal discharge, abnormal bleeding, and urinary tract symptoms. The diagnosis is made clinically, although ultrasound examination may provide additional information as to the extent of disease, including an associated tubo-ovarian abscess.

Patients with PID may have swelling and thickening of the fallopian tubes with heterogeneous material within the tubular lumen, which may be exudate or pus (**Fig. 12**). There may be a cogwheel sign (cross-section of tube) with thickened mucosa.[41] A normal ultrasound examination does not exclude PID.[42]

Beyond the focus of this article but important in the evaluation of the patient with pelvic pain are nongynecologic etiologies. These are discussed in Mahan Mathur and Leslie M. Scoutt's article, "Nongynecologic Causes of Pelvic Pain: Ultrasound First," in this issue. Nongynecologic etiologies include gastrointestinal conditions such as appendicitis and diverticulitis, as well as urologic etiologies such as acute cystitis and renal calculi. Pelvic congestion syndrome is an elusive disorder that has

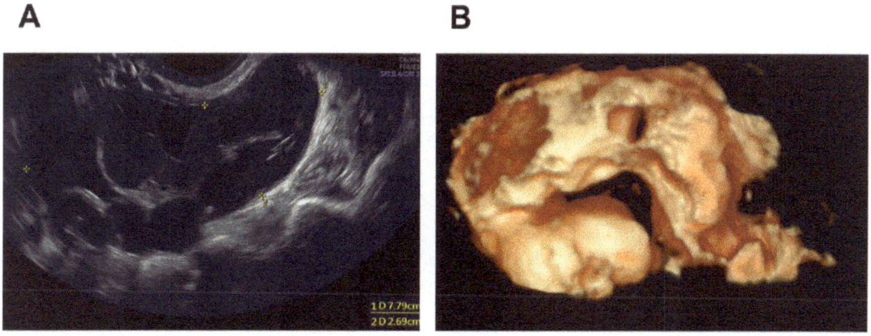


Fig. 12. (*A*) Transvaginal ultrasound of a heterogeneous tubular structure characteristic of a pyosalpinx in a patient with a history of PID. (*B*) Three-dimensional inversion mode of the tubo-ovarian structure demonstrating a dilated fallopian tube.

been reported as a cause of pain in premenopausal patients, exacerbated by standing and menses.[43,44] These entities should all be taken into consideration when primary gynecologic etiologies cannot be demonstrated.

## SUMMARY

Pelvic ultrasound examination should be the first-line imaging choice in evaluating the patient with pelvic pain. The differential diagnosis is broad; however ,a meticulous history along with a personally interactive tenderness-guided ultrasound examination looking for areas of pain and movement of organs will provide a wealth of information in identifying the etiology of the patient's pain. The use of 3D imaging and adjunctive color may help to narrow the differential diagnosis. Nongynecologic etiologies should be considered in the differential diagnosis when a primary gynecologic etiology is not apparent.

## SUPPLEMENTARY DATA

Supplementary data related to this article can be found online at https://doi.org/10.1016/j.ogc.2019.06.002.

## REFERENCES

1. Latthe P, Latthe M, Say L, et al. WHO systematic review of prevalence of chronic pelvic pain: a neglected reproductive health morbidity. BMC Public Health 2006; 6:177.
2. Mathias SD, Kuppermann M, Liberman RF, et al. Chronic pelvic pain: prevalence, health-related quality of life, and economic correlates. Obstet Gynecol 1996; 87(3):321–7.
3. Benacerraf BR, Abuhamad AZ, Bromley B, et al. Consider ultrasound first for imaging the female pelvis. Am J Obstet Gynecol 2015;212(4):450–5.
4. Steege JF, Siedhoff MT. Chronic pelvic pain. Obstet Gynecol 2014;124(3): 616–29.
5. Timor-Tritsch IE. Sliding organs sign in gynecological ultrasound. Ultrasound Obstet Gynecol 2015;46(1):125–6.
6. Timor-Tritsch IE, Monteagudo A, Rebarber A, et al. Transrectal scanning: an alternative when transvaginal scanning is not feasible. Ultrasound Obstet Gynecol 2003;21(5):473–9.
7. Jain KA. Sonographic spectrum of hemorrhagic ovarian cysts. J Ultrasound Med 2002;21(8):879–86.
8. Van Holsbeke C, Van Calster B, Guerriero S, et al. Endometriomas: their ultrasound characteristics. Ultrasound Obstet Gynecol 2010;35(6):730–40.
9. Van den Bosch T, Van Schoubroeck D. Ultrasound diagnosis of endometriosis and adenomyosis: state of the art. Best Pract Res Clin Obstet Gynaecol 2018; 51:16–24.
10. Guerriero S, Condous G, van den Bosch T, et al. Systematic approach to sonographic evaluation of the pelvis in women with suspected endometriosis, including terms, definitions and measurements: a consensus opinion from the International Deep Endometriosis Analysis (IDEA) group. Ultrasound Obstet Gynecol 2016;48(3):318–32.
11. Feng JL, Lei T, Xie HN, et al. Spectrums and outcomes of adnexal torsion at different ages. J Ultrasound Med 2017;36(9):1859–66.
12. Hibbard LT. Adnexal torsion. Am J Obstet Gynecol 1985;152(4):456–61.

13. Huchon C, Fauconnier A. Adnexal torsion: a literature review. Eur J Obstet Gynecol Reprod Biol 2010;150(1):8–12.
14. Shadinger LL, Andreotti RF, Kurian RL. Preoperative sonographic and clinical characteristics as predictors of ovarian torsion. J Ultrasound Med 2008; 27(1):7–13.
15. Melcer Y, Maymon R, Pekar-Zlotin M, et al. Does she have adnexal torsion? Prediction of adnexal torsion in reproductive age women. Arch Gynecol Obstet 2018; 297(3):685–90.
16. Smorgick N, Maymon R, Mendelovic S, et al. Torsion of normal adnexa in postmenarcheal women: can ultrasound indicate an ischemic process? Ultrasound Obstet Gynecol 2008;31(3):338–41.
17. Mashiach R, Melamed N, Gilad N, et al. Sonographic diagnosis of ovarian torsion: accuracy and predictive factors. J Ultrasound Med 2011;30(9):1205–10.
18. Lee EJ, Kwon HC, Joo HJ, et al. Diagnosis of ovarian torsion with color Doppler sonography: depiction of twisted vascular pedicle. J Ultrasound Med 1998; 17(2):83–9.
19. Navve D, Hershkovitz R, Zetounie E, et al. Medial or lateral location of the whirlpool sign in adnexal torsion: clinical importance. J Ultrasound Med 2013;32(9): 1631–4.
20. Valsky DV, Esh-Broder E, Cohen SM, et al. Added value of the gray-scale whirlpool sign in the diagnosis of adnexal torsion. Ultrasound Obstet Gynecol 2010; 36(5):630–4.
21. Grunau GL, Harris A, Buckley J, et al. Diagnosis of ovarian torsion: is it time to forget about Doppler? J Obstet Gynaecol Can 2018;40(7):871–5.
22. Bar-On S, Mashiach R, Stockheim D, et al. Emergency laparoscopy for suspected ovarian torsion: are we too hasty to operate? Fertil Steril 2010;93(6): 2012–5.
23. Testa AC, Di Legge A, Bonatti M, et al. Imaging techniques for evaluation of uterine myomas. Best Pract Res Clin Obstet Gynaecol 2016;34:37–53.
24. Lethaby A, Penninx J, Hickey M, et al. Endometrial resection and ablation techniques for heavy menstrual bleeding. Cochrane Database Syst Rev 2013;(8):CD001501.
25. Carey FT, El-Nashar SA, Hopkins MR, et al. Pathologic characteristics of hysterectomy specimens in women undergoing hysterectomy after global endometrial ablation. J Minim Invasive Gynecol 2011;18(1):96–9.
26. Wishall KM, Price J, Pereira N, et al. Postablation risk factors for pain and subsequent hysterectomy. Obstet Gynecol 2014;124(5):904–10.
27. Naftalin J, Hoo W, Pateman K, et al. How common is adenomyosis? A prospective study of prevalence using transvaginal ultrasound in a gynaecology clinic. Hum Reprod 2012;27(12):3432–9.
28. Andres MP, Borrelli GM, Ribeiro J, et al. Transvaginal ultrasound for the diagnosis of adenomyosis: systematic review and meta-analysis. J Minim Invasive Gynecol 2018;25(2):257–64.
29. Lazzeri L, Di Giovanni A, Exacoustos C, et al. Preoperative and postoperative clinical and transvaginal ultrasound findings of adenomyosis in patients with deep infiltrating endometriosis. Reprod Sci 2014;21(8):1027–33.
30. Lazzeri L, Morosetti G, Centini G, et al. A sonographic classification of adenomyosis: interobserver reproducibility in the evaluation of type and degree of the myometrial involvement. Fertil Steril 2018;110(6):1154–61.e3.
31. Sakhel K, Abuhamad A. Sonography of adenomyosis. J Ultrasound Med 2012; 31(5):805–8.

32. Bazot M, Darai E. Role of transvaginal sonography and magnetic resonance imaging in the diagnosis of uterine adenomyosis. Fertil Steril 2018;109(3):389–97.
33. Van den Bosch T, Dueholm M, Leone FP, et al. Terms, definitions and measurements to describe sonographic features of myometrium and uterine masses: a consensus opinion from the Morphological Uterus Sonographic Assessment (MUSA) group. Ultrasound Obstet Gynecol 2015;46(3):284–98.
34. Naftalin J, Hoo W, Nunes N, et al. Association between ultrasound features of adenomyosis and severity of menstrual pain. Ultrasound Obstet Gynecol 2016; 47(6):779–83.
35. Kavanaugh ML, Jerman J, Finer LB. Changes in use of long-acting reversible contraceptive methods among U.S. women, 2009-2012. Obstet Gynecol 2015; 126(5):917–27.
36. Grunloh DS, Casner T, Secura GM, et al. Characteristics associated with discontinuation of long-acting reversible contraception within the first 6 months of use. Obstet Gynecol 2013;122(6):1214–21.
37. Braaten KP, Benson CB, Maurer R, et al. Malpositioned intrauterine contraceptive devices: risk factors, outcomes, and future pregnancies. Obstet Gynecol 2011; 118(5):1014–20.
38. Gerkowicz SA, Fiorentino DG, Kovacs AP, et al. Uterine structural abnormality and intrauterine device malposition: analysis of ultrasonographic and demographic variables of 517 patients. Am J Obstet Gynecol 2019;220(2):183.e1–8.
39. Benacerraf BR, Shipp TD, Bromley B. Three-dimensional ultrasound detection of abnormally located intrauterine contraceptive devices which are a source of pelvic pain and abnormal bleeding. Ultrasound Obstet Gynecol 2009;34(1):110–5.
40. Inal MM, Ertopcu K, Ozelmas I. The evaluation of 318 intrauterine pregnancy cases with an intrauterine device. Eur J Contracept Reprod Health Care 2005; 10(4):266–71.
41. Timor-Tritsch IE, Lerner JP, Monteagudo A, et al. Transvaginal sonographic markers of tubal inflammatory disease. Ultrasound Obstet Gynecol 1998;12(1): 56–66.
42. Romosan G, Valentin L. The sensitivity and specificity of transvaginal ultrasound with regard to acute pelvic inflammatory disease: a review of the literature. Arch Gynecol Obstet 2014;289(4):705–14.
43. Borghi C, Dell'Atti L. Pelvic congestion syndrome: the current state of the literature. Arch Gynecol Obstet 2016;293(2):291–301.
44. Steenbeek MP, van der Vleuten CJM, Schultze Kool LJ, et al. Noninvasive diagnostic tools for pelvic congestion syndrome: a systematic review. Acta Obstet Gynecol Scand 2018;97(7):776–86.

# Abnormal Uterine Bleeding

Ashraf Khafaga, MBBCh[a,1], Steven R. Goldstein, MD[b,*]

**KEYWORDS**

- Abnormal uterine bleeding • Postmenopause • Perimenopause
- Endometrial biopsy • Transvaginal ultrasonography • Sonohysterography (SIS)
- PALM-COEIN system • Endometrial carcinoma

**KEY POINTS**

- Abnormal uterine bleeding (AUB) is an extremely common medical problem encountered in women, with a direct influence on their quality of life, utilization of the health care resources, and costs.
- AUB in women older than 40 years and especially in postmenopausal women requires a prompt and efficient evaluation, mainly to exclude the presence of malignant or premalignant lesions of the endometrium.
- Cancer of the endometrium is the most common gynecologic malignancy, with an incidence in the United States of more than 60,000 cases and mortality estimated at 10,000 women annually.

**Video content accompanies this article at http://www.obgyn.theclinics.com.**

## INTRODUCTION

Abnormal uterine bleeding (AUB) is a common gynecologic complaint that accounts for one-third of outpatient visits to gynecologists and accounts of more than 70% of all gynecologic consults in the perimenopausal and postmenopausal years.[1] A US population-based survey of women ages 18 to 50 years reported an annual prevalence rate of AUB as 53 per 1000 women.[2] The estimated annual direct cost of AUB in 2007 was approximately $1 billion, with indirect economic costs of $12 billion.[3]

---

A. Khafaga: No disclosures to report. S.R. Goldstein: GYN Advisory Board for AbbVie, Amag, and Therapeutics MD; Consultant for Cook OB/GYN, Cooper Surgical, and IBSA; Speakers Bureau for Amag, Duchesnay, Therapeutics MD; Equipment loan from GE Ultrasound.

[a] Icahn School of Medicine at Mount Sinai, 1 Gustave L. Levy Pl, New York, NY 10029, USA; [b] New York University School of Medicine, 530 First Avenue, Suite 10N, New York, NY 10016, USA
[1] Present address: 96-02 57th Avenue, unit 15A, Corona, NY 11368.
* Corresponding author.
*E-mail address:* steven.goldstein@nyumc.org

Obstet Gynecol Clin N Am 46 (2019) 595–605
https://doi.org/10.1016/j.ogc.2019.07.001
0889-8545/19/

In addition, vaginal bleeding is the presenting sign in more than 90% of postmenopausal women with cancer of the endometrium.[4] Cancer of the endometrium is the most common gynecologic malignancy in the United States, and worldwide as well. In 2018, the estimated incidence of uterine cancer in the United States was 63,230 new cases with an estimated mortality of 11,350 deaths.[5] Therefore, the management of AUB needs to be undertaken seriously.

The availability of newer diagnostic tools has made it possible to promptly diagnose and treat an increasing number of such AUBs in an office setting. Once a proper diagnosis has been established, appropriate management must be implemented. Thus, the primary aims in evaluation of patients with AUB are as follows:

1. Early detection of serious underlying pathology, such as carcinoma, or precancerous lesions, such as complex atypical endometrial hyperplasia, and
2. To diagnose the anatomic cause of bleeding so an appropriate treatment plan can be carried out.

## *Etiology*

The definition of AUB is "flow outside of normal volume, duration, regularity, or frequency."[1] AUB can be caused by anatomic uterine abnormalities or nonstructural causes. In 2011, the International Federation of Gynecology and Obstetrics (FIGO) introduced a new classification system for abnormal uterine bleeding that was endorsed by the American Congress of Obstetrics and Gynecology (ACOG) in 2012, in attempt to standardize the terminology used to describe AUB.[6] This system, known by the acronym PALM-COEIN, distinguishes abnormal uterine bleeding based on the suspected etiology: *p*olyp; *a*denomyosis; *l*eiomyoma; *m*alignancy and hyperplasia; *c*oagulopathy; *o*vulatory dysfunction; *e*ndometrial; *i*atrogenic; and *n*ot yet classified.[6] The PALM portion of the PALM-COEIN covers the structural causes of abnormal uterine bleeding. In contrast, The COEIN acronym represents the nonstructural, hormonal, or systemic causes of abnormal uterine bleeding.

Descriptive terms are paired with AUB to indicate the bleeding patterns. Heavy menstrual bleeding (AUB/HMB) is now used instead of the term menorrhagia and intermenstrual bleeding (AUB/IMB) has replaced the term metrorrhagia.[1] AUB is further denoted by the qualified letter or letters to indicated the underlying etiology such as AUB-P for AUB-POLYP, AUB-L for AUB- Leiomyoma, and so forth. Leiomyomas may be subclassified as either submucosal (AUB-$L_{SM}$) or those that do not affect the uterine cavity (AUB-$L_O$). Abnormal bleeding associated with the use of exogenous steroids (ie, hormonal treatments), intrauterine systems (IUSs) or devices, or other systemic or local agents are classified as iatrogenic, whereas the remainder of rare or ill-defined causes are categorized as not yet classified. Ovulatory dysfunction (AUB-O) is usually related to exposure to unopposed estrogen by different mechanisms such as polycystic ovary syndrome (PCOS), or oligo-ovulation, which is common in the perimenopausal years.

The term dysfunctional uterine bleeding is usually used to indicate AUB, which is caused by nonstructural abnormalities, and is not a part of the PALM-COEIN, so the ACOG recommended to discontinue using this term.[1]

## *Postmenopausal Bleeding*

Postmenopausal bleeding (PMB) is defined by any uterine bleeding in a menopausal woman who is not taking cycling postmenopausal hormone therapy. It represents 5% of office gynecology visits.[7] PMB should be considered as endometrial cancer until proven otherwise.[8] Any patient who is post menopause and presenting with any vaginal bleeding, staining, or spotting must be evaluated to rule out the presence of cancer. Studies have shown the incidence of malignancy in such patients ranges from 1% to 14% depending on the presence of coexisting risk factors, such as obesity, hypertension, diabetes, and low parity, so even though the most common underlying pathology of PMB is the atrophy of the vaginal mucosa or endometrium, cancer must be excluded.[8]

### *Diagnosis in Women Presenting with Abnormal Uterine Bleeding*

The evaluation of women with AUB starts with a through medical history and physical examination and appropriate laboratory and imaging tests as indicated. A medical history should be guided by the PALM-COEIN system and include inquiries about the menstrual bleeding pattern, the amount, the presence of pain, and family history of AUB or underlying bleeding disorders, medication or herbal preparation that might affect bleeding in general, such as ginseng, ginkgo, motherwort, contraceptives, nonsteroidal anti-inflammatory drugs, and warfarin or heparin derivatives.[9,10] One of the most important aspects of the medical history will be careful assessment of the bleeding pattern. For instance, very cyclic heavy menstrual bleeding without any intermenstrual bleeding would be unlikely to be carcinoma or even hyperplasia. Most often, an irregular bleeding pattern is associated with no endometrial pathology.

The physical examination also may reveal findings that contribute to AUB. Physical signs suggestive of the underlying disease include excessive weight, hyperprolactinemia (galactorrhea), signs of PCOS (eg, acne, hirsutism), signs of thyroid disease (eg, thyroid nodule or goiter), and signs of bleeding disorders (eg, ecchymosis and petechiae). In addition, a pelvic examination using a speculum should be performed to exclude lower genital tract causes as cervical or vaginal etiologies of bleeding, and bimanual assessment of size and contour of the uterus should be performed as well.

Laboratory testing should be ordered depending on the patient history and physical examination. In general, the initial laboratory assessment of AUB should include the following:

- Complete blood count in attempt to assess the presence of anemia and severity of bleeding
- Pregnancy test
- Thyroid-stimulating hormone level assessment
- Testing for *Chlamydia trachomatis*
- Cervical cancer screening if there are associated concerning symptoms also may be appropriate
- Endometrial sampling, if indicated
- Assessment of underlying bleeding disorders if concerning or suspected
- Pelvic imaging

The best initial imaging test of the uterus to assess AUB is transvaginal ultrasound (TVU). If TVU images are not adequate or further evaluation is required, then sonohysterography, also known as saline infusion sonography (SIS), or hysteroscopy is recommended. These procedures leverage the instillation of fluid or gel into the endometrial cavity to better delineate endometrial anatomy, with visualization via ultrasound in SIS, or directly via camera in hysteroscopy. Hysteroscopy is more expensive, requires more anesthesia, and, if performed, is preferably done in an office setting.[1] Newer disposable hysteroscopy, recently developed, makes this recommendation easier to follow.

One study of 443 women[8] between the ages of 37 and menopause used TVU, with SIS when necessary, as the first step in triage (**Fig. 1**). The investigators reported 79%

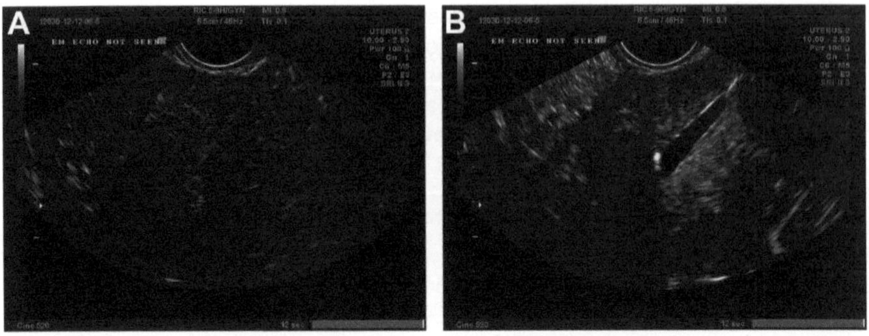


**Fig. 1.** (*A*) TVU of a perimenopausal patient with AUB. An endometrial echo is not well visualized. The uterus is somewhat axial and there is a suspicion of adenomyosis. (*B*) SIS on the patient in (*A*). The sonolucent area in the center is fluid that has been instilled through an SIS catheter. The endometrium surrounding the fluid is thin, compatible with lack of significant tissue. This was performed on the day after the bleeding cycle ended. This is indicative of dysfunctional anovulatory bleeding in this perimenopausal woman.

of women between 37 years old and menopause with AUB had no anatomic pathology, presumably secondary to dysfunctional anovulatory bleeding (**Fig. 2**). Some of these women with AUB/HMB may have an enlarged cavity with increased surface area due to increasing parity, uterine hypertrophy secondary to leiomyoma with no submucous component, or adenomyosis without endometrial abnormality. In that study, endometrial abnormalities included hyperplasia, polyps, and submucous myomas (**Figs. 3** and **4**).

### *Endometrial Sampling*

ACOG currently recommends performing endometrial sampling in patients presenting with AUB who are older than 45 years as their initial evaluation test. In addition, it should be done in patients who are younger than 45 years if there are additional risk factors, such as the following:

- Risk for unopposed estrogen, such as obesity and PCOS
- Failed medical management

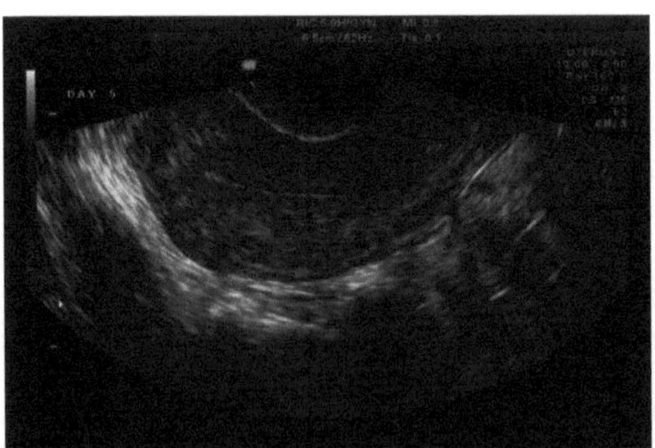


**Fig. 2.** TVU of a long-axis view of the uterus in a perimenopausal patient with AUB. This is done on day 5 of the cycle, the day after the bleeding has ended. Endometrial echo is a thin, white echogenic line down the center of the uterus. This is indicative of a lack of any significant tissue and is compatible with her diagnosis of dysfunctional anovulatory bleeding.

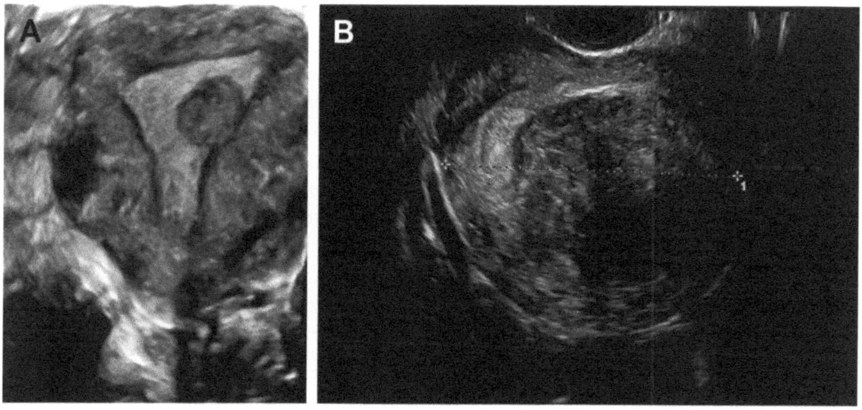


**Fig. 3.** (*A*) This recreated "Z-plane" from a 3-dimensional transvaginal scan in a perimenopausal patient with AUB. This was done in the luteal phase of the cycle and a submucous myoma is clearly visualized extending into the cavity approximately 90%. (*B*) Transvaginal pelvic ultrasound of a perimenopausal woman with AUB. This is a transverse view of the uterus. There is a large intramural myoma extending almost from the serosa deviating the echogenic endometrium, indicating some degree of submucous component.

- Persistent AUB or those who have any irregularity in the appearance of endometrium on TVU
- High risk of endometrial cancer (eg, tamoxifen therapy, Lynch or Cowden syndrome)[1]

Choosing 45 years old as the cutoff point for increased concern regarding endometrial neoplasia is supported by evidence that the risk of endometrial hyperplasia and carcinoma is quite low before age 45 years and increases with advancing age, as the incidence rate of 16.3% was reported in women aged 45 to 54 years compared with an incidence rate of 5.4% in those aged 35 to 44 years.[5,11]

*In postmenopausal women*, the endometrial evaluation is essential in triaging patients to no anatomic pathology or anatomic pathology and then, furthermore, whether such pathology Is focal in nature and needs to be distinguished from more global

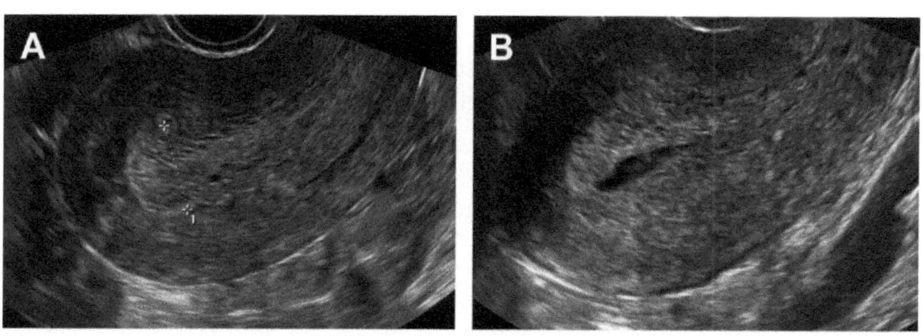


**Fig. 4.** (*A*) Transvaginal pelvic sonogram of a long-axis view of a patient with AUB. The endometrial echo is thickened. This measured 12 mm maximum anteroposterior thickness. The patient has just ended a bleeding cycle. (*B*) SIS of the patient from (*A*). There is a small amount of fluid expanding the endometrial cavity. This is some endometrial fluid in the cul-de-sac, indicating tubal patency. The tissue surrounding the fluid is thick and symmetric. Thus, blind endometrial sampling is appropriate, as the process is indeed global. Final pathology revealed complex hyperplasia without atypia.

processes. Historically, dilation and curettage was the primary diagnostic test for AUB, and was in fact, the most common surgical procedure in women during much of the twentieth century. Subsequently, endometrial sampling in an outpatient setting gained widespread acceptance as a modality to include or exclude the presence of carcinoma or premalignant lesions. The trend for blind endometrial sampling with disposable suction piston devices began after a single study by Stovall and colleagues.[12] Stovall and colleagues[12] performed an outpatient biopsy on 40 patients with known carcinoma in the week before their hysterectomy and obtained endometrial carcinoma in 39 of the 40 samples, thus reporting a 97.5% accuracy. This was widely publicized, marketed, and promoted, and was rapidly accepted as "standard of care." However, in a similar study, Guido and colleagues[13] performed similar blind endometrial sampling in 65 patients with known carcinoma in the operating room just before their hysterectomy. They missed 11 of 65 cancers (sensitivity only 83%) but, on opening all those uteri, they reported that, when the cancers occupied 50% or more of the endometrial surface, the biopsy was 100% accurate. These studies have been repeated, and in women with known carcinomas, the sensitivity of blind sampling was only 84%[14] and 68%[15] in those studies, yielding a false-negative rate of 16% and 32%, respectively. Rodriguez and colleagues[16] explained this poor performance characteristic by showing that the one brand of endometrial biopsy device managed to sample an average of only 4% of the endometrial surface area (range 0%–12%).

Finally, in 2012, ACOG acknowledged "the primary role of endometrial sampling in patients with AUB is to determine if carcinoma or premalignant lesions are present."[1] The Practice Bulletin goes on to state that endometrial biopsy has "high overall accuracy in diagnosing endometrial cancer when an adequate specimen is obtained and when the endometrial process is global. If the cancer occupies less than 50% of the surface area of the endometrial cavity, the cancer can be missed by blind endometrial biopsy. Therefore, these tests are only an endpoint when they reveal cancer or atypical complex hyperplasia." This statement has tremendous ramifications for clinical practice. Certainly, health care providers, especially in low-resource areas, can begin the evaluation with a blind biopsy, but, if the results do not indicate cancer or atypical hyperplasia, the evaluation is not adequate and cannot be accepted as an endpoint, especially if bleeding persists. In these cases without an endpoint, further testing, such as hysteroscopy with dilation and curettage is an appropriate choice.[4] Thus, the concept of distinguishing "global" from "focal" pathologies by using SIS is becoming increasingly understood.

To conclude, the shortcomings of blind endometrial biopsy and ACOG's acknowledgment of this nontrivial problem, represents a major shift in how blind endometrial sampling should be reviewed and has led to a fundamental change in the standard care of patients with AUB.

### *Imaging Techniques*

#### *Transvaginal ultrasonography*

TVU is an appropriate imaging study in women presenting with AUB, as it is a safe and cost-effective method of diagnosing structural causes of abnormal uterine bleeding by examining the uterine cavity. It is an integral diagnostic tool to exclude the PALM portion of the PALM-COEIN system. Vaginal probes for ultrasonography were introduced in the 1980s providing a degree of image magnification as if we were doing ultrasound through a low-power microscope, and can be considered a form of "sonomicroscopy."[17]

At its most elementary level, TVU is able to measure endometrial thickness. However, the use of TVU in the assessment of endometrial thickness is not an optimal tool to assess abnormalities in premenopausal woman, as compared with its use in exclusion of malignancy in postmenopausal women.[18–20] Endometrial thickness varies during the menstrual cycle as a result of the dynamic hormonal changes, leading to a limited application of endometrial thickness as a diagnostic tool in premenopausal women. Thus, the timing of the ultrasonography evaluation is crucial, as it must be done after the bleeding cycle ceases, when the endometrium is as thin as it can be without any hormonal influences.[8] In addition, the presence of endometrial moguls (**Fig. 5**), which are endometrial asymmetry and irregularities induced by dilation and curettage, normal vaginal deliveries, cesarean deliveries, and myomectomies, could be misinterpreted as polyps or focal hyperplasia.[8]

There are insufficient data collected on *perimenopausal* women with AUB. Perimenopause is defined as "the period around the onset of menopause that is often marked by various physical signs such as hot flushes and menstrual irregularities."[21] One potential pitfall in perimenopausal women is that their cycling of the endometrium is dependent on erratic estrogen production of perimenopausal ovaries. In the previously cited study of 433 perimenopausal patients[22] aged 37 to 54, 10.2% required sonohysterography (see **Fig. 1**) because the unenhanced TVU done at the end of a bleeding cycle was inadequate to effectively characterize and measure the endometrium.

*In postmenopausal women*, however, TVU is a reliable alternative to endometrial sampling as an initial evaluation tool, especially in women presenting with their initial episode of bleeding. The earliest reports comparing TVU with endometrial sampling in women with PMB consistently showed an endometrial thickness 4 mm to 5 mm or less reliably excluded endometrial cancer.[23] (**Fig. 6**, Video 1).

Multicentered clinical trials have been conducted to confirm the test characteristics of using endometrial echo thickness to exclude cancer. In 2016, Wong and colleagues[24] conducted a retrospective cohort study of 4383 postmenopausal bleeding women, stratified according to their endometrial thickness on TVU evaluation. They revealed that of 1915 patients with endometrial thickness of 3 mm or less, only 5 patients were reported to have cancer, representing a negative predictive value (NPV) of 99.7%. An endometrial thickness cutoff of 4 mm or less (n = 2,825, with 10 cases of cancer) had a 99.6% NPV, whereas 5 mm or less (n = 3131, with 11 cases of cancer)

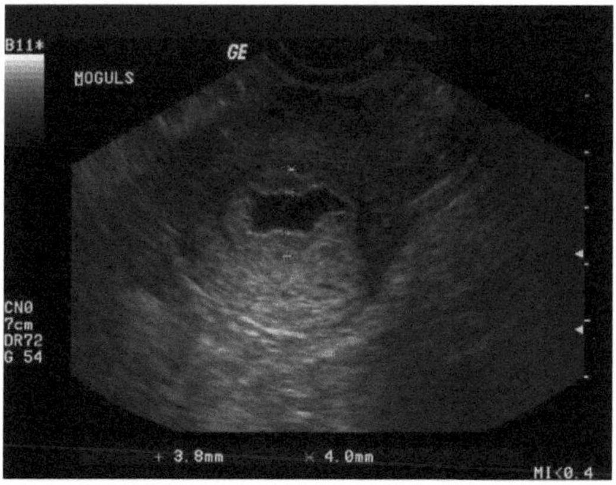


**Fig. 5.** Saline infusion sonohysterography done in the second half of the cycle showing topographic irregularities to the surface of the endometrium that have been called "moguls." (*Adapted from* Goldstein SR. Modern evaluation of the endometrium. Obstet Gynecol 2010;116(1):173; with permission.)

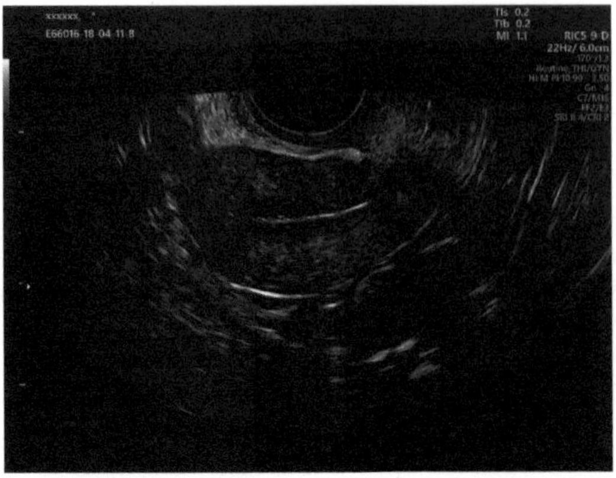

**Fig. 6.** Example of a long-axis transvaginal view in a patient with postmenopausal bleeding. The endometrial echo is seen to be thin and can be easily seen from the internal cervical os to the fundus. There is an intact hypoechoic zone surrounding it. This patient's endometrial echo measures 1.4 mm.

had a 99.6% NPV. Similar results were reported by Gull and colleagues,[25] who studied 1138 postmenopausal women with bleeding. In this study, a cutoff of 4 mm or less (n = 518, with no cancers) had a 100% NPV.

In cases of failure to identify a thin and distinct endometrial echo, further evaluation is needed by performing SIS, office hysteroscopy, or endometrial sampling. In a patient with recurrent or persistent bleeding despite absence of abnormal endometrial histology on endometrial sampling, hysteroscopy with dilation and curettage should be considered, irrespective of the endometrial thickness.[4] Conversely, an endometrial thickness more than 4 mm in an asymptomatic postmenopausal woman should not prompt further evaluation, unless the clinician's assessment is concerning for other cancer risk factors.[4] Clinical risk factors of endometrial cancer include age, obesity, use of unopposed estrogen, type 2 diabetes mellitus, PCOS, and family history of gynecologic cancer or cancer syndromes.[4]

Accordingly, ACOG states that when TVU images a thin, distinct endometrial echo measuring 4 mm or less, endometrial sampling is not required.[4] Thus, the initial evaluation of women with PMB may begin with a TVU, and if sufficiently distinct and thin, no further workup is necessary. In fact, if one does attempt endometrial sampling in such women, often no tissue is present, and if present, it is often insufficient for histologic evaluation.[26]

***Limitation of transvaginal ultrasonography***

Unfortunately, the main drawbacks of using TVU are the low sensitivity and specificity for assessing the intracavity lesions, reported as only 56% and 73%, respectively.[27] Although the endometrial cavity is a 3-dimensional structure, each frozen sonographic image is a 2-dimensional "snapshot," and a single long-axis view may not be completely reflective of the entire uterine cavity.[8] Three-dimensional assessment may be useful in ensuring that the entire endometrial cavity is interrogated; however, not all uteri lend themselves to a meaningful unenhanced TVU (**Fig. 7**). An axial uterus, marked obesity, coexisting myomas, adenomyosis, or previous uterine surgery can preclude satisfactory endometrial evaluation. In such cases, SIS will be extremely helpful in better delineating endometrial contents. Failure to adequately identify a thin, distinct endometrial echo in a postmenopausal woman with bleeding should

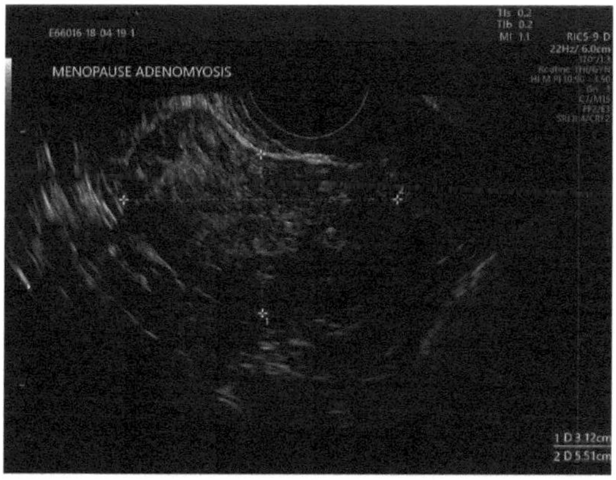


**Fig. 7.** A menopausal patient with a history of postmenopausal bleeding. This is a long-axis view of the uterus. An endometrial echo is not visualized, secondary to the presence of adenomyotic changes. This underscores the concept that not all uteri lend themselves to a meaningful unenhanced TVU.

trigger such an alternative method of evaluation. In some cases, endometrial fluid, which may result from atrophic changes or cervical stenosis or may represent blood, can serve as a physiologic sonohysterogram and can rule out pathology if the surrounding tissue is thin. However, if the surrounding tissue is not thin or there are focal abnormalities, further evaluation with direct visualization via hysteroscopy is indicated.

## SUMMARY

AUB is a common occurrence in perimenopausal and even postmenopausal women. Their evaluation has evolved over time with more data. Newer understanding of the shortcomings of blind endometrial biopsy and abundant data on the utility of TVU, and SIS when indicated, has radically changed the approach to these women.

## SUPPLEMENTARY DATA

Supplementary data related to this article can be found online at https://doi.org/10.1016/j.ogc.2019.07.001.

## REFERENCES

1. American College of Obstetricians and Gynecologists. Practice bulletin no. 128: diagnosis of abnormal uterine bleeding in reproductive-aged women. Obstet Gynecol 2012;120:197–206.
2. Kjerulff KH, Erickson BA, Langenberg PW. Chronic gynecological conditions reported by US women: findings from the National Health Interview Survey, 1984 to 1992. Am J Public Health 1996;86:195–9.
3. Liu Z, Doan QV, Blumenthal P, et al. A systematic review evaluating health-related quality of life, work impairment, and health-care costs and utilization in abnormal uterine bleeding. Value Health 2007;10:183–94.
4. American College of Obstetricians and Gynecologists Committee Opinion No. 734: the role of transvaginal ultrasonography in evaluating the endometrium of women with postmenopausal bleeding. Obstet Gynecol 2018;131:e124–9.

5. National Cancer Institute Surveillance, epidemiology, and end results program. Cancer stat facts: uterine cancer. Available at: https://seer.cancer.gov/statfacts/html/corp.html. Accessed October 2, 2018.
6. Munro MG, Critchley HO, Broder MS, et al. FIGO classification system (PALM-COEIN) for causes of abnormal uterine bleeding in nongravid women of reproductive age. Int J Gynecol Obstet 2011;113:3–13.
7. Moodley M, Roberts C. Clinical pathway for the evaluation of postmenopausal bleeding with an emphasis on endometrial cancer detection. J Obstet Gynaecol 2004;24:736.
8. Goldstein SR. Modern evaluation of the endometrium. Obstet Gynecol 2010;116: 168–76.
9. Basila D, Yuan CS. Effects of dietary supplements on coagulation and platelet function. Thromb Res 2005;117:49–53.
10. Wittkowsky AK. A systematic review and inventory of supplemental effects on warfarin and other anticoagulants. Thromb Res 2005;117:81–6.
11. Reed SD, Newton KM, Clinton WL, et al. Incidence of endometrial hyperplasia. Am J Obstet Gynecol 2009;200:678.e1.
12. Stovall TG, Photopulos GJ, Poston WM, et al. Pipelle endometrial sampling in patients with known endometrial carcinoma. Obstet Gynecol 1991;77:954–6.
13. Guido RS, Kanbour-Shakir A, Rulin MC, et al. Pipelle endometrial sampling. Sensitivity in the detection of endometrial cancer. J Reprod Med 1995;40:553–5.
14. Larson DM, Krawisz BR, Johnson KK, et al. Comparison of the Z-Sampler and Novak endometrial biopsy instruments for in-office diagnosis of endometrial cancer. Gynecol Oncol 1994;54:64–7.
15. Ferry J, Farnsworth A, Webster M, et al. The efficacy of the pipelle endometrial biopsy in detecting endometrial carcinoma. Aust N Z J Obstet Gynaecol 1993; 33:76–8.
16. Rodriguez MH, Platt LD, Medearis AL, et al. The use of transvaginal sonography for evaluation of postmenopausal size and morphology. Am J Obstet Gynecol 1988;159:810–4.
17. Goldstein SR. Pregnancy I: embryo. In: Goldstein SR, editor. Endovaginal ultrasound. 2nd edition. New York: Wiley-Liss; Inc; 1991. p. 55–70.
18. Dueholm M, Jensen ML, Laursen H, et al. Can the endometrial thickness as measured by trans-vaginal sonography be used to exclude polyps or hyperplasia in pre-menopausal patients with abnormal uterine bleeding? Acta Obstet Gynecol Scand 2001;80:645–51.
19. Breitkopf DM, Frederickson RA, Snyder RR. Detection of benign endometrial masses by endometrial stripe measurement in premenopausal women. Obstet Gynecol 2004;104:120–5.
20. Dijkhuizen FP, De Vries LD, Mol BW, et al. Comparison of transvaginal ultrasonography and saline infusion sonography for the detection of intracavitary abnormalities in premenopausal women. Ultrasound Obstet Gynecol 2000;15:372–6.
21. Meriam-Webster Dictionary. Perimenopause. Available at: https://www.merriam-webster.com/dictionary/perimenopause. Accessed June 09, 2018.
22. Goldstein SR. Use of ultrasonohysterography for triage of perimenopausal patients with unexplained uterine bleeding. Am J Obstet Gynecol 1994;170:565–70.
23. Goldstein SR, Nachtigall M, Snyder JR, et al. Endometrial assessment by vaginal ultrasonography before endometrial sampling in patients with postmenopausal bleeding. Am J Obstet Gynecol 1990;163:119–23.

24. Wong AW, Lao TH, Cheung CW, et al. Reappraisal of endometrial thickness for the detection of endometrial cancer in postmenopausal bleeding: a retrospective cohort study. BJOG 2016;123:439–46.
25. Gull B, Karlsson B, Milsom I, et al. Can ultrasound replace dilation and curettage? A longitudinal evaluation of postmenopausal bleeding and transvaginal sonographic measurement of the endometrium as predictors of endometrial cancer. Am J Obstet Gynecol 2003;188:401–8.
26. Elsandabesee D, Greenwood P. The performance of Pipelle endometrial sampling in a dedicated postmenopausal bleeding clinic. J Obstet Gynaecol 2005;25:32–4.
27. Kelekci S, Kaya E, Alan M, et al. Comparison of transvaginal sonography, saline infusion sonography, and office hysteroscopy in reproductive-aged women with or without abnormal uterine bleeding. Fertil Steril 2005;84:682–6.

# The Abnormal Ovary

## Evolving Concepts in Diagnosis and Management

Kalesha Hack, MD, FRCPC*, Phyllis Glanc, MD, FRCPC

**KEYWORDS**

• Ovary • Adnexa • Ovarian carcinoma • IOTA • O-RADS • Ultrasound • Ultrasound screening

**KEY POINTS**

- Over the past 20 years, there has been evidence of an evolving approach to diagnosis and management of abnormal ovarian lesions with several important changes in thinking.
- There is a shift toward more conservative management in benign-appearing lesions, such as simple cysts under 10 cm, and classic benign-appearing lesions, such as dermoids and endometriomas.
- There is a growing body of evidence that simple cysts are unlikely to be precursors to the more aggressive forms of epithelial ovarian cancers.
- Current evidence-based recommended practices include use of standardized lexicon, such as O-RADS, in reporting; use of conservative management strategies, including serial surveillance, as an alternative to surgery in low-risk lesions; use of second-step evaluation, including referral to an expert sonographer when diagnosis is uncertain; and preoperative risk of malignancy assessments and management recommendations in the imaging report.
- Although there is some evidence that transvaginal ultrasound may help detect ovarian cancers at an earlier stage, routine transvaginal ultrasound screening in patients at average risk is not yet recommended.

## INTRODUCTION

Ovarian lesions are common in women of all ages, with reported incidence ranging between 6% and 17%.[1,2] A majority, regardless of initial appearance, are benign lesions, which are destined to resolve spontaneously. The goal of an ultrasound evaluation is to help stratify these lesions into groups, such as likely benign, indeterminate, or highly suspicious for malignancy. The likely benign group may go on to conservative

Department of Medical Imaging, Sunnybrook Health Sciences Centre, 2075 Bayview Avenue, Toronto, ON M4N 3M5, Canada
* Corresponding author.
*E-mail address:* Kalesha.hack@sunnybrook.ca

Obstet Gynecol Clin N Am 46 (2019) 607–624
https://doi.org/10.1016/j.ogc.2019.07.002
obgyn.theclinics.com

management, the indeterminate group to second-stage evaluations, and the highly suspicious for malignancy group to management by specialized gynecologist-oncologists.[3]

Ovarian cancer has a low disease prevalence but remains a leading cause of mortality related to gynecologic cancer in the United States.[4] The high mortality rate is related to late stage at diagnosis in most cases. Given the overall poor prognosis of ovarian cancer, most ovarian lesions, especially in the postmenopausal age group, were historically advised to undergo surgical excision.[5] Since the early 2000s, however, there has been a progressive shift in approach to the abnormal ovary, with increasing emphasis on reducing the number of surgeries for benign disease, standardizing terminology, assessing risk of malignancy through the use of evidence-based scoring systems, and triaging suspicious abnormalities to dedicated oncology centers.[3,6–11]

Although pattern recognition by an expert examiner has long been established as the optimal method for discriminating between benign and malignant ovarian lesions,[12–16] there has been a strong push to translate the evidence-based literature and the collective knowledge of recognized experts into simple practical tools that can be used by imagers with varying levels of expertise to accurately assess risk of malignancy.[10,11,17–19] This change did not happen overnight but rather has been a gradual iterative process influenced by multiple research groups and organizations across several countries. These efforts include, but are not limited to, significant and additive contributions from the International Ovarian Tumor Analysis (IOTA) group[7,20] the Society for Radiologists in Ultrasound (SRU) consensus statement on cystic adnexal lesions,[9] the First International Consensus Report on Adnexal Masses,[3] and most recently the Ovarian-Adnexal Reporting and Data Systems (O-RADS) working group[11] (**Fig. 1**). This article focuses on some of the major changes in knowledge and management of ovarian lesions, including the evolution of the approach to simple cysts, the historical framework and current state of ovarian lesion lexicon, the growing role of serial sonography, the current tools for assessing risk of malignancy, and lastly the potential role for ovarian cancer screening with ultrasound.

## THE SIMPLE CYST: PRECURSOR TO MALIGNANCY OR SIMPLY BENIGN?

Traditionally, it was believed that a cyst in the postmenopausal ovary was a rare occurrence to be regarded with caution as a possible sign of early or developing malignancy. This idea has been challenged by more recent findings, including data from large-scale ovarian cancer screening trials. In an ovarian cancer screening population of more than 15,000 women over the age of 50, Modesitt and colleagues[21] reported the occurrence of a simple cyst less than 10 cm in 18%. At short-term follow-up imaging, a majority (70%) resolved, regardless of initial cyst volume or appearance. Of the 117 persistent lesions that went on to surgical excision, the commonest pathologic diagnosis was a serous cystadenoma (52%), none with malignant or borderline features. No woman with an isolated unilocular cystic ovarian tumor developed an ovarian cancer, albeit the overall risk of malignancy was reported as less than 0.1%.[3,21] In the Prostate, Lung, Colorectal and Ovarian (PLCO) Cancer Screening Trial, which included women from 55 years old to 74 years old, simple cysts were present in approximately 14% of women. Half of these cysts persisted at 1-year follow-up[22] but with no associated increased risk for developing invasive ovarian cancer. The United Kingdom Collaborative Trial of Ovarian Cancer Screening (UKCTOCS) found unilocular cysts in approximately 5% of postmenopausal women with a rate of malignancy of 4/2531 (0.16%).[23] The association between unilocular cysts and

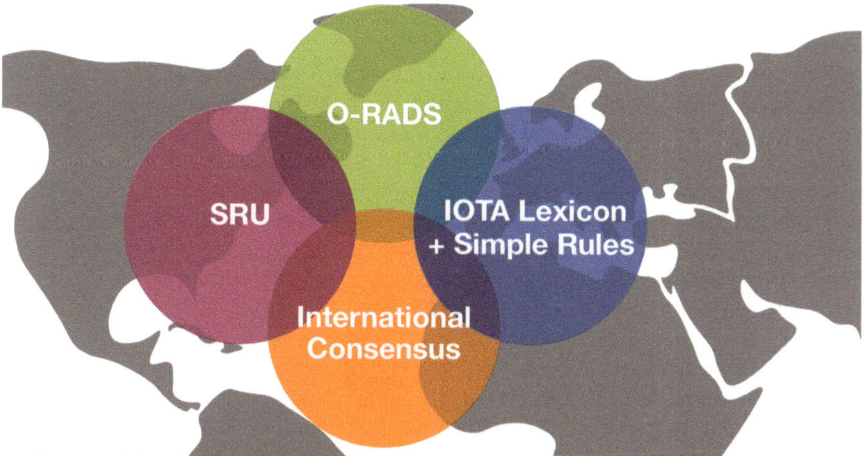


**SRU**

- Primarily North American
- Summary of pattern recognition with descriptors with focus on cystic and benign lesions
- Introduced management guidelines based on lesion size and menstrual status
- Eliminated follow up for physiologic lesions
- Introduced serial follow-up protocol for indeterminate lesions

**IOTA Lexicon + Simple Rules**

- Primarily European
- Standardized lexicon and terminology
- Subsequent iterations included risk assessment tools
- Extensively validated in literature
- Mainly tested in expert centres

**International Consensus**

- Collaboration of European and North American approaches
- Promoted use of either pattern recognition or algorithm approach (Simple Rules)
- Discouraged surgery for likely benign disease including simple cysts < 10 cm and emphasized appropriate triage to gynecology-oncology
- Introduced second-step evaluation including concept of expert imager

**O-RADS**

- Collaboration of Canadian, American and European societies
- Universal lexicon incorporating IOTA terminology with new additions
- Includes risk of malignancy assessment
- Includes standardized management recommendations in radiology report

**Fig. 1.** Historical and geographic evolution of the approach to adnexal masses in 2019, highlighting some of the important contributions of IOTA lexicon and Simple Rules, SRU consensus statement on cystic adnexal lesions, First International Consensus Report on Adnexal Lesions, and O-RADS.

risk of invasive ovarian cancer in this population went up to 0.35% if borderline tumors were included along with type 2 high-grade serous carcinomas (HGSCs). A recent meta-analysis by Parazzini and colleagues[24] reported the rate of malignancy of simple cysts to be 0.5% in premenopausal women (3/657) and 1.5% in postmenopausal women (7/469). Smith-Bindman and colleagues[25] in 2019 concluded that women with simple adnexal cysts had a low incidence of cancer similar to that of women without adnexal cysts in a retrospective study composed of 142 pelvic ultrasounds from women with cancers and 901 women without cancer. The data were then extrapolated to a population of more than 72,000 women. Although this study has some clear limitations, it does provide additional support that simple adnexal cysts are unlikely to be a source of malignancy, regardless of size and patient menopausal status.

When discussing the risk of malignancy in women with simple-appearing cysts, an important question to ask is whether serous cystadenomas have the potential to transform into malignant high-grade cystadenocarcinomas? Based on a growing understanding of the dualistic model of ovarian carcinoma and current research into the histologic origin of the more aggressive type 2 subtype, this does not seem to be the case. There is a growing body of evidence to support a nonovarian origin of type 2 high-grade ovarian cancers from precursor lesions that occur in the fimbriated end of the fallopian tube.[26–28] Molecular studies also do not support the idea that serous cystadenomas can transform into HGSCs.[29] A majority of studies that comment on the potential transformation of simple cysts into malignant lesions are retrospective in nature, therefore only describing a potential association rather than establishing a causal relationship.

Nonetheless, despite the growing evidence that unilocular cysts are highly likely to be benign, experts have struggled to agree on a size cutoff below which simple cysts in the postmenopausal women can be safely ignored. Groups such as the First International Consensus panel and American College of Obstetricians and Gynecologists (ACOG) in its 2016 practice bulletin have recommended conservative management of simple cysts but have not prescribed the duration or intervals for a surveillance program.[30] The O-RADS risk stratification and management system, available from the American College of Radiology (ACR) online resources, advises a minimum of 1-year follow-up for simple cyst greater than 5 and less than 10 cm in postmenopausal women, with suggested annual follow-up duration of 5 years,[31] but acknowledges a paucity of evidence for this recommendation. Future research and practice guidelines no doubt will be focused on determining evidence-based timing and duration of imaging follow-up for simple cysts in postmenopausal women.

## WHAT IS IN A NAME? THE EVOLUTION OF A STANDARDIZED LEXICON FOR OVARIAN LESIONS

There exists marked heterogeneity regarding terms, definitions, morphologic descriptors and color Doppler assessment for adnexal masses both between institutions and within single imaging centers. For example, the use of vague terminology, such as describing a "complex cyst," provides neither clinicians nor imagers with useful information regarding risk stratification of an ovarian lesion, given that both a benign hemorrhagic cyst and a high-grade ovarian cystadenocarcinoma can be described as complex.

Recognizing the need for a standardized lexicon, the IOTA group provided one of the earliest and most validated lexicons for describing adnexal masses.[7] This was a basis for the IOTA-derived Simple Rules[20] and Assessment of Different Neoplasias in the Adnexa (ADNEX) model[19,32] risk assessment tools for differentiating benign and malignant masses. The University of Kentucky group published the Kentucky Morphology Index, which demonstrated very high institutional accuracy for predicting risk of malignancy[33] in ovarian lesions. Amor and colleagues[10] proposed the Gynecologic Imaging Reporting and Data System (GIRADS), which grouped ovarian lesions into 1 of 5 categories based on estimated risk of malignancy; however, the system did not incorporate standardized descriptors. Each of these systems provided incremental steps toward improving communication and consistency in diagnosis and management of ovarian masses on ultrasound. Ultimately, in 2018, a white paper of the ACR was published, entitled "Ovarian-Adnexal Reporting Lexicon for Ultrasound,"[11] with the express goal of providing an internationally accepted nomenclature for the description of ovarian masses. Because the IOTA group lexicon was strongly evidence based, this was incorporated into the lexicon as a package. A summary of the O-RADS lexicon in modified table format is available at the referenced link on the ACR Web site.[31]

## ASK THE EXPERTS: THE EMERGING CONCEPT OF A SECOND-STEP EVALUATION FOR OVARIAN LESIONS

It is well accepted that subjective lesion assessment by an expert sonographer is the most accurate way to discriminate benign from malignant ovarian masses.[3,6,9,11–13,15,16] It is also recognized that gynecology ultrasound often is performed and interpreted by imagers with varying levels of expertise and diagnostic confidence.[3,20,34] This leaves nonexperts in a challenging position with respect to deciding next best steps.

Historically, options were limited between short-term follow-up imaging and surgical excision. Gynecologic surgery is not without risk, however, with reported major complication rates ranging from 2% to 15%.[23,35] The First International Consensus panel drew attention to the relatively large number of surgeries being performed in US centers for benign diseases[3] compared with European centers. In an effort to reduce the number surgeries for benign disease and to optimize patient outcomes among imagers of all levels of experience, they proposed several second-step options when a lesion could not be classified as either almost certainly benign or highly suspicious for malignancy. These included referral to an expert sonologist, serial sonography, utilization of established risk models with an emphasis on the IOTA-derived Simple Rules, correlation with serum biomarkers, magnetic resonance imaging (MRI), or referral to a gynecologic oncologist. The rationale for these steps is detailed in **Table 1**.

Equally important, The First International Consensus group noted that patients with malignant ovarian tumors have better outcomes when their treatment is managed by a gynecology oncologist, likely due to optimal initial staging, debulking surgery, and adjuvant treatment.[36–40] The concept of second-step evaluation by an expert sonographer or MRI as well as appropriate involvement of gynecology-oncology when malignancy is suspected has been incorporated into subsequent management strategies, including the O-RADS ultrasound risk stratification and management system.[31]

Recently, the IOTA group has developed the ADNEX model, the first risk model to statistically predict between benign, borderline, stage 1 invasive, stages 2 to 4 invasive, and secondary metastatic disease. It is based on 3 clinical and 6 ultrasound features and is predicated on a 2-step approach. It demonstrates good to excellent results in the hands of expert imagers and thus also could be utilized as a second-step process to evaluate challenging lesions.[19] The ADNEX model is available online (www.iotagroup.org/ adnexmodel/).

## ONLY TIME WILL TELL: THE GROWING ROLE OF SERIAL ULTRASOUND IN MANAGEMENT OF ADNEXAL LESIONS

Serial sonography can be considered a longitudinal biomarker, which permits those lesions that are destined to resolve over time to undergo conservative management

**Table 1**
**Potential second step options in the setting of an indeterminate mass**

| Second-Stage Step | Rationale |
|---|---|
| Referral to an expert sonologist | In expert hands, subjective pattern recognition remains the most sensitive and specific method of differentiating benign and malignant ovarian lesions. This expertise is not easily transferred between individuals or institution; thus, referral to an expert sonologist may be beneficial. |
| Serial sonography | The majority of adnexal lesions resolve spontaneously over time; thus, serial evaluation provides an opportunity to determine which lesions are destined to resolve or remain stable over time. It was acknowledged that appropriate interval and duration remain uncertain. |
| Established risk-prediction models | IOTA Simple Rules was considered the best evidence-based risk prediction model for preoperative characterization of ovarian masses, particularly in premenopausal women. |
| Serum biomarkers | Role is not yet clearly established. The RMI, which combines 2 biomarkers, is currently outperformed by subjective assessment. |
| MRI | Decreases the risk of both misdiagnosing a benign lesion as malignant and increases the specificity of benign diagnosis when the sonographic appearance is not classic. MRI is also highly sensitive for the diagnosis of malignancy. |
| Referral to a gynecologist-oncologist | Appropriate to use the oncologist's expertise to determine the next most appropriate step |

*Data from* Glanc P, Benacerraf B, Bourne T, et al. First International Consensus Report on Adnexal Masses: management recommendations. J Ultrasound Med 2017;36(5):849-863.

versus those with aggressive growth patterns, which should be referred for appropriate surgical intervention. Lesions that remain stable may be triaged to a serial surveillance group, the exact schedule of which will require additional research in order to be evidence based.

Data from ovarian cancer screening trials have provided a unique window to examine the natural evolution, incidence, and prevalence of abnormal ovarian lesions in large populations of healthy asymptomatic women. In 2013, Pavlik and colleagues[2] published the results of a University of Kentucky ovarian screening trial of 221,576 baseline and follow-up transvaginal ultrasounds examining the frequency and natural history of ovarian abnormalities at follow-up ultrasound. Of the 46.7% of patients with an initial abnormal ultrasound finding in the ovary, approximately two-thirds resolved on serial follow-up ultrasounds performed at intervals ranging between 6 weeks to 6 months, regardless of their initial appearance. The average length of follow-up in lesions that resolved spontaneously was approximately 9 months. Surgery was performed on 557 women, of whom 85 were found to have an ovarian malignancy. The positive predictive value was 8.1% without the use of serial ultrasound but progressively increased to 24.7% as serial sonography was introduced. The conclusions of this influential article helped to popularize the concept that serial ultrasound for abnormal lesions in the ovary is a valuable clinical tool that may obviate surgery in lesions that demonstrate long-term stability, size reduction, or complete resolution while reducing the false-positive rate of those who undergo surgical resection of ovarian lesions.

In 2015, Ormsby and colleagues[41] published a systematic literature review, which ultimately incorporated 30 peer-reviewed articles published after the year 2000 and concluded that serial ultrasound leads to improved positive predictive value for ovarian malignancy and a shift to detection at earlier stages. Suh-Bergmann and colleagues[42] recently published “Outcomes from Ultrasound Follow-up of Small Complex Adnexal Masses in Women over 50” and reported that repeat monitoring of stable persistent indeterminate lesions measuring between 1 cm and 6 cm is of questionable benefit and that follow-up beyond 7 months was unnecessary because all epithelial and borderline tumors in this group demonstrated interim growth within this time period.[42] This retrospective study was limited due to the inclusion criteria of complex lesion, which is considered vague and a potentially inappropriate descriptor on which to base the conclusions. Nonetheless, the study provides supportive evidence that short-term initial observation of isolated small adnexal masses is of benefit in preoperative triage of surgical cases.

Stability over time, unfortunately, does not equate to benignity, in particular for the so-called type 1 tumors, which demonstrate a stepwise progression originating from a benign precursor, borderline tumor, or endometriosis.[26] These include the low-grade serous carcinoma, endometroid carcinoma, and clear cell carcinoma. In contrast, the type 2 cancers demonstrate highly aggressive behavior and include HGSC, high-grade endometrioid carcinoma, undifferentiated carcinomas, and malignant mixed mesodermal carcinomas. HGSC accounts for approximately 75% of ovarian carcinomas and 90% of the related mortalities. As discussed previously, recent evidence indicates HGSCs originate from a precursor lesion, serous tubal intraepithelial carcinoma, arising in the fimbriated end of the fallopian tube. A TP53 mutation is present in greater than 90% cases.[27,29] Additionally, HGSCs are associated with BRCA gene inactivation.[26,43]

This heterogeneity in the biological behavior and origins of ovarian cancers makes it difficult to design an appropriate surveillance schedule. This dual model of ovarian cancer also helps explain some of the results from large ovarian screening trials, including the finding in the UKCTOCS trials that all cancers associated with normal appearance of the ovaries at ultrasound screening were type 2 whereas all cancers associated with ultrasound abnormalities were slow growing borderline tumors and type 1 epithelial ovarian carcinomas.[44] The strongest association between ovarian morphology and epithelial ovarian cancer is the presence of solid components.[23,44–46] Therefore, one of the principle features that is assessed for at serial ultrasound follow-up is the development of a solid component, which is considered worrisome and usually generates further work-up and/or referral.

Several groups now support serial ultrasound in cases for indeterminate cases. The ACOG practice bulletin on management of adnexal masses states that “repeat imaging is recommended if there is uncertainty of the diagnosis.”[30] An expert panel in 2017 also concluded that serial ultrasound is an appropriate next step in the management of indeterminate lesions.[3] Neither of these groups has provided a specific recommendation regarding frequency or duration of surveillance recommendations. There are several groups, however, which have proposed an initial follow-up interval of 3 months for such lesions.[2,47] In the absence of lesion growth or development of suspicious features, serial surveillance is a reasonable alternative to surgical excision and potential surgical morbidity. Although optimal timing and duration of serial sonography for ovarian lesions is difficult to define, a proposed schedule of follow-up was prescribed by Pavlik and colleagues[2] Unilocular cysts can be followed with an initial 6-month ultrasound, for example, whereas more indeterminate lesions can be assessed at 6 weeks to 3 months. For persistent lesions that demonstrate long-term stability, it seems reasonable to lengthen the time period between follow-up studies; however, more evidence is needed to determine what this interval should be and when cessation of follow-up can be safely considered. In order to ultimately determine appropriate surveillance protocols, it is critical that imaging reports clearly define with standardized descriptors the appearance of each lesion and whether there is equivocal or definite change in appearance of the adnexal lesion under surveillance. This will no doubt be an area of ongoing research as data from large screening trials continue to accumulate. The adoption of a universal ovarian lexicon may also help facilitate highly powered multicenter trials to investigate the outcomes of abnormal ovarian lesions assessed with serial ultrasound follow-up and provide further evidence-based guidelines for surveillance protocols.

## PUTTING IT ALL TOGETHER: ASSESSING RISK OF MALIGNANCY AND ESTABLISHING STANDARDIZED RISK-BASED MANAGEMENT PATHWAYS FOR ABNORMAL OVARIAN LESIONS WITH ULTRASOUND

Transvaginal ultrasound plays a key role in the assessment of ovarian masses and along with clinical factors, such as age, family history of malignancy, and laboratory work-up, helps to triage women into several risk management categories. These broad categories include benign findings requiring no further evaluation, indeterminate findings requiring either serial follow-up imaging or further diagnostic evaluation, and suspicious findings, which should be referred to a gynecology oncology service. Previous work referenced in this article has outlined the importance of establishing an accurate a priori risk of malignancy for ovarian lesions for optimal patient outcomes. These principle reasons are to reduce surgery and potential surgical complications in women with clearly benign lesions, to ensure management of suspicious lesions involves the care of a gynecology-oncologist, and to offer appropriate surveillance for women who have a small potential risk of malignancy as an alternative to surgery. Over the past 20 years, several groups have proposed risk assessment models for ovarian masses with varying levels of success and adoption. Although some models are based solely on ultrasound findings, such as the original IOTA Simple Rules[20] and GIRADS,[10] others rely on a combination of ultrasound features, clinical factors, and tumor marker levels, such as ADNEX[32] or the Risk of Malignancy Index[48] (RMI), which has gone through several iterations. Recent studies have shown that subjective assessment by ultrasound has greater accuracy than both the RMI and the Risk of Ovarian Malignancy Algorithm, which assesses serum cancer antigen 125 (CA-125) and human epididymis 4 levels.[32,49] Because the IOTA group Simple Rules and subsequent classification systems are detailed in Wouter Froyman and Dirk Timmerman's article, "Methods of Assessing Ovarian Masses: IOTA Approach," in this issue, the focus of this section is on the newly developed O-RADS Ultrasound Risk Stratification and Management System available through the ACR online resources.[31] This system consists of a 5-point scoring system based on ultrasound features described using the established O-RADS lexicon. Each category is associated with an estimated risk of malignancy in percentage and has accompanying management guidelines, which are divided into premenopausal and postmenopausal groups.

The O-RADS scoring system is briefly reviewed.

### *O-RADS 0: Incomplete Study*

Incomplete evaluation with either repeat study or alternate study required.

### *O-RADS 1: Normal Ovary*

The O-RADS 1 category includes physiologic follicles and the corpus luteum of the ovary, which may measure up to 3 cm and do not require further follow-up. The normal postmenopausal ovary should not demonstrate these physiologic findings (**Figs. 2–4**).

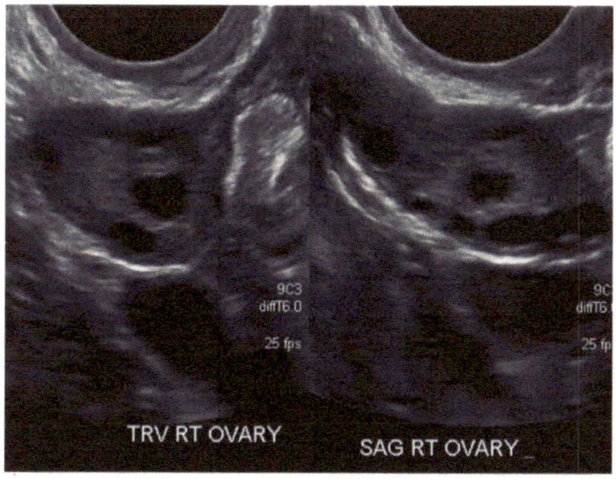


**Fig. 2.** Normal premenopausal (*right*) ovary in transverse and sagittal planes with developing follicles and homogeneous surrounding ovarian tissue.

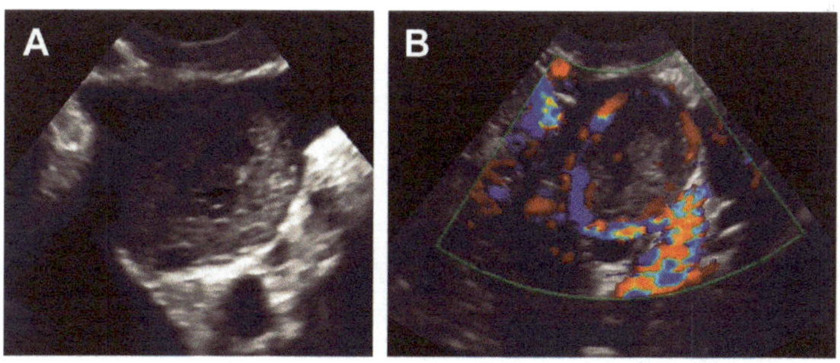


**Fig. 3.** Normal corpus luteum. (*A*) Thick-walled ovarian cyst with crenulated inner margin representing typical appearance of corpus luteum. (*B*) Color Doppler imaging shows peripheral vascularity with classic ring-of-fire appearance.

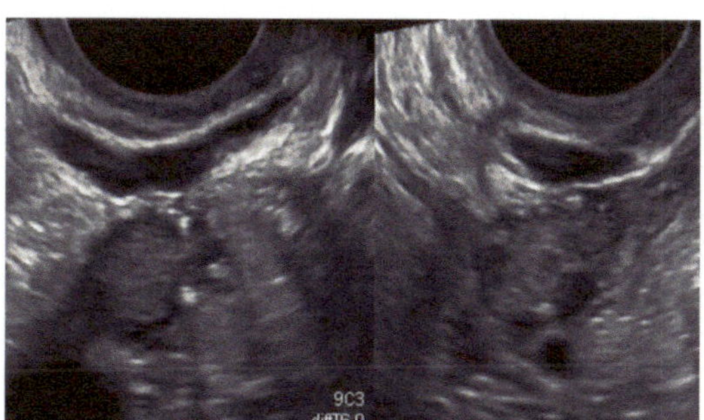


**Fig. 4.** Normal postmenopausal (right) ovary appears atrophic with paucity of follicles. A few small concretions noted.

### O-RADS 2: Almost Certainly Benign

The O-RADS 2 category refers to ovarian lesions that are almost certainly benign with a risk of malignancy less than 1%. This category includes the simple and unilocular cysts less than 10 cm; classic benign lesions, including hemorrhagic cysts; and endometriomas and dermoid cysts less than 10 cm as well as the peritoneal inclusion cyst, the paraovarian cyst, and the hydrosalpinx (**Figs. 5–9**).

Within this category, depending on size, level of diagnostic confidence, and menstrual status, the suggested management is variable, as published in ACR online tables. This group generally is managed by a gynecologist.

Serial follow-up is recommended and 5 years has been suggested as a reasonable benchmark to establish long-term stability,[45] with the caveat that there is a paucity of evidence to support this value. This likely will be an area of future discussion and research in subsequent iterations.

### O-RADS 3: Low Risk of Malignancy

The O-RADS 3 category refers to ovarian lesions with a low risk of malignancy, defined as 1% to less than 10%. This category includes the preceding group of simple and unilocular cysts, typical hemorrhagic cyst, dermoid cysts, and endometriomas when their largest dimension is greater than or equal to 10 cm. This category also includes unilocular cysts of any size with an irregular inner wall less than 3 mm in height and multilocular cysts less than 10 cm with smooth inner wall and color score 1-3. Lastly, a solid smooth lesion of any size with no color flow is also categorized as O-RADS 3. Ultrasound evaluation by an expert or magnetic resonance evaluation is suggested, and it is advised that patients may benefit from gynecology referral to facilitate thorough assessment of individual clinical and biochemical risk factors (**Fig. 10**).

### O-RADS 4: Intermediate Risk

The O-RADS 4 category refers to lesions with an intermediate risk of malignancy defined as 10% to less than 50%. Included are unilocular cysts with a solid component but no papillary projections and any color score, unilocular cysts with 1 to 3 papillary projections regardless of color score, multilocular cysts greater than or equal to10 cm with a smooth inner wall and demonstrating a range of no flow to mild or moderate color flow, multilocular cysts of any size with smooth wall but high color flow, multilocular cysts of any size with irregular inner walls or septations regardless of color score, multilocular cysts with a solid component but either no or mild color flow, and lastly a solid smooth mass with mild to moderate color flow.

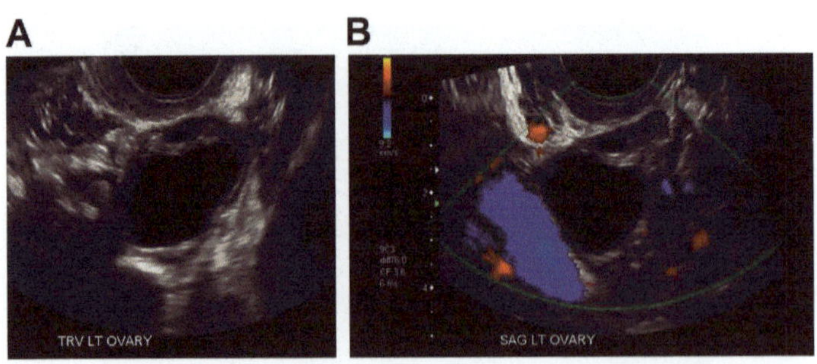


**Fig. 5.** Simple ovarian cyst. (*A*) Anechoic unilocular smooth thin-walled lesion with surrounding ovarian tissue representing simple ovarian cyst. (*B*) Note lack of internal vascularity on color Doppler imaging.

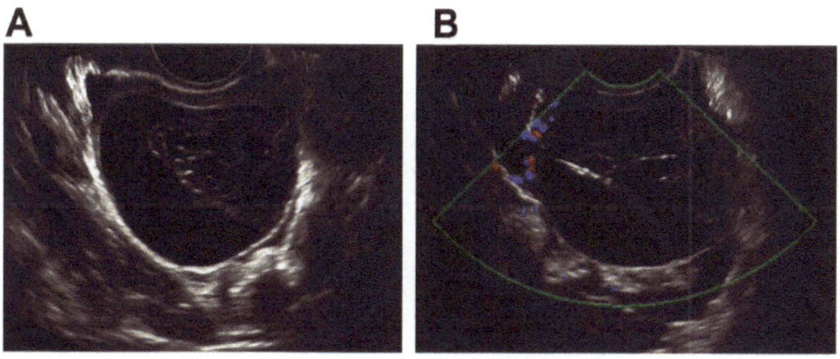


**Fig. 6.** Typical hemorrhagic cyst. (*A*) Cyst with internal reticular pattern. Note lacelike appearance. (*B*) Cyst contains echogenic avascular component representing retractile clot. Concave margins are demonstrated.

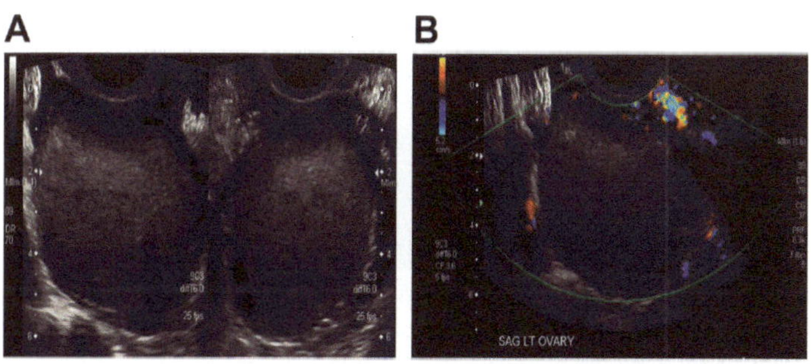


**Fig. 7.** Typical endometrioma. (*A*) Ovarian cyst with homogeneous low-level echoes/ground-glass appearance. A few peripheral follicles are seen confirming (*left*) intraovarian location. (*B*) No internal vascularity is seen.

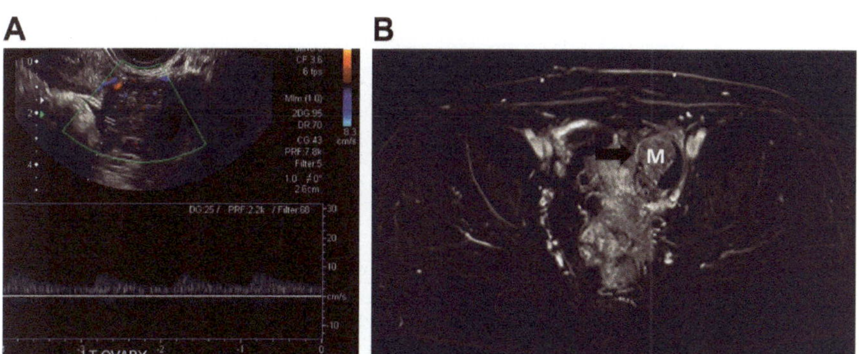


**Fig. 8.** Malignant degeneration of an endometrioma. (*A*) Development of a solid vascular component within an endometrioma in a 43-year-old woman with long-standing endometriosis. (*B*) MRI shows solid enhancing tissue suspicious for malignant degeneration (M).

A B C

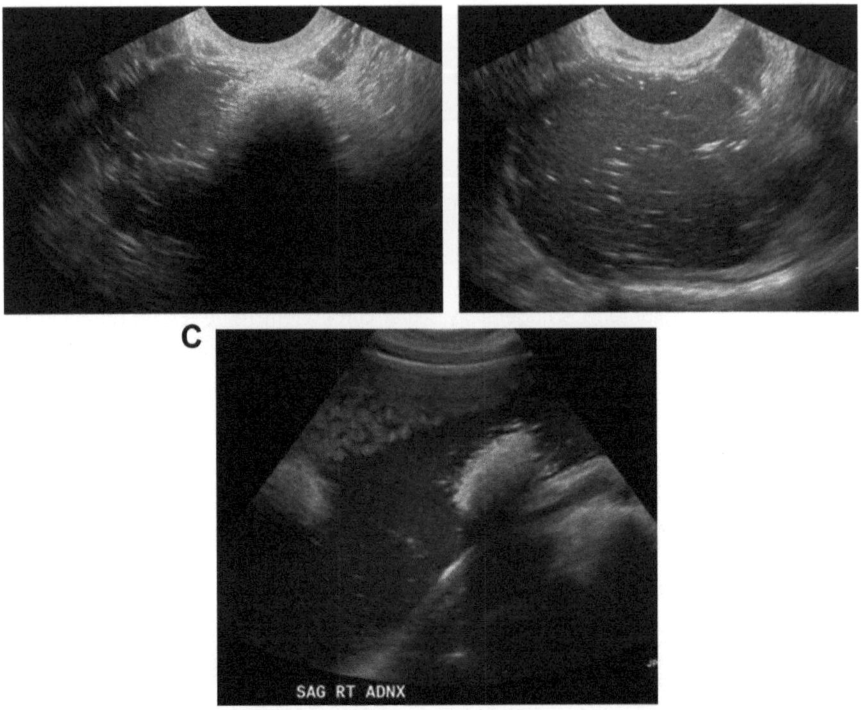


**Fig. 9.** Classic benign descriptors of ovarian dermoid. (*A*) Echogenic component with shadowing. (*B*) Hyperechoic lines and dots. (*C*) Floating echogenic structures.

Management recommendations include involvement of a gynecology oncologist and second-step evaluation of either referral to an ultrasound expert or additional characterization with MRI. Broadly speaking, this category refers to what subjective expert pattern assessment would historically grade as an indeterminate lesion (**Figs. 11** and **12**).

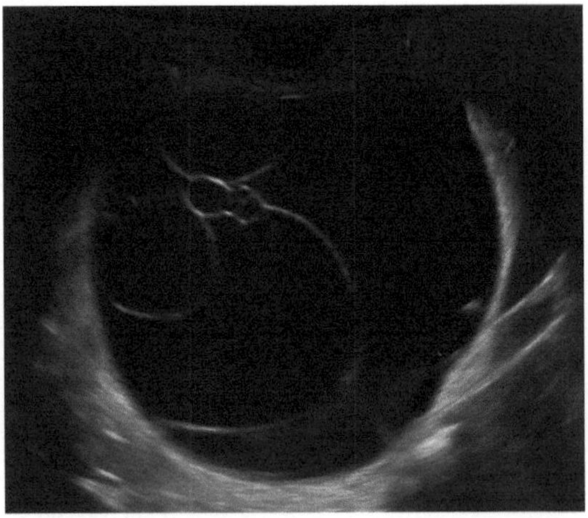

**Fig. 10.** O-RADS 3 low risk. Multilocular cyst less than 10 cm with thin avascular septations and no wall irregularities.

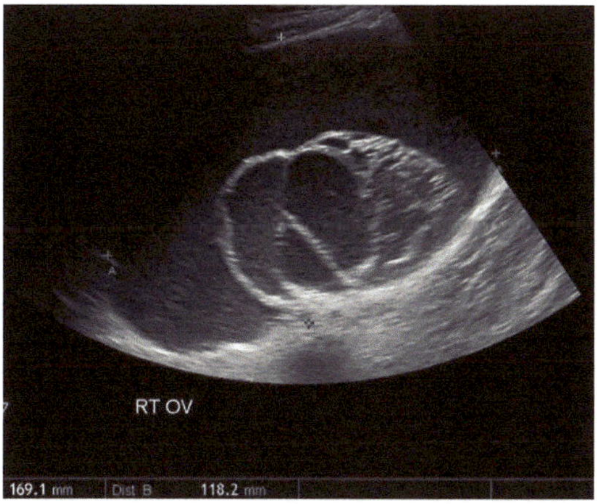


**Fig. 11.** O-RADS 4 intermediate risk. Multilocular smooth cyst greater than 10 cm with no internal flow found to represent mucinous borderline ovarian tumor. Note heterogeneous low-level echoes within lesion suggestive of mucinous origin.

### *O-RADS 5: High Risk of Malignancy*

The O-RADS 5 category refers to lesions with a high risk of malignancy defined as greater than 50%. Included are unilocular cysts with 4 or more papillary projections, multilocular cysts with solid component and moderate or high color score, solid smooth mass with high color score, solid irregular mass with any color score, and signs of metastatic disease, including ascites or peritoneal implants. In the setting of ascites and/or peritoneal nodules and a category 1 or 2 finding, other etiologies should be sought. O-RADS 5 lesions should be managed by a gynecologist-oncologist (**Figs. 13–15**).

## NIP IT IN THE BUD: IS EARLY DETECTION OF OVARIAN CANCER WITH TRANSVAGINAL ULTRASOUND POSSIBLE?

There is strong motivation to develop an effective screening test for ovarian cancer given its high mortality rate and significant drop-off in 5-year survival rates if diagnosed at a late stage (stage III/IV).[4] Sadly, metastatic disease is already present in as many as 60% of cases at initial diagnosis.[4,60] To prove effective, a screening test should demonstrate a shift to diagnosis at earlier stages of disease (ie, a stage shift) and should also demonstrate a mortality benefit from this stage shift that is not attributable to lead time bias. Several trials have evaluated the potential for ovarian cancer screening with transvaginal ultrasound mostly in postmenopausal women at average risk but with at least 1 trial including high-risk premenopausal women. The findings of some of the major trials are summarized.

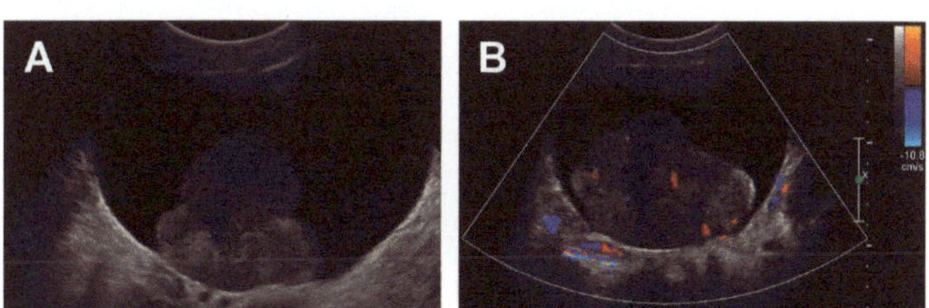


**Fig. 12.** O-RADS 4 intermediate risk. (*A*) Unilocular cyst with solid component found to represent clear cell carcinoma. (*B*) Color Doppler imaging shows mild flow, color score 2.

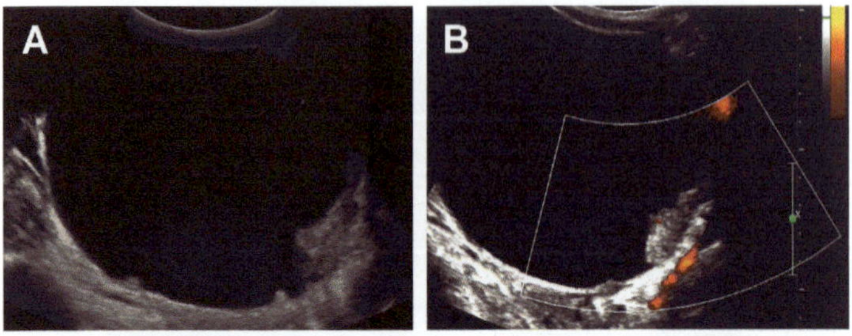


**Fig. 13.** O-RADS 5 high risk. (*A*) Unilocular cyst with greater than 4 papillary projections found to represent borderline tumor. (*B*) Color Doppler imaging shows mild flow, color score 2.

The 2011 University of Kentucky screening trial was a single-arm study of 37,293 women who voluntarily underwent annual ultrasound for a mean of 5.5 years.[46] This trial stands unique among ovarian screening trials in that it reported a potential stage shift in diagnosis with 70% of screen-detected cancers being stage I or II, in addition to a mortality reduction. The data are limited by the study design with no control group and a mixed risk population.[51,52]

The 2011 PLCO Cancer Screening Trial was a randomized-control trial of 78,216 postmenopausal women who were assigned to either control group or annual screen with CA-125 for 6 years and transvaginal ultrasound for 4 years.[35] No significant stage shift in ovarian cancer diagnosis and no statistically significant reduction in cancer-specific mortality was identified. This group reported a 15% (163/1080) major complication rate in those who underwent surgery for benign disease, indicating the potential for harm associated with false-positive screens.

A large Japanese randomized control trial of 82,487 published in 2008 also showed mixed results.[53] Patients were screened over a 13-year period in 212 hospitals with ultrasound and CA-125 using an absolute cutoff value of 35 U/mL. A stage shift was seen proportionally, with 63% of stage I cancers found in the screened population versus 38% in the control group; however, this was not statistically significant.

The UKCTOCS is the largest randomized controlled trial in a general population, with more than 200,000 postmenopausal women who were assigned to either a control group or annual screening with either ultrasound alone or a multimodal strategy (MMS), including ultrasound and serial CA-125 testing using the Risk of Cancer Algorithm.[54] The study showed a statistically significant stage shift within the MMS group,

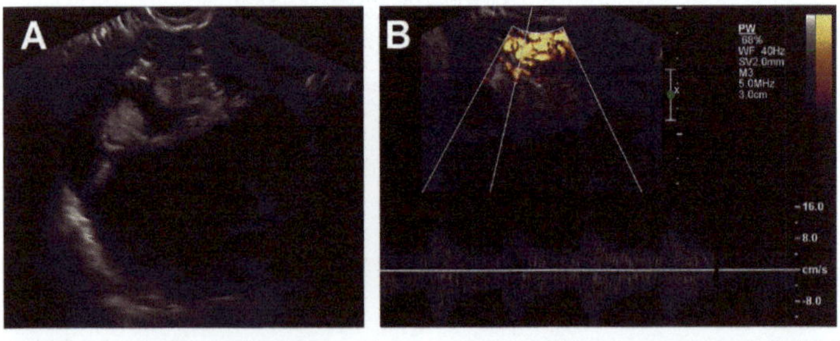


**Fig. 14.** O-RADS 5 high risk. (*A*) Multilocular cyst with solid components and thick irregular septations found to represent type 2 high-grade serous cystadenocarcinoma. (*B*) Color imaging shows strong flow, color score 4.

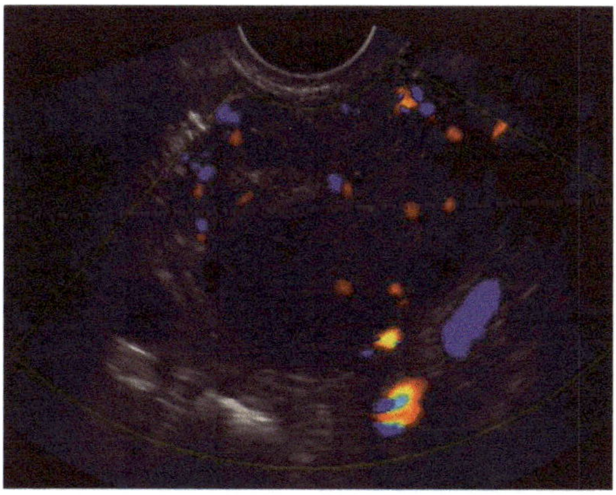

**Fig. 15.** O-RADS 5 high risk. Solid (>80%) mass with small cystic spaces and strong color flow found to represent a granulosa cell tumor.

with 46.1% of stage I/II cancers in the screened group compared with 23.9% in the control group but not in the ultrasound-only group. The primary analysis did not demonstrate a significant reduction in mortality; however, a subsequent analysis designed to account for late effect of screening has shown a late mortality effect in the MMS group, albeit insufficient to provide support for population screening. The trial is currently being extended for an additional 4 years, which may help provide clarity on whether a true reduction in late mortality can be shown.

Based on current available data, the ACR does not recommend routine use of ultrasound for ovarian cancer screening in women at average risk of developing the disease.[52]

## SUMMARY

Over the past 20 years, there has been evidence of an evolving approach to diagnosis and management of abnormal ovarian lesions with several important changes in thinking. There is a shift toward more conservative management in benign-appearing lesions, such as simple cysts under 10 cm, and classic benign-appearing lesions, such as dermoids and endometriomas. There is a growing body of evidence that simple cysts are unlikely to be precursors to the more aggressive forms of epithelial ovarian cancers. Current evidence-based recommended practices include use of standardized lexicon, such as O-RADS, in reporting; use of conservative management strategies, including serial surveillance as an alternative to surgery in low-risk lesions; use of second-step evaluation, including referral to an expert sonographer when diagnosis is uncertain; and preoperative risk of malignancy assessments and management recommendations in the imaging report. Although there is some evidence that transvaginal ultrasound may help detect ovarian cancers at an earlier stage, routine transvaginal ultrasound screening in patients at average risk is not yet recommended.

## REFERENCES

1. Borgfeldt C, Andolf E. Transvaginal sonographic ovarian findings in a random sample of women 25–40 years old. Ultrasound Obstet Gynecol 1999;13(5): 345–50.

2. Pavlik EJ, Ueland FR, Miller RW, et al. Frequency and disposition of ovarian abnormalities followed with serial transvaginal ultrasonography. Obstet Gynecol 2013;122(2 PART 1):210–7.
3. Glanc P, Benacerraf B, Bourne T, et al. First international consensus report on adnexal masses: management recommendations. J Ultrasound Med 2017; 36(5):849–63.
4. Torre LA, Trabert B, DeSantis CE, et al. Ovarian cancer statistics, 2018. CA Cancer J Clin 2018;68(4):284–96.
5. American College of Obstetricians and Gynecologists. Management of adnexal masses. Obstet Gynecol 2007;110(1):201.
6. Timmerman D, Schwärzler P, Collins WP, et al. Subjective assessment of adnexal masses with the use of ultrasonography: an analysis of interobserver variability and experience. Ultrasound Obstet Gynecol 1999;13(1):11–6.
7. Timmerman D, Valentin L, Bourne TH, et al. Terms, definitions and measurements to describe the sonographic features of adnexal tumors: a consensus opinion from the International Ovarian Tumor Analysis (IOTA) Group. Ultrasound Obstet Gynecol 2000;16(5):500–5.
8. Timmerman D. Lack of standardization in gynecological ultrasonography. Ultrasound Obstet Gynecol 2000;16(5):395–8.
9. Levine D, Brown DL, Andreotti RF, et al. Management of asymptomatic ovarian and other adnexal cysts imaged at US: Society of Radiologists in Ultrasound Consensus Conference Statement. Radiology 2010;256(3):943–54.
10. Amor F, Vaccaro H, Alcázar JL, et al. Gynecologic imaging reporting and data system: a new proposal for classifying adnexal masses on the basis of sonographic findings. J Ultrasound Med 2009;28(3):285–91.
11. Andreotti RF, Timmerman D, Benacerraf BR, et al. Ovarian-adnexal reporting lexicon for ultrasound: a white paper of the ACR ovarian-adnexal reporting and data system committee. J Am Coll Radiol 2018;15(10):1415–29.
12. Brown DL, Dudiak KM, Laing FC. Adnexal masses: US characterization and reporting. Radiology 2010;254(2):342–54.
13. Meys E, Kaijser J, Kruitwagen RF, et al. Subjective assessment versus ultrasound models to diagnose ovarian cancer: a systematic review and meta-analysis. Eur J Cancer 2016;58:17–29.
14. Timmerman D. The use of mathematical models to evaluate pelvic masses; can they beat an expert operator? Best Pract Res Clin Obstet Gynaecol 2004;18(1): 91–104.
15. Valentin L. Use of morphology to characterize and manage common adnexal masses. Best Pract Res Clin Obstet Gynaecol 2004;18(1):71–89.
16. Van Calster B, Timmerman D, Bourne T, et al. Discrimination between benign and malignant adnexal masses by specialist ultrasound examination versus serum CA-125. J Natl Cancer Inst 2007;99(22):1706–14.
17. Amor F, Alcázar JL, Vaccaro H, et al. GI-RADS reporting system for ultrasound evaluation of adnexal masses in clinical practice: a prospective multicenter study. Ultrasound Obstet Gynecol 2011;38(4):450–5.
18. Timmerman D, Ameye L, Fischerova D, et al. Simple ultrasound rules to distinguish between benign and malignant adnexal masses before surgery: prospective validation by IOTA group. BMJ 2010;341:c6839.
19. Van Calster B, Van Hoorde K, Valentin L, et al. Evaluating the risk of ovarian cancer before surgery using the ADNEX model to differentiate between benign, borderline, early and advanced stage invasive, and secondary metastatic tumours: prospective multicentre diagnostic study. BMJ 2014;349:g5920.

20. Timmerman D, Testa AC, Bourne T, et al. Simple ultrasound-based rules for the diagnosis of ovarian cancer. Ultrasound Obstet Gynecol 2008;31(6):681–90.
21. Modesitt SC, Pavlik EJ, Ueland FR, et al. Risk of malignancy in unilocular ovarian cystic tumors less than 10 centimeters in diameter. Obstet Gynecol 2003;102(3): 594–9.
22. Greenlee RT, Kessel B, Williams CR, et al. Prevalence, incidence, and natural history of simple ovarian cysts among women> 55 years old in a large cancer screening trial. Am J Obstet Gynecol 2010;202(4):373.e1-9.
23. Menon U, Gentry-Maharaj A, Hallett R, et al. Sensitivity and specificity of multimodal and ultrasound screening for ovarian cancer, and stage distribution of detected cancers: results of the prevalence screen of the UK Collaborative Trial of Ovarian Cancer Screening (UKCTOCS). Lancet Oncol 2009;10(4):327–40.
24. Parazzini F, Frattaruolo MP, Chiaffarino F, et al. The limited oncogenic potential of unilocular adnexal cysts: a systematic review and meta-analysis. Eur J Obstet Gynecol Reprod Biol 2018;225:101–9.
25. Smith-Bindman R, Poder L, Johnson E, et al. Risk of malignant ovarian cancer based on ultrasonography findings in a large unselected population. JAMA Intern Med 2019;179(1):71–7.
26. Shih I-M, Kurman RJ. Ovarian tumorigenesis: a proposed model based on morphological and molecular genetic analysis. Am J Pathol 2004;164(5):1511–8.
27. Kurman RJ, Shih I-M. Molecular pathogenesis and extraovarian origin of epithelial ovarian cancer—shifting the paradigm. Hum Pathol 2011;42(7):918–31.
28. Kurman RJ, Shih I-M. The dualistic model of ovarian carcinogenesis: revisited, revised, and expanded. Am J Pathol 2016;186(4):733–47.
29. Gilks CB, Irving J, Köbel M, et al. Incidental nonuterine high-grade serous carcinomas arise in the fallopian tube in most cases: further evidence for the tubal origin of high-grade serous carcinomas. Am J Surg Pathol 2015;39(3):357–64.
30. American College of Obstetricians and Gynecologists' Committee on Practice Bulletins—Gynecology. Practice bulletin No. 174: evaluation and management of adnexal masses. Obstet Gynecol 2016;128(5):e210.
31. Available at: http://www.acr.org/clinicalresources/reportinganddatasystems/ORADS.
32. Sayasneh A, Ferrara L, De Cock B, et al. Evaluating the risk of ovarian cancer before surgery using the ADNEX model: a multicentre external validation study. Br J Cancer 2016;115(5):542.
33. Ueland F, DePriest PD, Pavlik EJ, et al. Preoperative differentiation of malignant from benign ovarian tumors: the efficacy of morphology indexing and Doppler flow sonography. Gynecol Oncol 2003;91(1):46–50.
34. Froyman W, Wynants L, Landolfo C, et al. Validation of the performance of international ovarian tumor analysis (IOTA) methods in the diagnosis of early stage ovarian cancer in a non-screening population. Diagnostics (Basel) 2017;7(2):32.
35. Buys SS, Partridge E, Greene MH, et al. Ovarian cancer screening in the Prostate, Lung, Colorectal and Ovarian (PLCO) cancer screening trial: findings from the initial screen of a randomized trial. Am J Obstet Gynecol 2005;193(5):1630–9.
36. Covens AL, Dodge JE, Lacchetti C, et al. Surgical management of a suspicious adnexal mass: a systematic review. Gynecol Oncol 2012;126(1):149–56.
37. Earle CC, Schrag D, Neville BA, et al. Effect of surgeon specialty on processes of care and outcomes for ovarian cancer patients. J Natl Cancer Inst 2006;98(3): 172–80.

38. Engelen MJ, Kos HE, Willemse PH, et al. Surgery by consultant gynecologic oncologists improves survival in patients with ovarian carcinoma. Cancer 2006; 106(3):589–98.
39. Fung-Kee-Fung M, Kennedy EB, Biagi J, et al. The optimal organization of gynecologic oncology services: a systematic review. Curr Oncol 2015;22(4):e282.
40. Giede KC, Kieser K, Dodge J, et al. Who should operate on patients with ovarian cancer? An evidence-based review. Gynecol Oncol 2005;99(2):447–61.
41. Ormsby EL, Pavlik EJ, van Nagell JR. Ultrasound follow up of an adnexal mass has the potential to save lives. Am J Obstet Gynecol 2015;213(5):657.e1.
42. Suh-Burgmann E, Hung Y-Y, Kinney W. Outcomes from ultrasound follow-up of small complex adnexal masses in women over 50. Am J Obstet Gynecol 2014; 211(6):623.e1-7.
43. McCluggage WG. Morphological subtypes of ovarian carcinoma: a review with emphasis on new developments and pathogenesis. Pathology 2011;43(5): 420–32.
44. Sharma A, Apostolidou S, Burnell M, et al. Risk of epithelial ovarian cancer in asymptomatic women with ultrasound-detected ovarian masses: a prospective cohort study within the UK collaborative trial of ovarian cancer screening (UKCTOCS). Ultrasound Obstet Gynecol 2012;40(3):338–44.
45. Van Nagell JR, DePriest PD, Ueland FR, et al. Ovarian cancer screening with annual transvaginal sonography. Cancer 2007;109(9):1887–96.
46. Van Nagell JR, Miller RW, DeSimone CP, et al. Long-term survival of women with epithelial ovarian cancer detected by ultrasonographic screening. Obstet Gynecol 2011;118(6):1212–21.
47. Van Nagell J, DePriest P. Management of adnexal masses in postmenopausal women. Am J Obstet Gynecol 2005;193(1):30–5.
48. Jacobs I, Oram D, Fairbanks J, et al. A risk of malignancy index incorporating CA 125, ultrasound and menopausal status for the accurate preoperative diagnosis of ovarian cancer. Br J Obstet Gynaecol 1990;97(10):922–9.
49. Van Gorp T, Veldman J, Van Calster B, et al. Subjective assessment by ultrasound is superior to the risk of malignancy index (RMI) or the risk of ovarian malignancy algorithm (ROMA) in discriminating benign from malignant adnexal masses. Eur J Cancer 2012;48(11):1649–56.
50. Bankhead CR, Kehoe ST, Austoker J. Symptoms associated with diagnosis of ovarian cancer: a systematic review. BJOG 2005;112(7):857–65.
51. Campbell S, Gentry-Maharaj A. The role of transvaginal ultrasound in screening for ovarian cancer. Climacteric 2018;21(3):221–6.
52. Pandharipande PV, Lowry KP, Reinhold C, et al. ACR Appropriateness Criteria® Ovarian Cancer Screening. J Am Coll Radiol 2017;14(11):S490–9.
53. Kobayashi H, Yamada Y, Sado T, et al. A randomized study of screening for ovarian cancer: a multicenter study in Japan. Int J Gynecol Cancer 2008;18(3): 414–20.
54. Skates SJ, Menon U, MacDonald N, et al. Calculation of the risk of ovarian cancer from serial CA-125 values for preclinical detection in postmenopausal women. J Clin Oncol 2003;21(10 Suppl):206s–10s.

# Methods of Assessing Ovarian Masses

## International Ovarian Tumor Analysis Approach

Wouter Froyman, MD[a,b], Dirk Timmerman, MD, PhD[a,b,*]

**KEYWORDS**

• Adnexa • Diagnosis • International Ovarian Tumor Analysis • Ovarian cancer
• Ovarian neoplasms • Preoperative evaluation • Risk assessment • Ultrasonography

**KEY POINTS**

- Subjective assessment by an experienced ultrasound operator is known to be the best performing strategy to characterize adnexal masses.
- Ovarian lesions should be assessed according to standardized terms, definitions, and measurement techniques.
- Certain types of ovarian tumors, such as endometriomas or dermoid cysts, exhibit characteristic ultrasound features, which make them easy to recognize.
- International Ovarian Tumor Analysis (IOTA) approaches have been validated and show the best performance of currently available diagnostic tools to discriminate between benign and malignant adnexal pathology.
- The International Ovarian Tumor Analysis Assessment of Different Neoplasias in the adneXa (ADNEX) model includes clinical and ultrasound information to calculate the likelihood of malignancy and the likelihood of 4 subclasses of malignant tumors.

## INTRODUCTION

Despite the implementation of radical surgical approaches and the focus on development of new targeted therapy, the prognosis for patients with ovarian cancer has hardly improved during the last 3 decades.[1] Ovarian cancer is known to be the most lethal gynecologic malignancy, with almost 60% of patients diagnosed in advanced stages with regional or distant spread, corresponding with an unfavorable long-term prognosis. Five-year survival depends on the stage of the disease: 46% for all stages, but ranging from 90% at stage I to 4% at stage IV disease.[2]

[a] Department of Development and Regeneration, KU Leuven, Leuven, Belgium; [b] Department of Obstetrics and Gynecology, University Hospitals Leuven, Herestraat 49, Leuven 3000, Belgium
* Corresponding author. Department of Obstetrics and Gynecology, University Hospitals Leuven, Herestraat 49, Leuven 3000, Belgium.
*E-mail address:* dirk.timmerman@uzleuven.be

Obstet Gynecol Clin N Am 46 (2019) 625–641
https://doi.org/10.1016/j.ogc.2019.07.003
obgyn.theclinics.com
0889-8545/19/

With the aim of detecting the disease in early stages, several large ovarian cancer screening trials have been conducted. However, none of them has proven any clear benefit in terms of survival, when asymptomatic postmenopausal women are screened by means of serum testing with or without ultrasound examination.[3,4]

Moreover, because ultrasound-based screening algorithms have a high sensitivity for benign lesions, many patients would undergo surgical treatment for asymptomatic and innocent neoplasms, exposing them to possible surgical complications.

Correct differentiation between benign and malignant lesions is of high clinical relevance. On one hand, patients with a malignant adnexal tumor will benefit from being referred to gynecologic oncologists in tertiary hospitals for debulking surgery and appropriate systemic therapies.[5,6] On the other hand, patients with benign lesions may be followed conservatively,[7] or undergo minimally invasive surgery by general gynecologists, while preserving fertility or sparing ovarian function, depending on the clinical context.

Various diagnostic approaches have been introduced to characterize ovarian pathology before surgery. Most tests used in clinical practice incorporate findings of transvaginal ultrasound examination, because evidence shows this is the most appropriate first-line imaging technique for the preoperative assessment of women with adnexal pathology,[8] with subjective evaluation of ultrasound findings by an experienced examiner being the best method for discriminating between benign and malignant disease.[9–11]

In a randomized controlled trial, the management of patients with adnexal lesions has been shown to benefit from ultrasound assessment by experienced operators.[12] However, not all ultrasound operators are sufficiently exposed to adnexal pathology for them to gain a good level of experience to use subjective assessment. To help clinicians in obtaining a correct diagnosis, the International Ovarian Tumor Analysis (IOTA) study aims to develop diagnostic methods for characterizing adnexal pathology. The IOTA group initially published a consensus paper to standardize terms, definitions and measurements used to describe ovarian pathology (For educational material, see https://www.iotagroup.org/educational-material).[13] This agreement on a unified approach to report all possible ultrasound variables is a key element for the successful implementation of any ultrasound-based protocol for classifying ovarian pathology. It was the starting point for an ongoing international multicenter study, investigating a large number of patients presenting with an adnexal mass (ie, nonscreening population), thereby prospectively collecting information on gray scale ultrasound examination, Doppler imaging, biomarkers, and clinical characteristics.

In this article, we aim to describe the advances in the IOTA study, and we discuss newly available diagnostic algorithms, thereby providing guidance in choosing the best strategy for the preoperative characterization of ovarian masses and the diagnosis of ovarian cancer. We illustrate this as well with 4 case examples.

## INTERNATIONAL OVARIAN TUMOR ANALYSIS METHODS

### *Easy Descriptors*

Many common adnexal lesions (eg, mature teratomas, endometriomas) share typical characteristics that make them easy to be identified immediately, without the need to apply diagnostic rules or to perform risk calculations. Based on this knowledge, the IOTA group proposed 4 easy descriptors describing typical features of common benign lesions, and 2 Easy Descriptors suggestive of malignancy. These easy descriptors were applicable to about 43% of adnexal masses, where they proved to result in a positive predictive value of 93.4%, and a negative predictive value of 99.2%.[14] Recently, the Easy Descriptors were revised, with the largest diameter of the lesion <10 cm as an additional criterion for all Benign Descriptors (**Fig. 1**).

The idea is that application of these easy descriptors allows an instant diagnosis in a large proportion of cases, whereas nonclassifiable cases might be assessed using a more advanced diagnostic method.

### *Logistic Regression Models 1 and 2*

The IOTA group has created different prediction models based on logistic regression analysis.[15–17] The first clinically useful models were logistic regression models 1 and 2 (LR1 and LR2).[15] LR2 is easier to use than LR1 as it includes 6 instead of 12 variables. Because risk prediction models are based on a mathematical formula, their use requires the support of a computer (a calculator is freely available online at https://www.iotagroup.org/iota-models-software/lr2-risk-model-diagnose-ovarian-cancer), an application for smartphone, or integration into the ultrasound machine to acquire the individual risk of malignancy for an adnexal lesion.

Predictors used in LR2 are patient age (years), presence of ascites (yes/no), presence of blood flow within a papillary projection (yes/no), maximum diameter of the solid component (expressed in millimeters and truncated at 50 mm), irregular internal cyst walls (yes/no), and presence of acoustic shadows (yes/no).

The area under the receiver operating characteristic curve (AUC) reflects the overall test performance of a prediction model. An optimal probability level to indicate malignancy must be chosen depending on the individual clinical setting. In selecting this cut-off, there is always a compromise between sensitivity (true-positive rate) and

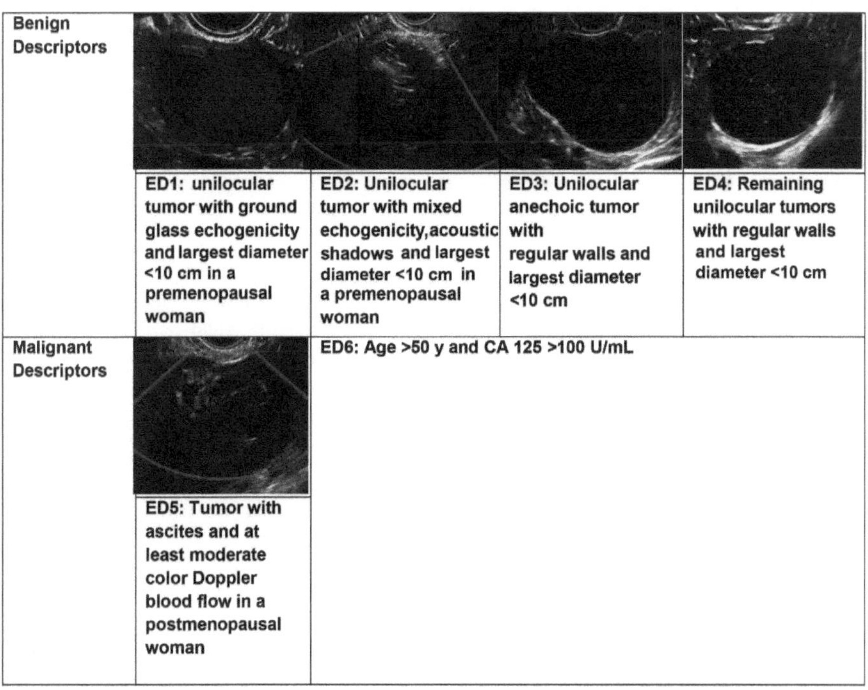


**Fig. 1.** Revised Easy Descriptors.

the number of false-positive test results.[15] In an external validation study, LR2 had an AUC of 0.95 and with an often suggested 10% cut-off, a sensitivity and specificity of 92% and 86%, respectively.[18]

### *Simple Rules*

The Simple Rules are a set of rules based on 5 ultrasound features suggesting a benign lesion (B-features) and 5 features that suggest a malignant lesion (M-features; **Fig. 2**).[19] The rules state that if at least one of the B-features is present without any M-feature, the lesion is classified as benign. Conversely, if at least one M-feature is present without any B-feature, the lesion is classified as malignant. However, in about 20% of cases, both B- and M-features are present, or no features are present (ie, not any of the B- and M-features are applicable to the adnexal tumor), resulting in an inconclusive diagnosis. For these patients, a second-stage diagnostic test is needed. A reasonable alternative strategy is to classify these cases as malignant and refer these patients to a gynecologic oncologist, because about 40% of these more complicated tumors will turn out to be malignant histologically.[20] Another limitation of the Simple Rules is that they provide a categorical outcome (benign–malignant–inconclusive) and so they lack an estimation of the likelihood of malignancy, although this information could be relevant for risk stratification and for individualizing patient management.

The IOTA Simple Rules have become very popular because they are easy to use, by memory or on a paper tick box. In 2011, The Royal College of Obstetricians and Gynecologists (RCOG) incorporated the Simple Rules into the Green-top Guideline (ie, a guideline produced by the RCOG as an aid to good clinical practice, presenting recognized methods and techniques, based on published evidence, for consideration by obstetricians/gynecologists and other relevant health professionals) on how to manage premenopausal women with adnexal masses.[21] This was followed in 2016 by the American College of Obstetrician and Gynecologists integrating the Simple Rules into their clinical guideline on the evaluation and management of adnexal

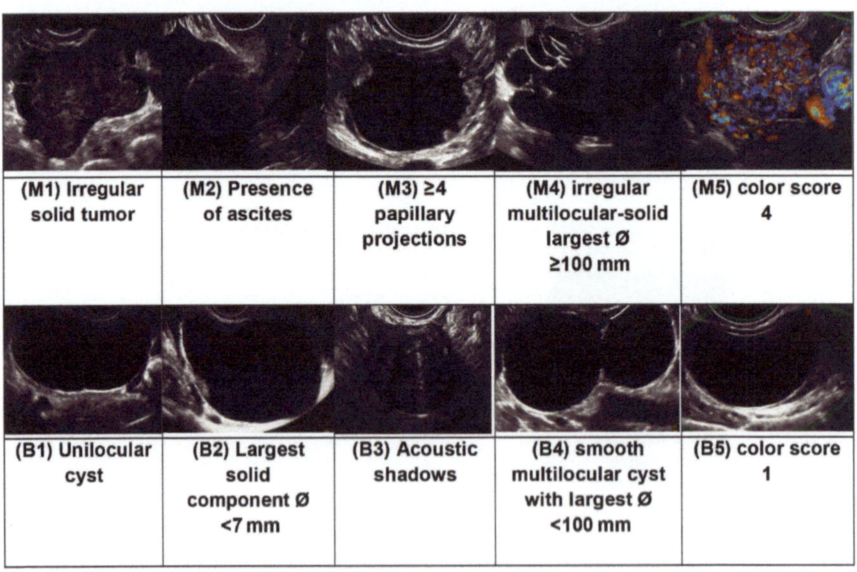


**Fig. 2.** Ultrasound features used in the Simple Rules. B, benign; M, malignant.

masses.[22] In 2017, the Simple Rules were considered as the main diagnostic strategy in a first international consensus report for the assessment of adnexal masses.[23]

In an external validation study, the Simple Rules achieved a sensitivity and specificity of 95% and 78% respectively, classifying the inconclusive cases (23% of all masses) as malignant.[20]

### *Simple Rules Risk Model*

To deal with the shortcomings of the original Simple Rules (the proportion of inconclusive cases and the absence of an estimated risk of malignancy), the IOTA group published a logistic regression model to estimate the individual risk of malignancy in all adnexal masses, based on the ultrasound features of the Simple Rules and the type of center (oncology or nononcology center). The Simple Rules risk model showed an AUC of 0.92 for discriminating between benign and malignant tumors. To make the model more user friendly in daily practice, a simple classification based on the risk estimates given has been proposed to form the basis of a clinical management system (**Fig. 3**).[16]

### *Assessment of the Different NEoplasias in the adneXa Model*

In gynecologic oncology, malignant adnexal masses are managed differently according to their subtype. For instance, borderline malignant ovarian tumors can be treated with fertility-sparing techniques, whereas the treatment of metastatic lesions depends on the origin of the primary tumor. Therefore, preoperative ovarian cancer characterization has become very important in clinical practice.

The recent Assessment of Different Neoplasias in the adneXa (ADNEX) model is the first multiclass prediction model for adnexal masses, not only calculating the likelihood of malignancy, but also the likelihood that the mass is borderline malignant, stage I primary invasive ovarian cancer, stages II to IV primary invasive ovarian cancer, or a metastasis in the ovary from another primary tumor.[17]

The model integrates 3 clinical predictors (age, serum CA-125 level and type of center: oncology center vs other hospital), and 6 ultrasound predictors (maximum diameter of the lesion, proportion of solid tissue, presence of >10 cyst locules, number of papillary projections, acoustic shadows, and ascites; **Fig. 4**). These ultrasound variables are very similar and perhaps even easier to obtain than variables used in both the IOTA LR2 model and the Simple Rules.

| Features | Observed malignancy rate | Estimated individual risk of malignancy | Classification |
|---|---|---|---|
| No M-features AND >2 B-features | 1/175 (0.6%) | <0.01–0.29% | Very low risk |
| - No M-features AND 2 B-features<br>- No M-features AND feature B1 present | 20/1560 (1.3%) | 0.19–2.7%<br>1.2–3.1% | Low risk |
| No M-features AND 1 B-feature present (except B1) | 60/722 (8.3%) | 2.4–15.2% | Intermediate risk |
| - No features<br>- Equal no. of M- and B-features<br>- >0 M-features, but more B- than M-features | 451/1096 (41.1%) | 27.5–48.7%<br>5.6–78.1%<br>1.3–28.4% | Elevated risk |
| More M- than B-features present | 1133/1295 (87.5%) | 42.0–>99.9% | Very high risk |

This simplified system only provides risk ranges for no. of B- and M-features present, but facilitates clinical triaging in absence of electronic devices. Personalized risk estimates can be obtained in second step.

*B-feature*, benign feature; *M-feature*, malignant feature.

**Fig. 3.** Summary classification of Simple Rules risk model. B, benign; M, malignant. (*From* Timmerman D, Van Calster B, Testa A, et al. Predicting the risk of malignancy in adnexal masses based on the Simple Rules from the International Ovarian Tumor Analysis group. Am J Obstet Gynecol 2016;214(4):435; with permission.)

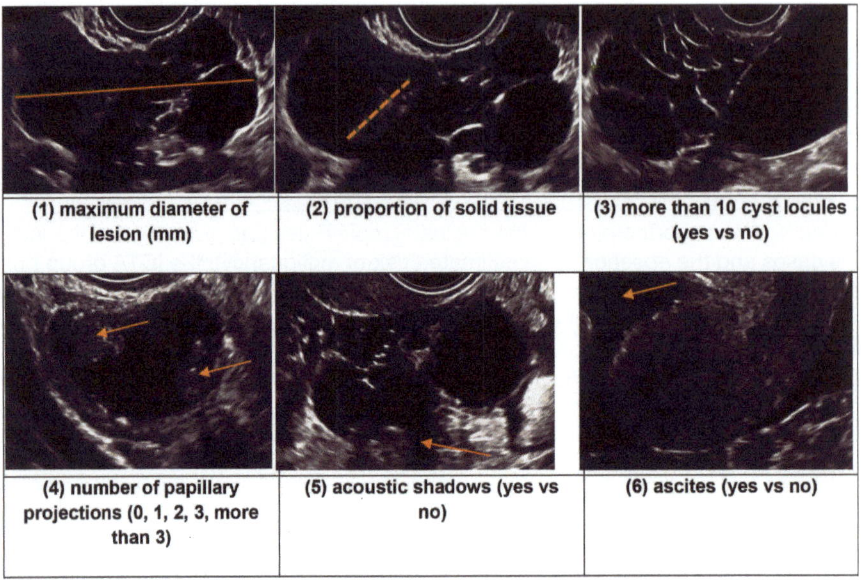


**Fig. 4.** Ultrasound features used in the ADNEX model.

ADNEX is available in a version with and without the CA-125 value. CA-125 will not aid much in differentiation between benign and malignant adnexal masses. However, when calculating the risks for the different subtypes of malignancy, knowing the CA-125 level will improve discrimination between late stage cancers and other types of malignancy.[17]

The AUC of the ADNEX model for the basic discrimination between benign and malignant tumors was 0.94 (IOTA phase 3 data). Moreover, the model was able to distinguish stages II to IV cancer from other malignancies (validation AUCs between 0.82 and 0.95) and showed fair discrimination between stage I cancer and borderline tumors (AUC, 0.75) and stage I cancer and secondary metastatic cancer (AUC, 0.71).[17] ADNEX has been validated by several research groups, including relatively inexperienced examiners. AUCs were always higher than 0.90.[24–28] We have published a practical guide to apply the ADNEX model, and provided some guidance for clinical management and some case examples. The risk cut-off to indicate malignancy is flexible, and can be adjusted depending on the individual setting. For example, for some centers it may be more important to have a high sensitivity, by choosing a low cut-off for malignancy (eg, 5%–10%). This leads to the appropriate referral of most malignancies to a gynecologic oncologist. For another center, it may be more important to have a high specificity, by choosing a much higher cut-off value for malignancy (eg, 30%). This practice limits the number of false-positive results, that is, patients with benign pathology who are referred to the gynecologic oncologist.

It must be emphasized that predicted risks should never be followed blindly using cut-offs alone, because it is important to integrate them with patient characteristics (eg, comorbidity, fertility wish) when making clinical decisions.[29]

ADNEX is freely available online (www.iotagroup.org/adnexmodel/ or https://www.evidencio.com/models/show/946) or can be downloaded as an application for smartphone. More recently, the model has been incorporated into ultrasound machines.

## COMPARISON OF DIFFERENT METHODS

### *International Ovarian Tumor Analysis Phase 3*

In IOTA phase 3, we compared different existing IOTA methods with the Risk of Malignancy Index (RMI) and subjective assessment on the same prospectively collected cohort of 2403 patients recruited from 2009 to 2012.[30]

The RMI is a multimodal scoring system based on a combination of ultrasound findings, serum CA-125 levels, and menopausal status.[31] Using the formula of the RMI results into a score, and a threshold is chosen to define a positive test result for cancer, leading to the woman being referred for specialist oncological treatment. The score is largely influenced by serum CA-125, often leading to a false-negative diagnosis for borderline or early invasive tumors, especially in premenopausal women. Conversely, CA-125 may trigger a false-positive diagnosis in numerous benign tumors or conditions that irritate the pelvic peritoneum (eg, endometriosis, fibroids, pregnancy, infection, and surgery).[32]

All IOTA strategies had excellent diagnostic performance in comparison with RMI. LR2 (AUC, 0.92) had a diagnostic performance similar to expert subjective assessment (AUC, 0.91), whereas for RMI, the AUC was only 0.88 (**Fig. 5**). The IOTA LR2 model and strategies using various combinations of Simple Rules, easy descriptors, and LR2 achieved sensitivities and specificities ranging from 90% to 96% and 74% to 79%, respectively. Classifying inconclusive cases (23%) as malignant, the sensitivity and specificity of the Simple Rules were 95% and 74%, respectively. Alternatively, inconclusive cases can be assessed by an expert, resulting into an increased specificity of 89% and a slightly decreased sensitivity of 92%. In comparison, the sensitivity of RMI was 67% and the specificity 91%, using a score of greater than 200 as an indication of malignancy.[30]

When validated on the same population, the ADNEX model attained the best performance for the basic discrimination between benign and malignant tumors, with an AUC of 0.94[17,33] (see **Fig. 5**).

Evaluation of calibration performance, that is, the extent to which the estimated risks of malignancy correspond with the observed prevalence of malignancy, shows that ADNEX is better calibrated than the LR2.[17]

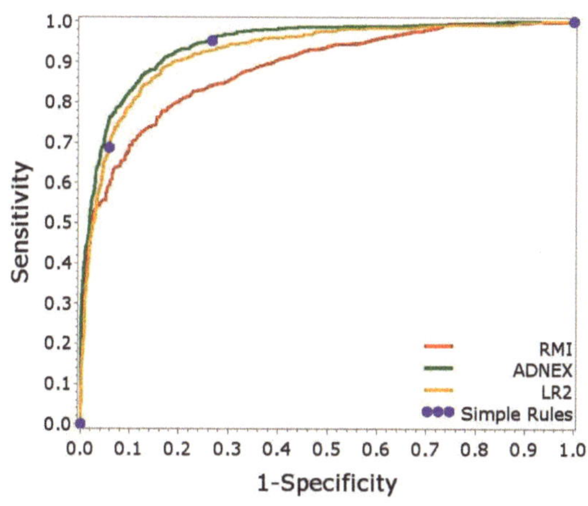


**Fig. 5.** Receiver operating characteristic curves for different diagnostic methods (IOTA phase 3 data; N = 2403). (*From* Kaijser J. Towards an evidence-based approach for diagnosis and management of adnexal masses: findings of the International Ovarian Tumour Analysis (IOTA) studies. Facts Views Vis Obgyn 2015;7(1):50; with permission.)

## Systematic Reviews, Meta-Analyses, and Randomized Trials

In 2014, the IOTA group performed a systematic review and meta-analysis, including evidence up to October 2013. Ninety-six validation studies met the predefined criteria for quantitative data analysis, including a total of 26,438 masses and 19 different diagnostic methods. The LR2 model (with a risk cut-off of 10%) and Simple Rules (classifying inconclusive cases as malignant) performed better than all other included models with a pooled sensitivity and specificity of 92% and 83% for LR2 and 93% and 81% for the Simple Rules. In contrast, for the RMI (cut-off 200), the pooled sensitivity and specificity were 72% and 92%, respectively. Compared with the RMI, the IOTA LR2 and Simple Rules had a higher sensitivity for cancer irrespective of menopausal status (**Fig. 6**).[34]

A more recent meta-analysis performed by Meys and colleagues[11] in 2016, comprising 47 studies on a total of 19,674 tumors, also included evidence on subjective assessment by an expert sonographer. The pooled sensitivity and specificity were 93% and 80% for the Simple Rules (classifying inconclusive cases as malignant), 93% and 84% for the LR2 (cut-off 10%), and 75% and 92% for the RMI (cut-off 200), respectively. Besides confirming that the Simple Rules and LR2 outperformed RMI, they concluded that a 2-step approach with the Simple Rules as the first step and subjective assessment by an expert for inconclusive tumors as a second step matched the test performance of expert ultrasound examiners[11] (see **Fig. 6**).

Because they have been published more recently, the IOTA Simple Rules Risk and ADNEX model were not included in previously mentioned meta-analyses.

In 2017, a diagnostic assessment report has been commissioned by the National Institute of Health Research on behalf of the National Institute for Health and Care Excellence. A systematic review with a cost-effectiveness analysis has been

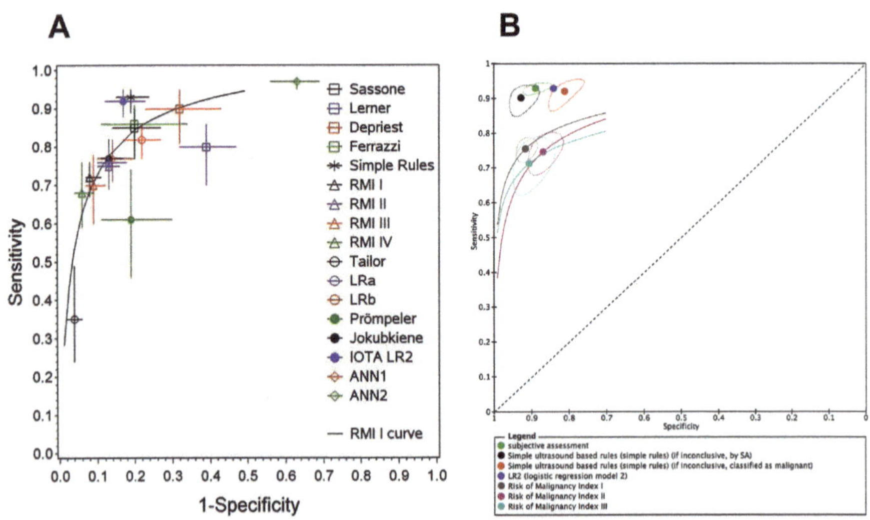


**Fig. 6.** (*A, B*) Summary receiver operating characteristic plots from meta-analysis. ([*A*] *From* Kaijser J, Sayasneh A, Van Hoorde K, et al. Presurgical diagnosis of adnexal tumours using mathematical models and scoring systems: a systematic review and meta-analysis. Hum Reprod Update 2014;20(3):457; with permission; [*B*] *From* Meys EM, Kaijser J, Kruitwagen RF, et al. Subjective assessment versus ultrasound models to diagnose ovarian cancer: A systematic review and meta-analysis. Eur J Cancer 2016;58:24; with permission.)

performed aiming at tests in secondary care to identify people at high risk of ovarian cancer, including the ADNEX model. Summary estimates for sensitivity and specificity for ADNEX (with a 10% cut-off) were 96% and 69%, for the Simple Rules (classifying inconclusive cases as malignant) 94% and 76%, and for the Simple Rules (classifying inconclusive cases by expert subjective assessment) 88% and 93%, respectively. Menopausal status did not significantly affect the performance of either the ADNEX model or the Simple Rules. For the RMI (cut-off 250), the summary estimates of sensitivity and specificity were 64% and 92%, respectively. The report concluded that the use of Simple Rules or ADNEX instead of RMI would be likely to decrease the numbers of cases that would be falsely classified as low-risk (increased sensitivity), with the trade-off of an increased number of patients with benign disease unnecessarily referred for specialist gynecologic oncology treatment (decreased specificity). It must also be mentioned that this report showed that Simple Rules and more importantly ADNEX were the most cost effective compared with other assessed methods.[35]

Despite these findings, we could comment that, from a methodological point of view, it is not ideal to compare the RMI with ADNEX on the basis of their sensitivity and specificity, because both methods use different cut-offs to indicate malignancy. Instead, there should be a comparison of AUCs, because with the changing risk cut-offs, there will be a different balance of sensitivity and specificity.

### *Randomized, Controlled Trials*

Nunes and colleagues[36] performed a randomized, controlled trial in 148 asymptomatic postmenopausal women to assess surgical intervention rates using a RCOG protocol based on the RMI versus IOTA Simple Rules–based triage. They concluded that the Simple Rules–based triage protocol resulted in lower surgical intervention rates compared with the standard RMI/RCOG protocol, without an increase in delayed diagnosis of malignancy.[36]

## CASE EXAMPLES

The diagnostic methods used in these case examples are limited to the easy descriptors, Simple Rules, and ADNEX model, because we believe these are the most useful in clinical practice, while having an excellent diagnostic performance.

### *Case 1*

A 67-year-old woman presented with a unilateral multilocular-solid lesion on the right ovary. The lesion has an irregular contour. Size is 135 × 110 × 100 mm. The diameter of the largest solid component is 88 × 56 × 50 mm, but there are no papillary projections. The number of locules is less than 10. There is subtle acoustic shadowing present (see white arrow in **Fig. 7**A). The IOTA color score is 2. There is no ascites. CA-125 is 28 U/mL (**Fig. 7**A).

The IOTA Easy Descriptors are not applicable in this case. Using the Simple Rules, there is one M-feature (irregular multilocular-solid tumor ≥100 mm in maximal diameter) and one B-feature (presence of acoustic shadowing). Applying the Simple Rules, the diagnosis is inconclusive (**Fig. 7**B).

Using the ADNEX model with CA-125, the absolute risk of malignancy is 27%. Using a threshold of 10% to define malignancy, we classify this lesion as malignant and we will refer the patient to a gynecologic oncologist. In a second step, we can look at the risks of the different subtypes of malignant tumors. The highest absolute risk is that of stage I invasive tumor (14.1%). Compared with the baseline IOTA population, the risk

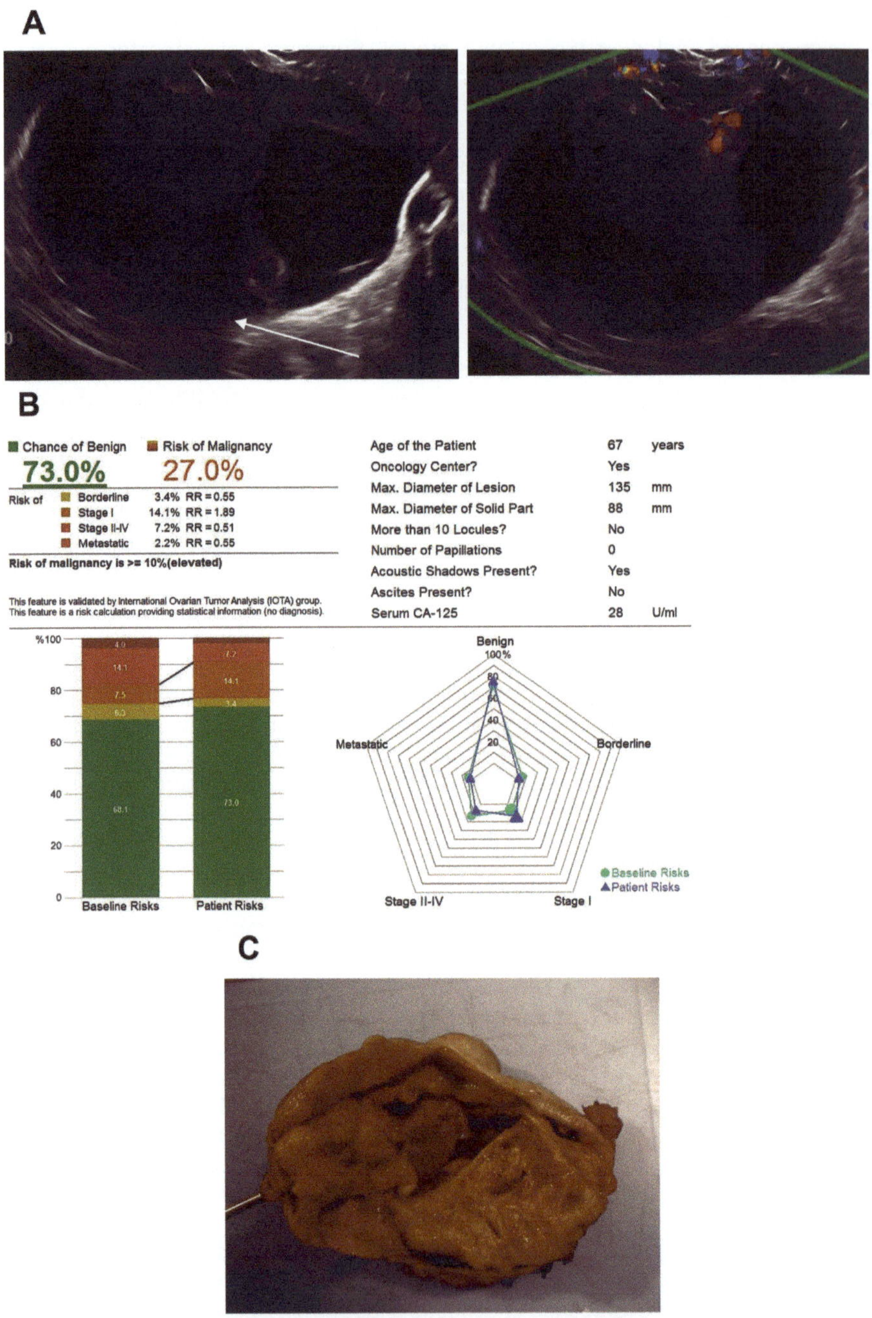


**Fig. 7.** Case 1. (*A*) Ultrasound images: left panel grayscale, right panel color Doppler. (*B*) ADNEX calculation results. (*C*) Macroscopic image of adnexal tumor after surgery. RR, relative risk. ([*C*] *Courtesy of* A.S. Van Rompuy, MD, PhD, Leuven, Belgium.)

of a stage I invasive tumor has also increased most strongly (from 7.5% to 14.1%; relative risk, 1.89). This patient underwent debulking surgery and was ultimately diagnosed with a primary invasive mucinous cystadenocarcinoma, stage I (**Fig. 7**C).

### *Case 2*

A 23-year-old woman presented with a unilocular solid lesion on the right ovary. Size is 31 × 30 × 25 mm. There are 2 papillary projections, the largest measures 13 × 10 × 10 mm. Acoustic shadowing is not present. The IOTA color score is 3. There is no ascites. Serum CA-125 is 21 U/mL (**Fig. 8**A).

The IOTA Easy Descriptors are not applicable in this case. Using the Simple Rules, there are no M-features and no B-features present, resulting into an inconclusive diagnosis (**Fig. 8**B).

Using the ADNEX model with CA-125, the absolute risk of malignancy is 32.4%. Using a threshold of 10% to define malignancy, we classify this lesion as malignant and we will refer the patient to a gynecologic oncologist. In a second step, we can look at the risks of the different subtypes of malignant tumors. The highest absolute risk is that of borderline malignant tumor (23.6%). Compared with the baseline IOTA population, the risk of borderline tumor has also increased most strongly (from 6.3% to 23.6%; relative risk, 3.76). This patient underwent fertility-sparing surgery and was ultimately diagnosed with a borderline serous papillary cystadenoma, stage IIIB (**Fig. 8**C).

### *Case 3*

A 58-year-old patient presented with a unilateral solid lesion on the left ovary. The lesion has a regular contour. Size is 26 × 22 × 20 mm. There is acoustic shadowing present. The IOTA color score 3. There is no ascites. CA-125 is 9 U/mL (**Fig. 9**A).

The IOTA Easy Descriptors are not applicable in this case. Using the Simple Rules, there are no M-features and 1 B-feature (presence of acoustic shadowing). Applying the Simple Rules, the diagnosis is benign (**Fig. 9**B).

Using the ADNEX model without CA-125, the absolute risk of malignancy is 6.7%. Using a threshold of 10% to define malignancy, we classify this lesion as benign. The patient underwent surgery and was ultimately diagnosed with a benign Leydig cell tumor (**Fig. 9**C).

### *Case 4*

A 30-year-old woman presented with a unilocular lesion in the right ovary. Size is 53 × 48 × 45 mm. The lesion has a mixed echogenicity and an IOTA color score of 1. There is acoustic shadowing. There is no ascites (**Fig. 10**).

The benign easy descriptors are applicable, because this patients is premenopausal with a unilocular lesion with mixed echogenicity (suggestive for dermoid cyst). There is no need to apply any other method such as the Simple Rules or ADNEX model in this case. The patient underwent surgery and a mature teratoma was confirmed histologically.

## FUTURE CONSIDERATIONS

### *Value of MRI for Difficult Tumors*

An interesting research subject is the management of adnexal masses that are "difficult to classify" by ultrasound examination. In a systematic review and meta-analysis, Anthoulakis and Nikoloudis[37] concluded that pelvic MRI with intravenous contrast administration should be considered as an option in all diagnostic protocols investigating adnexal masses that remain unclassified after assessment by

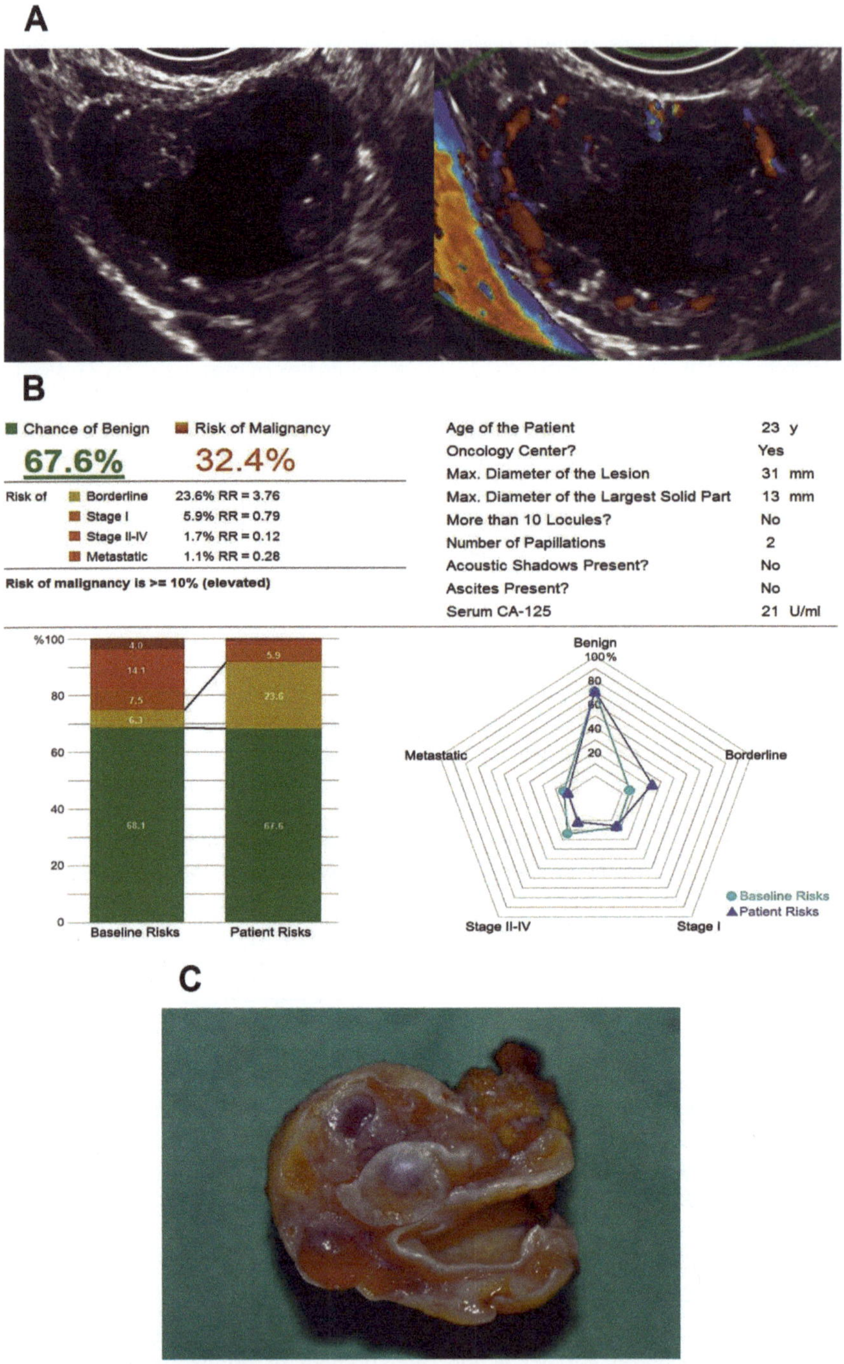


**Fig. 8.** Case 2. (*A*) Ultrasound images: left panel grayscale, right panel color Doppler. (*B*) ADNEX calculation results. (*C*) Macroscopic image of adnexal tumor after surgery. RR, relative risk. ([*C*] *Courtesy of* A.S. Van Rompuy, MD, PhD, Leuven, Belgium.)

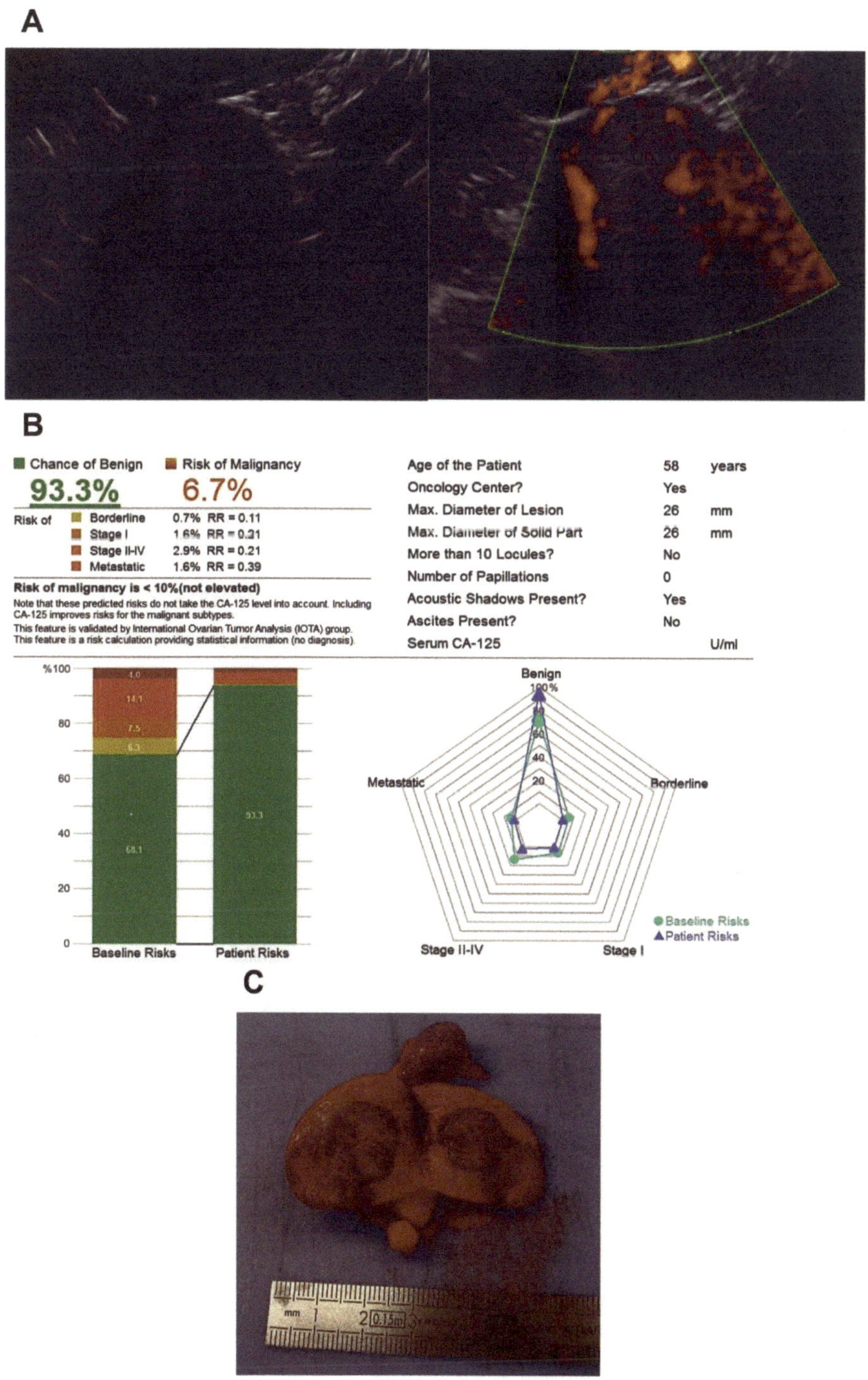


**Fig. 9.** Case 3. (*A*) Ultrasound images: left panel grayscale, right panel color Doppler. (*B*) ADNEX calculation results. (*C*) Macroscopic image of adnexal tumor after surgery. RR, relative risk. ([*C*] *Courtesy of* A.S. Van Rompuy, MD, PhD, Leuven, Belgium.)

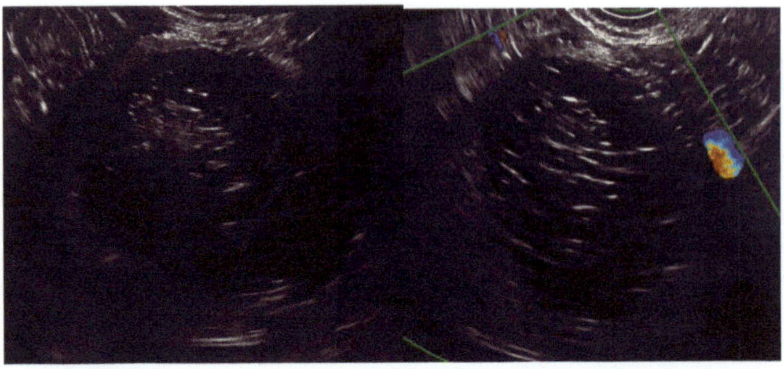

Fig. 10. Case 4. Ultrasound images: left panel grayscale, right panel color Doppler.

ultrasound. This strategy outperformed other imaging modalities, including computed tomography scans.[37]

However, most studies lack uniformity in describing the exact features used to define such difficult masses. A benefit of using the IOTA strategies is that they offer straightforward criteria that can be used to define a difficult mass (eg, when the Simple Rules do not apply).

The ongoing IOTA-MRI study (ClinicalTrials.gov Identifier: NCT02836275) evaluates the performance of MRI in the assessment of this well-defined group of tumors.[8] Until results are available, the subjective interpretation of ultrasound images by an expert clinician with a special interest in gynecologic ultrasonography offers the best available second-stage test in this group of masses.[38]

### *Expectant Management of Ovarian Tumors*

The majority of studies involving the development and validation of diagnostic tests and models designed to assess ovarian tumors use final histology after surgery as a clear end point to verify the index test results. This is a reflection of clinical practice, where the traditional management of patients with adnexal lesions has been surgery, also when the presumed diagnosis was benign.

Possible explanations are the fear of a false-negative diagnosis and the lack of knowledge about the natural behavior of cysts in long-term follow-up (with the presumed risk of complications as cyst torsion or rupture, and the potential risk of malignant transformation).

Consequently, many patients are exposed to surgical risks. In the literature, perioperative complication rates of gynecologic surgery for benign disease are reported to be as high as 15%.[3] It may jeopardize fertility in women of reproductive age, and in the long term in the case of bilateral oophorectomy in a premenopausal patient, a negative impact on overall mortality may be expected.[39] Moreover, every surgical intervention and hospitalization have a financial cost.

The ongoing IOTA5 study (ClinicalTrials.gov Identifier: NCT01698632) is the first multicenter prospective study recruiting not only patients scheduled for surgical management, but also patients selected for ultrasound follow-up. In a recently published 2-year interim analysis, we described the outcomes during the first 2 years of follow-up of 1919 newly diagnosed adnexal masses with benign ultrasound morphology. Our results showed that the risk of complications in conservatively managed adnexal masses is very low. The 2-year cumulative incidence of spontaneous resolution was 20.2% and for surgical intervention was 16.1%, and the 2-year cumulative incidence of major complications, including invasive malignancy, torsion, and cyst rupture, were each less than 0.5%. These reassuring results could lead to a paradigm shift in recommended management of benign adnexal masses resulting in less surgery.[7]

Besides evaluating complications during longer term follow-up, we will further investigate the performance of previously established diagnostic methods on all patients, including patients selected for conservative management. We will also explore the possibility to improve the safe selection of patients for conservative management, perhaps by using a risk prediction model (eg, ADNEX) with a low risk cut-off.

## SUMMARY

Many diagnostic methods exist for preoperative evaluation of adnexal masses. Based on standardized definitions and measurement techniques, recent IOTA methods such as the Simple Rules and the ADNEX model are the best of available methods, as suggested by direct comparison on IOTA phase 3 data, as well as recent systematic reviews with meta-analysis. ADNEX does not only show the best performance to discriminate between benign and malignant lesions, but is the first multiclass prediction model, giving risk estimates for different types of malignant tumors. As shown by the case examples, this is very relevant to guide patient management.

In contrast, 2-year interim analysis results of the IOTA phase 5 study have shown that expectant management of adnexal masses with benign ultrasound morphology could be safe. Future research further needs to explore the longer term follow-up of conservatively managed adnexal masses, the performance of diagnostic methods when applied on all patients, as well as the role of MRI for lesions difficult to characterize on ultrasound examination.

## ACKNOWLEDGMENTS

The IOTA5 study is supported by the Research Foundation–Flanders (FWO) projects G049312N/G0B4716N/12F3114N, and Internal Funds KU Leuven (project C24/15/037). Wouter Froyman is doctoral fellow (1701819N) and Dirk Timmerman is senior clinical investigator of FWO (1803415N).

## REFERENCES

1. Vaughan S, Coward JI, Bast RC Jr, et al. Rethinking ovarian cancer: recommendations for improving outcomes. Nat Rev Cancer 2011;11(10):719–25.
2. Cancer Research UK. 2018. Available at: www.cancerresearchuk.org. Accessed December 24, 2018.
3. Buys SS, Partridge E, Black A, et al. Effect of screening on ovarian cancer mortality: the prostate, lung, colorectal and ovarian (PLCO) cancer screening randomized controlled trial. JAMA 2011;305(22):2295.
4. Jacobs IJ, Menon U, Ryan A, et al. Ovarian cancer screening and mortality in the UK Collaborative Trial of Ovarian Cancer Screening (UKCTOCS): a randomised controlled trial. Lancet 2016;387(10022):945–56.
5. Woo YL, Kyrgiou M, Bryant A, et al. Centralisation of services for gynaecological cancer. Cochrane Database Syst Rev 2012;(3):CD007945.
6. Engelen MJ, Kos HE, Willemse PH, et al. Surgery by consultant gynecologic oncologists improves survival in patients with ovarian carcinoma. Cancer 2006; 106(3):589–98.
7. Froyman W, Landolfo C, De Cock B, et al. Risk of complications in patients with conservatively managed ovarian tumours (IOTA5): a 2-year interim analysis of a multicentre, prospective, cohort study. Lancet Oncol 2019;20(3):448–58.

8. Kaijser J, Vandecaveye V, Deroose CM, et al. Imaging techniques for the pre-surgical diagnosis of adnexal tumours. Best Pract Res Clin Obstet Gynaecol 2014;28(5):683–95.
9. Valentin L, Hagen B, Tingulstad S, et al. Comparison of 'pattern recognition' and logistic regression models for discrimination between benign and malignant pelvic masses: a prospective cross validation. Ultrasound Obstet Gynecol 2001;18:357–65.
10. Timmerman D. The use of mathematical models to evaluate pelvic masses; can they beat an expert operator? Best Pract Res Clin Obstet Gynaecol 2004;18(1):91–104.
11. Meys EM, Kaijser J, Kruitwagen RF, et al. Subjective assessment versus ultrasound models to diagnose ovarian cancer: a systematic review and meta-analysis. Eur J Cancer 2016;58:17–29.
12. Yazbek J, Raju SK, Ben-Nagi J, et al. Effect of quality of gynaecological ultrasonography on management of patients with suspected ovarian cancer: a randomised controlled trial. Lancet Oncol 2008;9(2):124–31.
13. Timmerman D, Valentin L, Bourne T, et al. Terms, definitions and measurements to describe the sonographic features of adnexal tumors: a consensus opinion from the International Ovarian Tumor Analysis (IOTA) group. Ultrasound Obstet Gynecol 2000;16:500–5.
14. Ameye L, Timmerman D, Valentin L, et al. Clinically oriented three-step strategy for assessment of adnexal pathology. Ultrasound Obstet Gynecol 2012;40(5):582–91.
15. Timmerman D, Testa AC, Bourne T, et al. Logistic regression model to distinguish between the benign and malignant adnexal mass before surgery: a multicenter study by the International Ovarian Tumor Analysis Group. J Clin Oncol 2005;23(34):8794–801.
16. Timmerman D, Van Calster B, Testa A, et al. Predicting the risk of malignancy in adnexal masses based on the Simple Rules from the International Ovarian Tumor Analysis group. Am J Obstet Gynecol 2016;214(4):424–37.
17. Van Calster B, Van Hoorde K, Valentin L, et al. Evaluating the risk of ovarian cancer before surgery using the ADNEX model to differentiate between benign, borderline, early and advanced stage invasive, and secondary metastatic tumours: prospective multicentre diagnostic study. BMJ 2014;349:g5920.
18. Van Holsbeke C, Van Calster B, Bourne T, et al. External validation of diagnostic models to estimate the risk of malignancy in adnexal masses. Clin Cancer Res 2012;18(3):815–25.
19. Timmerman D, Testa AC, Bourne T, et al. Simple ultrasound-based rules for the diagnosis of ovarian cancer. Ultrasound Obstet Gynecol 2008;31(6):681–90.
20. Timmerman D, Ameye L, Fischerova D, et al. Simple ultrasound rules to distinguish between benign and malignant adnexal masses before surgery: prospective validation by IOTA group. BMJ 2010;341:c6839.
21. Royal College of Obstetricians and Gynaecologists. Management of suspected ovarian masses in premenopausal women. Green-top Guideline No. 62. 2011.
22. The American College of Obstetricians and Gynecologists. Practice bulletin - evaluation and management of adnexal masses. Obstet Gynecol 2016;128(5):e210–26.
23. Glanc P, Benacerraf B, Bourne T, et al. First international consensus report on adnexal masses: management recommendations. J Ultrasound Med 2017;36(5):849–63.
24. Araujo KG, Jales RM, Pereira PN, et al. Performance of the IOTA ADNEX model in the preoperative discrimination of adnexal masses in a gynecologic oncology center. Ultrasound Obstet Gynecol 2017;49(6):778–83.

25. Szubert S, Wojtowicz A, Moszynski R, et al. External validation of the IOTA ADNEX model performed by two independent gynecologic centers. Gynecol Oncol 2016;142(3):490–5.
26. Sayasneh A, Ferrara L, De Cock B, et al. Evaluating the risk of ovarian cancer before surgery using the ADNEX model: a multicentre external validation study. Br J Cancer 2016;115(5):542–8.
27. Meys EM, Jeelof LS, Achten NM, et al. Estimating the risk of malignancy in adnexal masses: an external validation of the ADNEX model and comparison with other frequently used ultrasound methods. Ultrasound Obstet Gynecol 2017;49(6):784–92.
28. Joyeux E, Miras T, Masquin I, et al. Before surgery predictability of malignant ovarian tumors based on ADNEX model and its use in clinical practice. Gynecol Obstet Fertil 2016;44(10):557–64.
29. Van Calster B, Van Hoorde K, Froyman W, et al. Practical guidance for applying the ADNEX model from the IOTA group to discriminate between different subtypes of adnexal tumors. Facts Views Vis Obgyn 2015;7(1):32–41.
30. Testa A, Kaijser J, Wynants L, et al. Strategies to diagnose ovarian cancer: new evidence from phase 3 of the multicentre international IOTA study. Br J Cancer 2014;111(4):680–8.
31. Jacobs I, Oram D, Fairbanks J, et al. A Risk of Malignancy Index incorporating CA 125, ultrasound and menopausal status for the accurate preoperative diagnosis of ovarian cancer. Br J Obstet Gynaecol 1990;97(10):922–9.
32. Sevinc A, Adli M, Kalender ME, et al. Benign causes of increased serum CA-125 concentration. Lancet Oncol 2007;8(12):1054–5.
33. Kaijser J. Towards an evidence-based approach for diagnosis and management of adnexal masses: findings of the International Ovarian Tumour Analysis (IOTA) studies. Facts Views Vis Obgyn 2015;7(1):42–59.
34. Kaijser J, Sayasneh A, Van Hoorde K, et al. Presurgical diagnosis of adnexal tumours using mathematical models and scoring systems: a systematic review and meta-analysis. Hum Reprod Update 2014;20(3):449–62.
35. Westwood M, Ramaekers B, Lang S, et al. Risk scores to guide referral decisions for people with suspected ovarian cancer in secondary care: a systematic review and cost-effectiveness analysis. Health Technol Assess 2018;22(44):1–264.
36. Nunes N, Ambler G, Foo X, et al. Comparison of two protocols for the management of asymptomatic postmenopausal women with adnexal tumours - a randomised controlled trial of RMI/RCOG vs Simple Rules. Br J Cancer 2017;116(5): 584–91.
37. Anthoulakis C, Nikoloudis N. Pelvic MRI as the "gold standard" in the subsequent evaluation of ultrasound-indeterminate adnexal lesions: a systematic review. Gynecol Oncol 2014;132(3):661–8.
38. Van Holsbeke C, Van Calster B, Testa AC, et al. Prospective internal validation of mathematical models to predict malignancy in adnexal masses: results from the international ovarian tumor analysis study. Clin Cancer Res 2009;15(2):684–91.
39. Parker WH, Feskanich D, Broder MS, et al. Long-term mortality associated with oophorectomy compared with ovarian conservation in the nurses' health study. Obstet Gynecol 2013;121(4):709–16.

# Ultrasound Imaging in Endometriosis

Francesca Moro, MD, PhD[a], Martina Leombroni, MD[a,*],
Antonia Carla Testa, MD, PhD[a,b]

**KEYWORDS**

• Endometrioma • Ultrasonography • Endometriosis

**KEY POINTS**

- Ultrasound examination represents an indisputable imaging method in the diagnosis of endometriosis.
- Ultrasound evaluation of the pelvic endometriosis is fundamental in planning the appropriate timing and type of surgical procedure.
- The surveillance of menopausal women with history of endometriosis still represents a challenge.
- The ultrasound characteristics of malignant masses arising in endometriomas are the same features characterizing malignant ovarian masses.
- During pregnancy, endometriomas may undergo major morphologic changes, which are referred to as *decidualization*.

## INTRODUCTION

Endometriosis is defined as the presence of ectopic endometrial-like tissue outside the uterus correlated with a chronic and inflammatory reaction[1(p16)] Ultrasound examination represents an indisputable imaging method in the diagnosis of endometriosis as the first step in the detection, as the fundamental tool in planning the management, and as the best diagnostic instrument during surveillance of affected women.[2–7] Ultrasound is a noninvasive, commonly available, affordable method associated with minimal risk and discomfort to the patient. Moreover, it stands out from other diagnostic imaging modalities because of its dynamic and interactive nature. The careful manipulation of an endocavitary probe allows the operator to assess the mobility and elasticity of pelvic structures; this dynamic examination is able to provide a more accurate

Disclosure Statement: The authors declare no conflicts of interest.
[a] Fondazione Policlinico Universitario Agostino Gemelli, IRCCS, Dipartimento Scienze della Salute della Donna, del Bambino e di Sanità Pubblica, L.go A. Gemelli 8, Rome 00168, Italy; [b] Catholic University of the Sacred Heart, Department of Obstetrics and Gynecology, Rome, Italy
* Corresponding author.
*E-mail address:* martina.leombroni@gmail.com

Obstet Gynecol Clin N Am 46 (2019) 643–659
https://doi.org/10.1016/j.ogc.2019.07.004
obgyn.theclinics.com

diagnosis than the static visualization of the pelvic organs.[8] The accuracy reported in the literature in assessing pelvic endometriosis with the different manifestations and clinical phases of this pathology is very high.[4,9,10] The accuracy of ultrasound, however, is largely dependent on the operators, on their knowledge of the disease, and on the techniques they use to perform the examination.[8,11–13]

The key steps for a correct assessment of the pelvis have previously well reported.[8,13,14] First, all patients should be examined systematically and carefully using an endocavitary sonography, with a microconvex array probe inserted transvaginally or transrectally. Both techniques are optimal approaches for examining uterus (including the different uterine zones: cervix, endometrium, junctional zone, and myometrium), adnexa, paracolpium, parametrium, vesicocervical, vesicovaginal, and rectovaginal spaces as well as urinary bladder, ureters, and rectum.[13–15] Second, in order to ensure that no pathology is overlooked in the lower pelvis (eg, a nodule in the rectovaginal septum or vaginal pathology), it is important to begin the transvaginal gynecologic examination by looking at the structures at the point of insertion into the vagina so that, in addition to the actual vagina, the urethra, the anorectal canal, and the perineum as a whole can be studied. Then, having gently introduced the transvaginal probe, cervix, uterus, adnexa, and all the other pelvic structures can be assessed.

## ULTRASOUND AND DETECTION OF ENDOMETRIOSIS

The ultrasound scan, as with all diagnostic methods, should be preceded by an accurate medical history of the patient in order to correlate any morphologic signs to a patient's symptoms,[16] to interpret any eventual negative ultrasound findings, and to suggest the best treatment. After the classic schemes reported in the literature, the pelvic localization of endometriosis can be described according to 3 compartments (central, anterior, and posterior). In these 3 compartments, the endometriosis can appear on ultrasound as following:

- Cystic mass with ground-glass content (which can be located either in the ovary or within the myometrium)[9]
- Hyperechoic island(s) (in the myometrium)[17,18]
- Hypoechoic nodule(s), which can be found anywhere in the pelvis or in the entire body[7,16]
- Fixation of the pelvic organs,[19] which appear adherent when pushing one against the other (negative sliding sign).[16,20,21]

**Table 1** summarizes the ultrasounds findings in endometriosis, with detailed description in the following sections.

### *Central Compartment*

The central compartment includes uterus and adnexa. At the uterus level, the migration and proliferation of endometrial glands and stroma from the basal layer of the endometrium to deep within the myometrium is known as adenomyosis and gives origin to particular morphologic findings seen on ultrasound.[22–24] Recently, the ultrasound features of these morphologic aspects have been systematically described by the international Morphological Uterus Sonographic Assessment (MUSA) group[17] after a critical revision of previously reported data.[25–29]

In particular, on ultrasound, an adenomyotic uterus appears with a globular shape, enlarged dimensions, and uterine wall asymmetry unrelated to leiomyoma[7] (**Fig. 1**). The myometrium typically appears heterogeneous on gray-scale, characterized by the presence of an indistinctly defined area with either decreased or increased

**Table 1**
**Ultrasound features of endometriosis**

| Pathology | Ultrasonographic Characteristics |
|---|---|
| Adenomyosis | • Globular shape<br>• Enlarged dimensions of the uterus<br>• Uterine wall asymmetry unrelated to leiomyoma<br>• Presence of an indistinctly defined area with either decreased or increased echogenicity<br>• Hypoechoic linear striations<br>• Round anechoic areas of 1–7 mm diameter (myometrial cysts)<br>• Adenomyotic lesion<br>• Irregularities of the endometrial-myometrial junctional zone |
| Endometrioma | • Unilocular cyst (most commonly), multilocular, unilocular-solid, multilocular-solid (less commonly)<br>• Ground-glass content<br>• No vascularization on color Doppler |
| Deep infiltrating endometriosis | • Hypoechoic lesion with or without regular contours<br>• Hourglass-shaped or diabolo-like nodule appearance<br>• Comet nodule appearance<br>• Indian headdress sign<br>• Thickened and hyperechoic uterosacral ligaments |
| Decidualized endometrioma | • Unilocular-solid or multilocular-solid<br>• Ground-glass or low-level cyst content<br>• Rounded papillary projections with smooth surface<br>• Well vascularized |

echogenicity[30–33] (**Fig. 2**). Myometrial hypoechoic linear striations are thin acoustic shadows radiating out from the endometrium into the myometrium without a clear endomyometrial junction, due to the ectopic endometrial tissue[31,33] (**Fig. 3**). Round anechoic areas of 1-mm to 7-mm diameter, named *myometrial cysts*, also could be present within the myometrium.[30,33] In cases of focal adenomyosis, the adenomyotic lesion appears as a heterogeneous (**Fig. 4**) and hypoechogenic area within the myometrium,[30] usually with anechoic lacunae or cysts with ill-defined contours and fan-shaped shadowing. These hypoechogenic areas reflect muscular hypertrophy of the myometrial tissue.

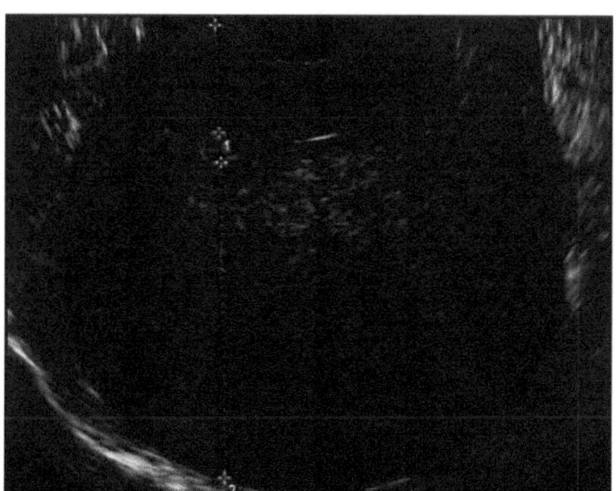

**Fig. 1.** Gray-scale ultrasound image of an adenomyotic uterus with a globous shape, enlarged dimension, and uterine wall asymmetry.

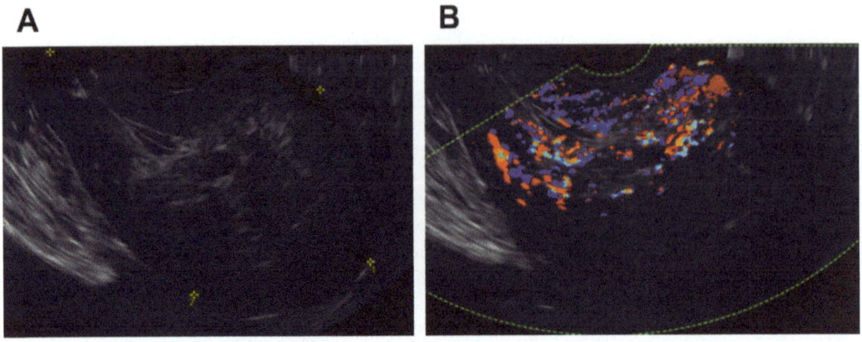


**Fig. 2.** (*A*) Gray-scale and (*B*) color Doppler ultrasound images of an adenomyotic uterus with heterogeneous myometrium.

Irregularities of the endometrial-myometrial junctional zone is another common ultrasound marker in the diagnosis of adenomyosis.[32,34] This endomyometrial interface is normally visualized as hypoechoic tissue layer seen beyond the endometrial basal layer. In women with adenomyosis, the diffuse or focal hyperplasia and hypertrophy of myocytes determine whether diffuse or focal thickening of this zone is seen.[24,29]

According to the MUSA consensus, adenomyosis should be described as localized and diffuse. Adenomyosis is classified as diffuse, if the total involvement of myometrium exceeds 50% of the corpus uteri (including in cases of multiple focal lesion), and localized when less than 50% of myometrium is involved.[17]

Demarcated focal adenomyosis surrounded by hypertrophic myometrium is defined adenomyoma.[35] The size of the adenomyosis lesion(s) should be measured (in particular the largest diameter of each focal lesion or the myometrial wall thickness in cases of a diffuse lesion).[18] The term, *cystic adenomyosis*, should be used in case of a measurable cysts (largest diameter $\geq$2 mm) with an echogenic rim.[16,18] Additional descriptors include the evaluation of the involvement of the uterine layers, such as the inner myometrium, middle myometrium, or outer myometrium, and of the extent of the disease, based on the estimated volume of the uterine corpus affected by adenomyosis (mild<25%, moderate 25%–50%, and severe >50%).[18,36–38]

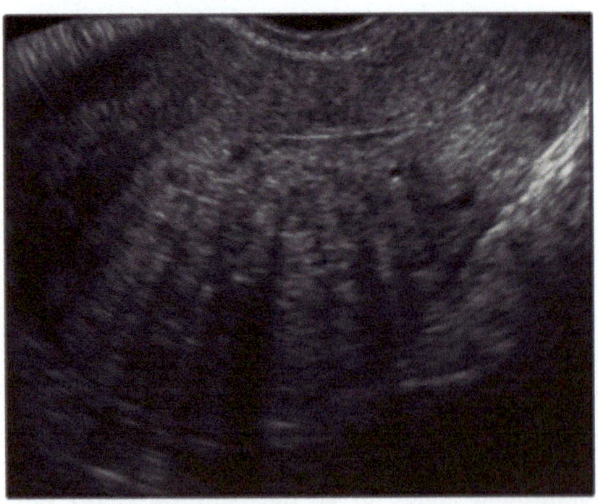

**Fig. 3.** Gray-scale ultrasound image of myometrial hypoechoic linear striations.

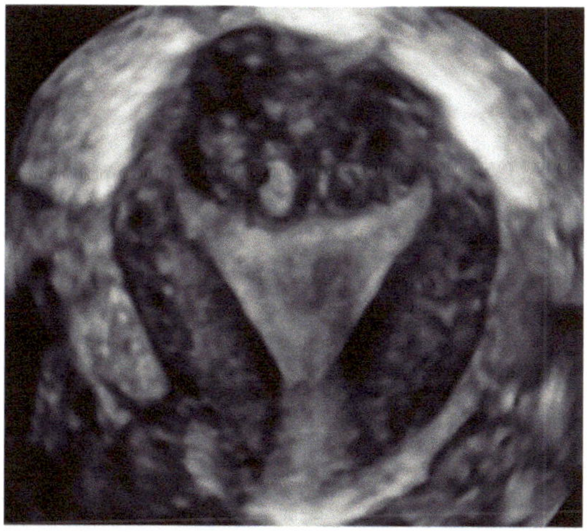

Fig. 4. 3-D ultrasound image of adenomyotic uterus with hyperechoic myometrial island.

Finally, the mobility of the uterus should be investigated and noted as normal, reduced, or fixed (question mark sign [**Fig. 5**]). Di Donato and colleagues[39] described this sign when the uterine corpus was flexed backward, the fundus of the uterus was facing the posterior pelvic compartment, and the cervix was directed anteriorly toward the urinary bladder. Investigators found 93% specificity and 75% sensitivity of this sign in detecting adenomyosis.

Once assessment of the uterus is completed, the evaluation of the adnexa includes the examination of the ovaries and Fallopian tubes. The typical ultrasound feature of an endometriotic cyst located within the ovary (endometrioma) is a unilocular cyst with ground-glass content with no vascularization on color Doppler (**Fig. 6**). It can appear, however, as unilocular-solid or multilocular-solid cysts with papillary projections or as multilocular cyst.[9,40] The presence of echoic material within the internal cyst wall, due to the accumulation of debris on the cyst wall, can falsely interpreted as papillary projections on ultrasound[3,41] (**Fig. 7**). The absence of vascularization using color Doppler, the localization of the echogenic

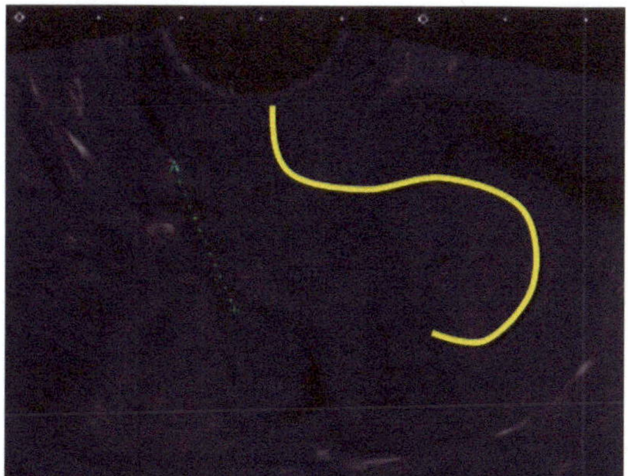

Fig. 5. Gray-scale ultrasound image of question mark sign (*yellow line*) of adenomyotic uterus.

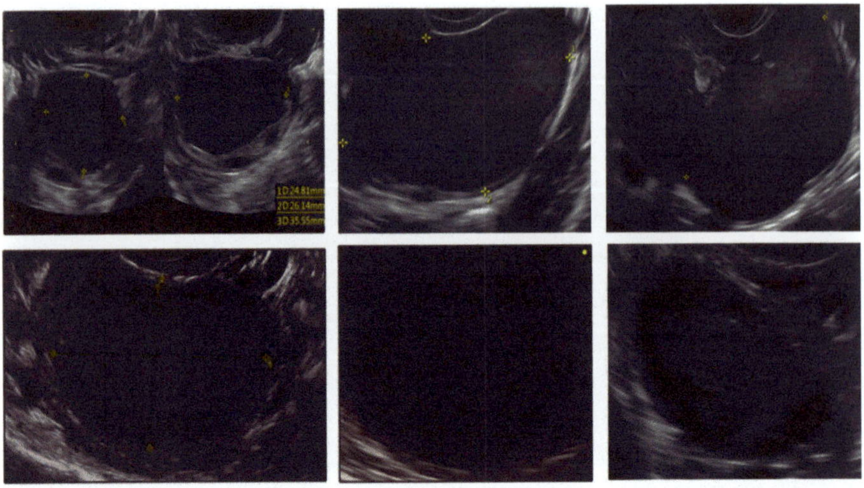

Fig. 6. Gray-scale images of typical ultrasound endometriomas: unilocular cysts with ground-glass content within the ovary.

intracystic material, and the movement during dynamic examination help an examiner in correctly discriminating between papillary projection and amorphous material. The multilocular morphology may originate by multiple endometriomas in the same ovary.[40] There is evidence that ovarian endometriomas originate from ovulatory events[42–44] and it is likely that the number of endometriomas may increase with age, and multiple endometriomas in the same ovary may assume a multilocular morphology.[40] Guerriero and colleagues[40] reported that ultrasound appearance of endometriomas differed between premenopausal and postmenopausal patients. The endometriomas in the postmenopausal patients were less often unilocular

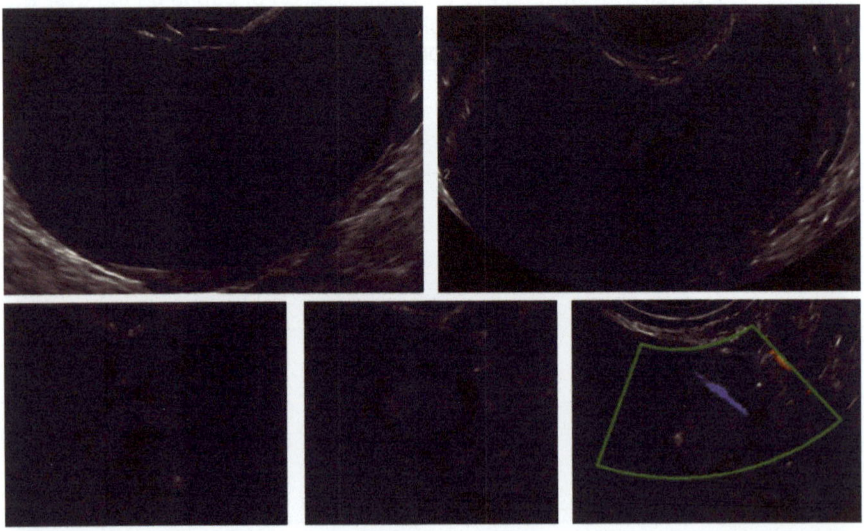

Fig. 7. Gray-scale and color Doppler images of atypical endometriomas with amorphous material.

cysts and less likely to exhibit ground-glass echogenicity.[3,9] The subjective assessment by an experienced sonologist is very accurate in the diagnosis of an endometrioma, with 81% sensitivity and 97% specificity.[9]

Ovarian mobility can be judged by applying pressure to the ovaries using the endocavitary probe and by concomitant application of an abdominal hand in bimanual examination. Nonmobile ovaries are considered a soft marker of pelvic endometriosis. The operator should observe the mobility of the ovaries against the pelvic side wall laterally, against the uterus medially, against uterosacral ligaments inferiorly, and against all the other pelvic organs.[16] The fixation of bilateral ovaries behind the uterus is known as kissing ovaries[45] (**Fig. 8**).

Finally, in the presence of endometriosis of the salpinx, a dilated tube with thick walls and incomplete septa can be detected, with fluid dense content (hematosalpinx) in cases of endoluminal pathology or with anechoic content (hydrosalpinx) in cases of obliteration by adhesions[46] (**Fig. 9**).

### *Anterior Compartment*

The anterior compartment is comprised of the urinary bladder, uterovesical septum, and ureters.

Involvement of the urinary tract occurs in approximately 1% to 2% of patients with endometriosis[47] and involves bladder in 85% of these cases.[48] Ureteric involvement is found in 4% of patients with rectovaginal endometriosis.[49,50]

On ultrasound, bladder endometriosis appears as hypoechoic lesion with or without regular contours bulging toward the lumen, involving the serosa, muscularis (most common), or (sub)mucosa of the bladder,[16,51–53] more frequently at the base and dome levels.[16,54,55] Obliteration of the uterovesical septum can be detected as the absence of the sliding sign between the uterus and the bladder. The term, *bladder endometriosis*, should be used only in cases of infiltration of the bladder wall and not in cases of adhesions or superficial peritoneal implants on the bladder serosa (**Fig. 10**).

During examination, from a longitudinal section through the cervix and moving the probe toward the lateral pelvic wall, it is possible to assess the distal part of the ureter adjacent to the bladder trigone, in order to evaluate the presence of stenosis and subsequent cephalad dilatation of the pelvic ureters.[50] This finding can suggest direct invasion or compression of the ureter by endometriotic nodules, ovarian endometriomas, or adhesions.[57] Mapping of ureteric involvement, including the site of obstruction and presence of hydroureter or hydronephrosis, facilitates preoperative assessment of renal function and improves preoperative counseling.

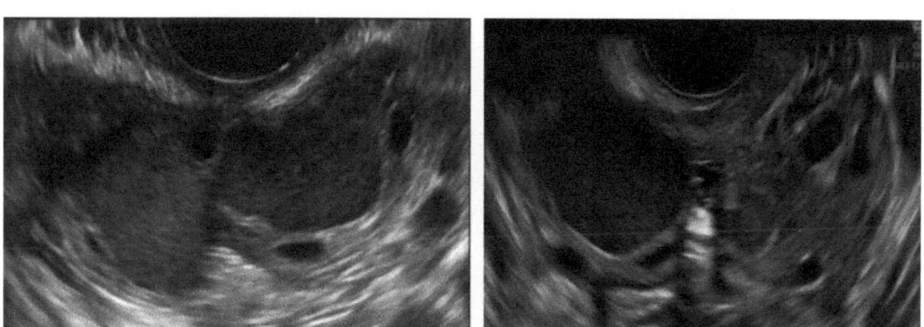

**Fig. 8.** Gray-scale images of kissing ovaries.

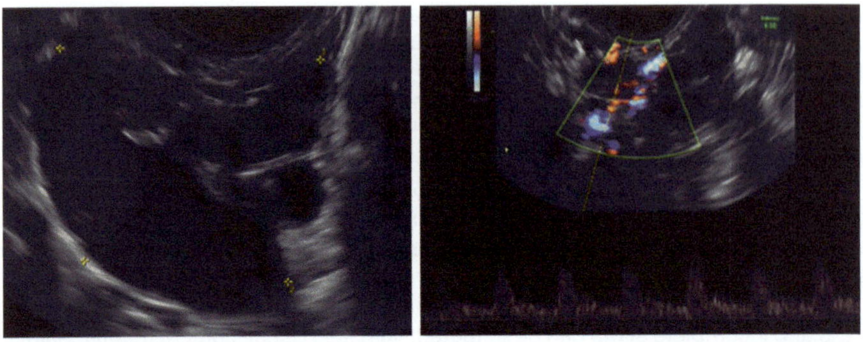

Fig. 9. Ultrasound images of endometriosis of the salpinx showing a dilated tube with thick walls and incomplete septa and fluid dense content.

### *Posterior Compartment*

According to Chapron and colleagues,[58] the most common sites of deep infiltrating endometriosis in the posterior compartment are posterior vaginal fornix/rectovaginal septum, uterosacral ligaments, anterior rectum/anterior rectosigmoid junction, and sigmoid colon.

Recently, the ultrasound features of the deep infiltrating endometriosis nodules have been systematically defined by the International Deep Endometriosis Analysis group.[16] According to this classification, involvement of the rectovaginal septum should be suspected when an endometriotic nodule, which appears as hypoechoic solid nodule with smooth or irregular contours, is seen in the rectovaginal space below the line passing along the lower border of the posterior lip of the cervix (under the peritoneum). Isolated rectovaginal septum nodule is rare, and it is usually an extension of posterior vaginal wall, anterior rectal wall, or both posterior vaginal wall and anterior rectal wall involvement. Hourglass-shaped or diabolo-like nodules can occur when endometriosis lesions from the posterior vaginal fornix extend to the anterior rectal wall.[59]

The uterosacral ligaments affected by deep infiltrating endometriosis are characterized by the presence of hypoechoic tissue, with regular/irregular margins within the peritoneal fat surrounding the uterosacral ligaments (**Fig. 11**). Sometimes, the uterosacral ligaments appear thickened and hyperechoic, probably as the morphologic expression of fibrosis, due to the chronic process of inflammation.

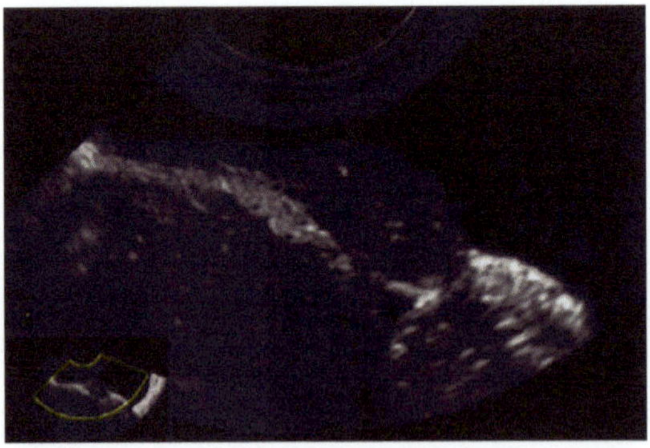

Fig. 10. Ultrasound image showing a hypoechoic nodule of the bladder wall.

The anterior rectum, rectosigmoid junction, and sigmoid colon are the most commonly affected posterior compartment areas.[58] The endometriosis affecting the bowel can appear as a thickening of the muscularis propria or as a hypoechoic nodule with blurred margins, sometimes a thinner section resembling a comet, usually associated with retraction and adhesion resulting in the so-called Indian headdress sign[51] (**Fig. 12**).Iin the presence of endometriotic nodule, a systematic evaluation is important, including details of the anatomic localizations, the size and number of nodules, the depth of infiltration of the nodules, and the degree of stenosis of the bowel lumen, which is important to plan the surgical procedures, to counsel accurately the patients, and to choose the appropriate surgical team (**Fig. 13**).

Finally, during the evaluation of posterior compartment, a negative sliding sign between the rectosigmoid and uterus could indicate an obliteration of the pouch of Douglas, whereas a hypoechoic tissue altering the hyperechoic layer between the vagina and rectum highlights the presence of deep infiltrating endometriosis in the rectovaginal septum.

Ultrasound features of endometriosis are summarized in **Table 1**.

## ULTRASOUND AND PLANNING OF MEDICAL AND SURGICAL TREATMENT

### *How Do Ultrasound Findings Have an Impact on the Medical and Surgical Treatment Planning in Women with Endometriosis?*

Regarding medical treatment, the description and the localization of pelvic endometriosis could triage a patient toward a local-release medical treatment (ie, levonorgestrel-releasing intrauterine system [LNG-IUS]) instead of an oral treatment. Although there are not specific guidelines, LNG-IUS showed reduction of symptoms in a higher prevalence of women with adenomyosis in comparison with women treated with combined oral contraceptives.[60]

As far as the impact on surgical treatment is concerned, the ultrasound evaluation of the pelvic endometriosis is fundamental in planning the appropriate timing and type of surgical procedure and potential need for subspecialty surgical involvement (eg, urology or colorectal consultants). The morphologic depiction, together with patients' characteristics (age, symptoms, and desire of pregnancy), allow clinicians to plan the best personalized treatment. For instance, in the presence of an endometrioma, ultrasound can provide the surgeon the exact localization within the ovary, especially in those cases of small size and in those patients with severe pelvic adhesions. Moreover, the assessment of residual normal ovarian parenchyma can allow a more appropriate preoperative counseling with the patient, in particular, in those women who want to preserve their fertility. It is known that 30% to 50% of patients affected by endometriosis suffer from infertility.[61]

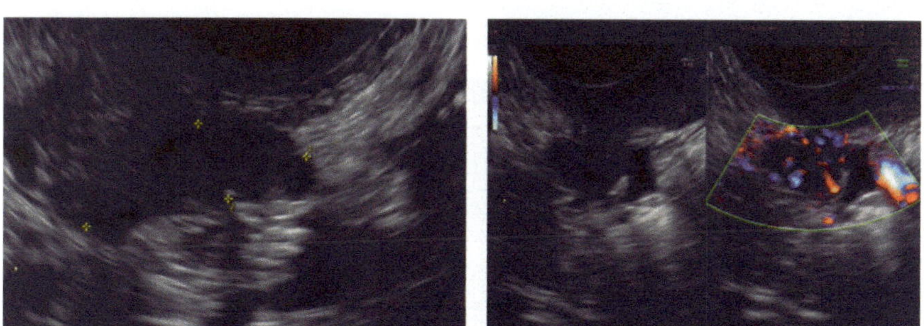

**Fig. 11.** Ultrasound images of endometriotic nodules involving the uterosacral ligaments.

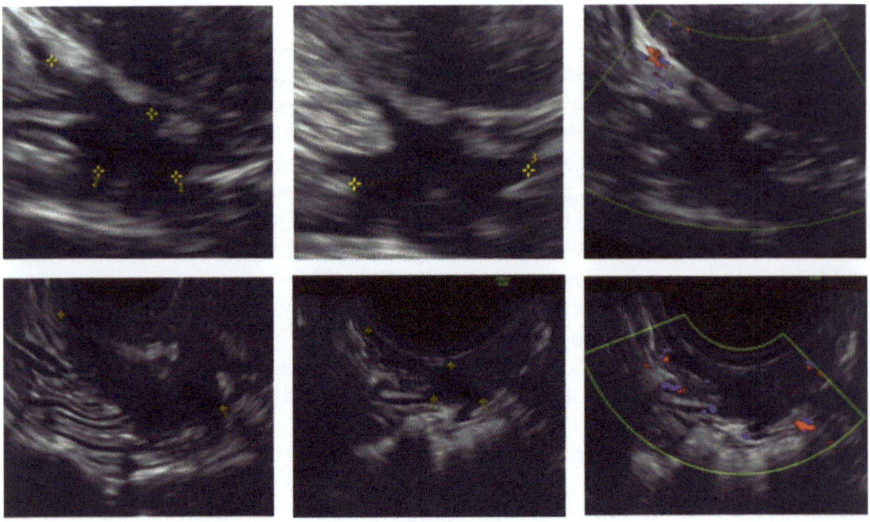

**Fig. 12.** Ultrasound images of endometriosis affecting the bowel.

In cases of deep pelvic endometriosis, the distribution of the pelvic disease is increasingly important. The diagnosis of endometriotic nodules infiltrating the urinary tract is a key example. If patients with bladder endometriosis are usually symptomatic (urinary frequency, urgency, and dysuria), women with ureteral endometriosis are more often asymptomatic, leading to silent urinary tract obstruction and loss of renal function. In this scenario, ultrasound diagnosis of ureteral endometriosis with hydroureter and hydronephrosis plays a fundamental role in planning the best surgical procedure.[62]

Moreover, the accurate assessment of endometriosis affecting the bowel, including the eventual infiltration of the submucosal layer, the presence of multifocal disease, the measurement of the largest nodule, and the distance between the more caudal

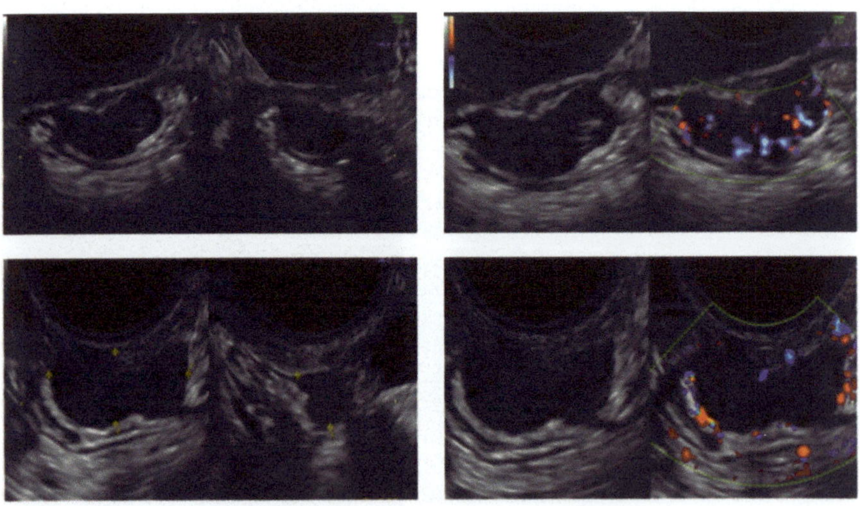

**Fig. 13.** Ultrasound images of endometriosis affecting the bowel.

nodule and the anal verge, allows a more precise definition of the type of surgical procedures.[63] In particular, some investigators suggested performing shaving or discoid resection of the bowel in cases of small nodules (diameter <30 mm) or in cases of muscularis involvement, whereas bowel resection is recommended in case of larger nodules.[64,65]

## ULTRASOUND AND SURVEILLANCE OF PATIENTS WITH ENDOMETRIOSIS

Ultrasound examination plays a fundamental role in the surveillance of women with endometriosis.

### *Surveillance in Premenopausal Women*

In young patients with a diagnosis of ovarian cysts showing morphologic characteristics indicative of endometriomas, serial ultrasound scans usually are recommended at 3 months to 6 months after first diagnosis and then yearly if there is no fast growth or change in sonographic features.[66]

In patients undergoing medical therapy for endometriosis, an ultrasound surveillance is usually performed without strong evidence on the clinical impact of such routine diagnostic method. In particular, there are no data about the reduction rate of the endometriotic cyst or the involution of the adenomyotic uterus according to the different medical strategies. Ultrasound changes of the endometriotic lesion(s), such as an increase in size and/or rising of vascularized solid component during hormonal therapy, are the only relevant recommendations indicating surgical excision.[67]

### *Surveillance in Menopausal Women*

The surveillance of menopausal women with history of endometriosis still represents a challenge for several reasons:

1. Lack of data about the natural history of endometriomas left in situ
2. Wide heterogeneous sonographic morphology of endometriomas in postmenopausal women[9]
3. Paucity of data regarding the morphologic appearance of borderline and invasive cancer arising in endometriosis[68]

Endometriomas affecting postmenopausal women appear more often as multilocular cysts or cysts with papillation and solid component, more frequently exhibiting anechoic cyst fluid or cyst with mixed echogenicity and less often having typical ground-glass echogenicity than endometriomas in premenopausal women.[9,40] The most probable explanation of changes in cyst content is ascribed to the effects of local degrading enzyme, leading to the conversion from ground-glass into low-level echogenicity and to the accumulation of debris from tissue degradation that appears as a nonvascularized solid component on ultrasound.[40]

The association between endometriosis and ovarian cancer has been widely reported, with an estimated prevalence of 0.2% to 0.7%.[68–70] The ultrasound characteristics of malignant masses arising in endometriomas are the same features characterizing malignant ovarian masses (ie, the presence of irregular vascularized solid component),[68,71,72] thus reassuring clinicians when these features are not visible during follow-up of ovarian endometriomas.

### *Surveillance in Pregnancy*

During pregnancy, endometriomas may undergo major morphologic changes, which are referred to as *decidualization*. Decidualization is the process of endometrial changes caused by high progesterone levels, which increase glandular epithelial secretion, accumulation of glycogen, and stromal vascularity. These changes create conditions that facilitate implantation and development of early gestation. Formation of ectopic decidua (deciduosis) during pregnancy is a well-documented phenomenon that is caused by the effect of progesterone on ectopic endometrium, such as in endometrioma or within foci of endometriosis.[73]

The most typical ultrasound appearance of decidualized endometriomas is a unilocular-solid or multilocular-solid ovarian mass with ground-glass or low-level cyst content and with well-vascularized, rounded papillary projections with smooth surface[74] (**Fig. 14**). This ultrasound appearance allows the clinician to distinguish a decidualized endometrioma from a borderline tumor, where papillary projections usually have an irregular surface.[74] These findings also were confirmed by the same investigators when analyzing the ultrasound appearances of ovarian masses with papillary projections surgically removed during pregnancy.[74]

Although the ultrasound features of decidualized endometriomas have been described, there is limited information regarding the behavior of endometriomas during pregnancy.[75] Pateman and colleagues[75] described the natural history of endometriosis in a retrospective series of 36 ovarian endometriomas, reporting that 12% of endometriomas undergo decidualization and a majority of decidualized endometriomas decrease in size during pregnancy. These data suggested that expectant management of decidualized endometrioma is likely to be safe with a fast regression rate.

Therefore, women with an ultrasound diagnosis of endometrioma before pregnancy are conservatively managed and an ultrasound follow-up is useful to reassure

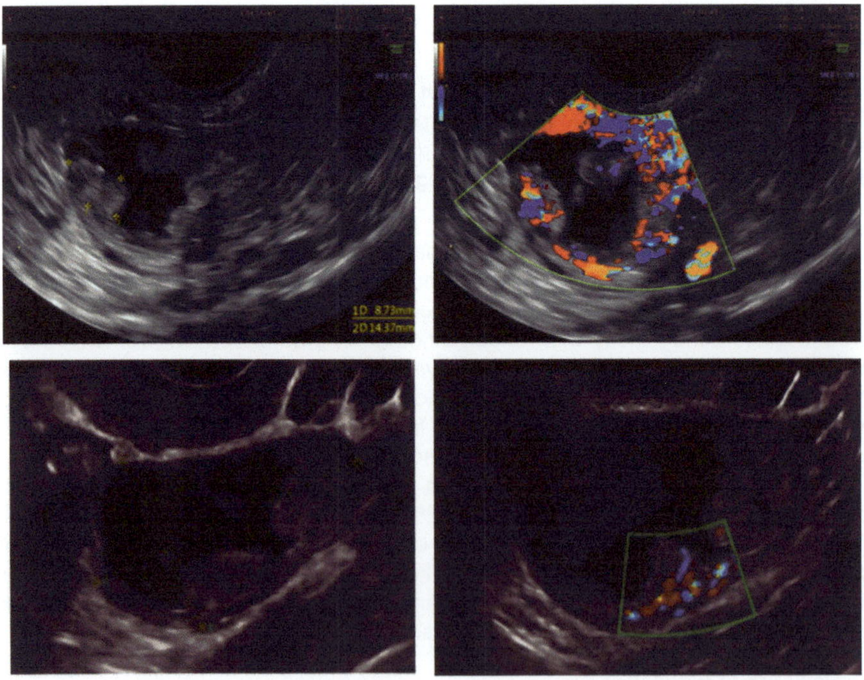

**Fig. 14.** Gray-scale and color Doppler images of ultrasound appearance of decidualized endometriomas. They appear as unilocular-solid ovarian masses with low-level cyst content and rounded papillary projections with smooth surface and rich vascularization.

clinicians and patients in cases of concerning or atypical morphology.[74] In cases of incidental findings of ovarian cyst with papillary projections diagnosed during pregnancy, however, the management of the cyst remains a challenge and the ultrasound diagnosis can be inconclusive.[74]

Deep infiltrating endometriotic nodules also undergo morphologic changes due to the process of decidualization, showing rich vascularization on color Doppler examination during second trimester and experiencing shrinkage after pregnancy.[76]

## SUMMARY

This review shows that ultrasound examination plays a fundamental role in the diagnosis of adenomyosis and endometrioma as well as in the identification and localization of pelvic endometriosis. The possibility of correctly recognizing and exactly mapping endometriosis in the pelvis allows personalizing treatment of patients. Finally, ultrasound examination plays an important role in the surveillance of premenopausal and postmenopausal patients as well as pregnant women with endometriosis, leading to the best management in these subgroups of patients.

## REFERENCES

1. Kennedy S, Bergqvist A, Chapron C, et al. ESHRE guideline for the diagnosis and treatment of endometriosis. Hum Reprod 2005;20:2698–704.
2. Mais V, Guerriero S, Ajossa S, et al. The efficiency of transvaginal ultrasonography in the diagnosis of endometrioma. Fertil Steril 1993;60:776–80.
3. Exacoustos C, Manganaro L, Zupi E. Imaging for the evaluation of endometriosis and adenomyosis. Best Pract Res Clin Obstet Gynaecol 2014;28:655–81.
4. Guerriero S, Ajossa S, Minguez JA, et al. Accuracy of transvaginal ultrasound for diagnosis of deep endometriosis in uterosacral ligaments, rectovaginal septum, vagina and bladder: systematic review and meta-analysis. Ultrasound Obstet Gynecol 2015;46:534–45.
5. Piketty M, Chopin N, Dousset B, et al. Preoperative work-up for patients with deeply infiltrating endometriosis: transvaginal ultrasonography must definitely be the first-line imaging examination. Hum Reprod 2009;24:602–7.
6. Moore J, Copley S, Morris J, et al. A systematic review of the accuracy of ultrasound in the diagnosis of endometriosis. Ultrasound Obstet Gynecol 2002;20:630–4.
7. Exacoustos C, Zupi E, Piccione E. Ultrasound Imaging for Ovarian and Deep Infiltrating Endometriosis. Semin Reprod Med 2017;35:5–24.
8. Testa AC, Van Holsbeke C, Mascilini F, et al. Dynamic and interactive gynecological ultrasound examination. Ultrasound Obstet Gynecol 2009;34:225–9.
9. Van Holsbeke C, Van Calster B, Guerriero S, et al. Endometriomas: their ultrasound characteristics. Ultrasound Obstet Gynecol 2010;35:730–40.
10. Holland TK, Yazbek J, Cutner A, et al. Value of transvaginal ultrasound in assessing severity of pelvic endometriosis. Ultrasound Obstet Gynecol 2010;36:241–8.
11. Valentin L. High-quality gynecological ultrasound can be highly beneficial, but poor-quality gynecological ultrasound can do harm. Ultrasound Obstet Gynecol 1999;13:1–7.
12. Testa AC, Di Legge A, Bonatti M, et al. Imaging techniques for evaluation of uterine myomas. Best Pract Res Clin Obstet Gynaecol 2016;34:37–53.
13. Fischerova D. Ultrasound scanning of the pelvis and abdomen for staging of gynecological tumors: a review. Ultrasound Obstet Gynecol 2011;38:246–66.

14. Pateman K, Mavrelos D, Hoo WL, et al. Visualization of ureters on standard gynecological transvaginal scan: a feasibility study. Ultrasound Obstet Gynecol 2013; 41:696–701.
15. Bean E, Naftalin J, Jurkovic D. How to assess the ureters during pelvic ultrasound. Ultrasound Obstet Gynecol 2019;53(6):729–33.
16. Guerriero S, Condous G, Bosch T, et al. Systematic approach to sonographic evaluation of the pelvis in women with suspected endometriosis, including terms, definitions and measurements: a consensus opinion from the International Deep Endometriosis Analysis (IDEA) group. Ultrasound Obstet Gynecol 2016;48: 318–32.
17. Van den Bosch T, Dueholm M, Leone FP, et al. Terms, definitions and measurements to describe sonographic features of myometrium and uterine masses: a consensus opinion from the Morphological Uterus Sonographic Assessment (MUSA) group. Ultrasound Obstet Gynecol 2015;46:284–98.
18. Van den Bosch T, de Bruijn AM, de Leeuw RA, et al. A sonographic classification and reporting system for diagnosing adenomyosis. Ultrasound Obstet Gynecol 2019;53(5):576–82.
19. Guerriero S, Ajossa S, Garau N, et al. Diagnosis of pelvic adhesions in patients with endometrioma: the role of transvaginal ultrasonography. Fertil Steril 2010; 94:742–6.
20. Hudelist G, Fritzer N, Staettner S, et al. Uterine sliding sign: a simple sonographic predictor for presence of deep infiltrating endometriosis of the rectum. Ultrasound Obstet Gynecol 2013;41:692–5.
21. Reid S, Lu C, Casikar I, et al. Prediction of pouch of Douglas obliteration in women with suspected endometriosis using a new real-time dynamic transvaginal ultrasound technique: the sliding sign. Ultrasound Obstet Gynecol 2013;41: 685–91.
22. Ferenczy A. Pathophysiology of adenomyosis. Hum Reprod Update 1998;4: 312–22.
23. Zaloudek C, Norris HJ. Mesenchymal tumors of the uterus. In: Kurmann RJ, editor. Blaustein's pathology of the female genital tract. New York: Springer-Velag; 1994. p. 487–627.
24. Exacoustos C, Brienza L, Di Giovanni A, et al. Adenomyosis: three-dimensional sonographic findings of the junctional zone and correlation with histology. Ultrasound Obstet Gynecol 2011;37:471–9.
25. Dueholm M. Transvaginal ultrasound for diagnosis of adenomyosis: a review. Best Pract Res Clin Obstet Gynaecol 2006;20:569–82.
26. Reinhold C, Tafazoli F, Wang L. Imaging features of adenomyosis. Hum Reprod Update 1998;4:337–49.
27. Dueholm M, Lundorf E, Hansen ES, et al. Magnetic resonance imaging and transvaginal ultrasonography for the diagnosis of adenomyosis. Fertil Steril 2001;76: 588–94.
28. Bazot M, Cortez A, Darai E, et al. Ultrasonography compared with magnetic resonance imaging for the diagnosis of adenomyosis: correlation with histopathology. Hum Reprod 2001;16:2427–33.
29. Kepkep K, Tuncay YA, Goynumer G, et al. Transvaginal sonography in the diagnosis of adenomyosis: which findings are most accurate? Ultrasound Obstet Gynecol 2007;30:341–5.
30. Reinhold C, Atri M, Mehio A, et al. Diffuse uterine adenomyosis: morphologic criteria and diagnostic accuracy of endovaginal sonography. Radiology 1995; 197:609–14.

31. Bazot M, Daraï E, Rouger J, et al. Limitations of transvaginal sonography for the diagnosis of adenomyosis, with histopathological correlation. Ultrasound Obstet Gynecol 2002;20:605–11.
32. Reinhold C, McCarthy S, Bret PM, et al. Diffuse adenomyosis: comparison of endovaginal US and MR imaging with histopathologic correlation. Radiology 1996; 199:151–8.
33. Vercellini P, Cortesi I, De Giorgi O, et al. Transvaginal ultrasonography versus uterine needle biopsy in the diagnosis of diffuse adenomyosis. Hum Reprod 1998;13:2884–7.
34. Fedele L, Bianchi S, Dorta M, et al. Transvaginal ultrasonography in the diagnosis of diffuse adenomyosis. Fertil Steril 1992;58:94–7.
35. Exacoustos C. Adenomyosis and ultrasound: the role of ultrasound and its impact on understanding the disease. In: Habiba M, Benegiano G, editors. Uterine adenomyosis. Cham (Switzerland): Springer; 2016. p. 141–52.
36. Sammour A, Pirwany I, Usubutun A, et al. Correlations between extent and spread of adenomyosis and clinical symptoms. Gynecol Obstet Invest 2002;54: 213–6.
37. Brosens JJ, de Souza NM, Barker FG. Uterine junctional zone: function and disease. Lancet 1995;346:558–60.
38. Aguilar HN, Mitchell BF. Physiological pathways and molecular mechanisms regulating uterine contractility. Hum Reprod Update 2010;16:725–44.
39. Di Donato N, Bertoldo V, Montanari G, et al. Question mark form of uterus: a simple sonographic sign associated with the presence of adenomyosis. Ultrasound Obstet Gynecol 2015;46:126–7.
40. Guerriero S, Van Calster B, Somigliana E, et al. Age-related differences in the sonographic characteristics of endometriomas. Hum Reprod 2016;31:1723–31.
41. Guerriero S, Ajossa S, Mais V, et al. The diagnosis of endometriomas using color Doppler energy imaging. Hum Reprod 1998;6:1691–5.
42. Jain S, Dalton ME. Chocolate cysts from ovarian follicles. Fertil Steril 1999;72: 852–6.
43. Vercellini P, Somigliana E, Vigano P, et al. 'BloodOn The Tracks' from corpora lutea to endometriomas. BJOG 2009;116:366–71.
44. Vercellini P, Somigliana E, Vigano' P, et al. Post-operative endometriosis recurrence: a plea for prevention based on pathogenetic, epidemiological and clinical evidence. Reprod Biomed Online 2010;21:259–65.
45. Ghezzi F, Raio L, Cromi A, et al. "Kissing ovaries": a sonographic sign of moderate to severe endometriosis. Fertil Steril 2005;83:143–7.
46. Timor-Tritsch IE, Lerner JP, Monteagudo A, et al. Transvaginal sonographic markers of tubal inflammatory disease. Ultrasound Obstet Gynecol 1998;12: 56–66.
47. Yohannes P. Ureteral endometriosis. J Urol 2003;170:20–5.
48. Maccagnano C, Pellucchi F, Rocchini L, et al. Diagnosis and treatment of bladder endometriosis: state of the art. Urol Int 2012;89:249–58.
49. Donnez J, Nisolle M, Squifflet J. Ureteral endometriosis: a complication of rectovaginal endometriotic (adenomyotic) nodules. Fertil Steril 2002;77:32–7.
50. Pateman K, Holland TK, Knez J, et al. Should a detailed ultrasound examination of the complete urinary tract be routinely performed in women with suspected pelvic endometriosis? Hum Reprod 2015;30:2802–7.
51. Guerriero S, Ajossa S, Gerada M, et al. "Tenderness-guided" transvaginal ultrasonography: a new method for the detection of deep endometriosis in patients with chronic pelvic pain. Fertil Steril 2007;88:1293–7.

52. Hudelist G, Ballard K, English J, et al. Transvaginal sonography vs. clinical examination in the preoperative diagnosis of deep infiltrating endometriosis. Ultrasound Obstet Gynecol 2011;37:480–7.
53. Fedele L, Bianchi S, Raffaelli R, et al. Pre-operative assessment of bladder endometriosis. Hum Reprod 1997;12:2519–22.
54. Bazot M, Thomassin I, Hourani R, et al. Diagnostic accuracy of transvaginal sonography for deep pelvic endometriosis. Ultrasound Obstet Gynecol 2004;24: 180–5.
55. Savelli L, Manuzzi L, Pollastri P, et al. Diagnostic accuracy and potential limitations of transvaginal sonography for bladder endometriosis. Ultrasound Obstet Gynecol 2009;34:595–600.
56. Carfagna P, De Cicco Nardone C, De Cicco Nardone A, et al. Role of transvaginal ultrasound in evaluation of ureteral involvement in deep infiltrating endometriosis. Ultrasound Obstet Gynecol 2018;51:550–5.
57. Gambadauro P, Olovsson M, Persson P. Unusually rapid growth of bilateral endometriomas and acute bilateral hydronephrosis. Gynecol Endocrinol 2011;27: 948–50.
58. Chapron C, Chopin N, Borghese B, et al. Deeply infiltrating endometriosis: pathogenetic implications of the anatomical distribution. Hum Reprod 2006;21: 1839–45.
59. Squifflet J, Feger C, Donnez J. Diagnosis and imaging of adenomyotic disease of the retroperitoneal space. Gynecol Obstet Invest 2002;54:43–51.
60. Missmer SA, Hankinson SE, Spiegelman D, et al. Incidence of laparoscopically confirmed endometriosis by demo- graphic, anthropometric, and lifestyle factors. Am J Epidemiol 2004;160:784–96.
61. Shaaban OM, Ali MK, Sabra AM, et al. Levonorgestrel-releasing intrauterine system versus a low-dose combined oral contraceptive for treatment of adenomyotic uteri: a randomized clinical trial. Contraception 2015;92:301–7.
62. Darwish B, Stochino-Loi E, Pasquier G, et al. Surgical Outcomes of Urinary Tract Deep Infiltrating Endometriosis. J Minim Invasive Gynecol 2017;24:998–1006.
63. Ferrero S, Scala C, Stabilini C, et al. Transvaginal sonography with vs without bowel preparation in diagnosis of rectosigmoid endometriosis: prospective study. Ultrasound Obstet Gynecol 2019;53(3):402–9.
64. Davalos ML, De Cicco C, D'Hoore A, et al. Outcome after rectum or sigmoid resection: a review for gynecologists. J Minim Invasive Gynecol 2007;14:33–8.
65. Fanfani F, Fagotti A, Gagliardi ML, et al. Discoid or segmental rectosigmoid resection for deep infiltrating endometriosis: a case-control study. Fertil Steril 2010;94:444–9.
66. Froyman W, Landolfo C, De Cock B, et al. Risk of complications in patients with conservatively managed ovarian tumours (IOTA5): a 2-year interim analysis of a multicentre, prospective, cohort study. Lancet Oncol 2019;20(3):448–58.
67. Nezhat F, Apostol R, Mahmoud M, et al. Malignant transformation of endometriosis and its clinical significance. Fertil Steril 2014;102:342–4.
68. Testa AC, Timmerman D, Van Holsbeke C, et al. Ovarian cancer arising in endometrioid cysts: ultrasound findings. Ultrasound Obstet Gynecol 2011;38:99–106.
69. Nishida M, Watanabe K, Sato N, et al. Malignant transformation of ovarian endometriosis. Gynecol Obstet Invest 2000;50:18–25.
70. Gemmil JA, Stratton P, Cleary SD, et al. Cancers, infections, and endocrine diseases in women with endometriosis. Fertil Steril 2010;94:1627–31.

71. Moro F, Magoga G, Pasciuto T, et al. Imaging in gynecological disease (13): clinical and ultrasound characteristics of endometrioid ovarian cancer. Ultrasound Obstet Gynecol 2018;52:535–43.
72. Pozzati F, Moro F, Pasciuto T, et al. Imaging in gynecological disease (14): clinical and ultrasound characteristics of ovarian clear cell carcinoma. Ultrasound Obstet Gynecol 2018;52(6).792–800.
73. Miyakoshi K, Tanaka M, Gabionza D, et al. Decidualized ovarian endometriosis mimicking malignancy. Am J Roentgenol 1998;171:1625–6.
74. Mascilini F, Moruzzi C, Giansiracusa C, et al. Imaging of gynecological disease: clinical and ultrasound characteristics of decidualized endometriomas surgically removed during pregnancy. Ultrasound Obstet Gynecol 2014;44:354–60.
75. Pateman K, Moro F, Mavrelos D, et al. Natural history of ovarian endometrioma in pregnancy. BMC Womens Health 2014;14:128.
76. De Blasis I. Ultrasound appearance of decidualised deep endometriosis during pregnancy OP31.05, ISUOG World Congress. Vienna, Austria, September 16–19, 2017.

# Ultrasound Assessment of the Intrauterine Device

Adam T. Evans, MD[a], Kam Szlachetka, RDMS, RDCS, RVT[b], Loralei L. Thornburg, MD[a,*]

**KEYWORDS**

- Intrauterine device • IUD • Ultrasound • 3D • Coronal • Rendering

**KEY POINTS**

- Ultrasound imaging of intrauterine devices (IUDs) should include assessment of body, arms, and endometrial cavity in relationship to each other, both abdominally and transvaginally.
- Coronal imaging using 3-dimensional rendering or omniplane may be especially helpful for imaging IUD locations in retroverted or scarred uteruses.
- Although there are limited data, ultrasound guidance for IUD placement may be most helpful in women with malpositioned uterus, immediately postpartum, or with uterine anomalies.
- Although most modern IUDs are "T" shaped, double S, ring, and linear IUDs may also be visualized in some circumstances.

## INTRODUCTION

Intrauterine devices (IUDs) have been widely used throughout the world for more than 2 centuries in various forms. However, the materials and mechanisms of IUDs have evolved dramatically. In the early twentieth century Ernst Gräfenberg demonstrated that a silver ring placed in the uterine cavity provided highly effective contraceptive.[1] Since then IUDs have taken a wide variety of shapes and sizes, from rings, to shields, to the curving "double S" of the Lippes Loop, eventually culminating in the currently used "T"-shaped design.

## PART I: CLINICAL USES OF INTRAUTERINE DEVICES AND PREVALENCE OF USE

IUDs are widely regarded as one of the most effective means of preventing unplanned pregnancy. As a result of their efficacy, due in part to elimination of user error,

Disclosure Statement: The authors have nothing to disclose.

[a] Department of Obstetrics and Gynecology, University of Rochester Medical Center, 601 Elmwood Avenue, Box 668, Rochester, NY 14642, USA; [b] Department of Obstetrics and Gynecology, University of Rochester Medical Center, 601 Elmwood Avenue, Box 685, Rochester, NY 14642, USA
* Corresponding author.
*E-mail address:* Loralei_Thornburg@urmc.rochester.edu
twitter: @KamSzlachetka (K.S.); @drloralei (L.L.T.)

Obstet Gynecol Clin N Am 46 (2019) 661–681
https://doi.org/10.1016/j.ogc.2019.07.005

long-acting reversible contraceptive devices—including IUDs—are recommended as first-line birth control for all patients, including nulliparas and adolescents.[2,3] IUDs also serve as first-line contraceptive for women with specific medical conditions, such as migraines with aura, cardiovascular disease, breast cancer, or history of venous thromboembolism. In addition, levonorgestrel (LNG) IUDs have noncontraceptive benefits and can be used to reduce or eliminate menstrual symptoms and effectively manage gynecologic conditions such as abnormal uterine bleeding and endometrial hyperplasia without the risks of systemic medications or surgery.[4]

As a result of the number of ways IUDs can be used, the prevalence in the United States has increased from 5.6% to 11.6% between 2008 and 2014.[5] This trend underscores the need for education regarding the best practices of imaging IUDs and how these findings should influence patient care. Ultrasound is one of the most accessible, safest, and cost-effective imaging solutions for the evaluation of the female pelvis.[6] The same principles apply to imaging of IUDs with the added benefit of real-time evaluation of pelvic anatomy. In clinical practice, there remain several questions that arise surrounding use of ultrasound for placement and evaluation of IUDs including the following: when is insertion under ultrasound guidance indicated? Is universal imaging indicated after IUD placement? What defines a "malpositioned IUD" and when should they be removed? How are IUDs assessed and removed during active pregnancy?

## PART II: IMAGING THE INTRAUTERINE DEVICES

### *Radiolucency and the Basics of IUD Ultrasonography*

In the United States, women have the option for either a nonhormonal copper-based IUD or 1 or 2 IUDs containing the synthetic progestin LNG. All 3 of these devices feature a "T" shape with a straight vertical stem/shaft and extending crossbars or arms (**Fig. 1**). By ultrasound, the copper IUD is strongly echogenic with posterior acoustic shadowing of the central shaft and sidearms, attributable to the coils of copper wire in these areas[7] (**Fig. 2**). However, the density of the device stem may also create a "ring-down" artifact when imaging in the transverse plane, which appears as a series of parallel bands radiating away from the IUD.[8] In contrast, the orientation and position of LNG-IUDs is more challenging, as visualization is often limited to the superior and inferior aspects of the vertical stem in the sagittal plan and posterior shadowing at the junction of the stem and the side arms.[9] LNG-IUDs will have a typical "laminar" or 3-layered appearance due to the medication reservoir around the shaft,

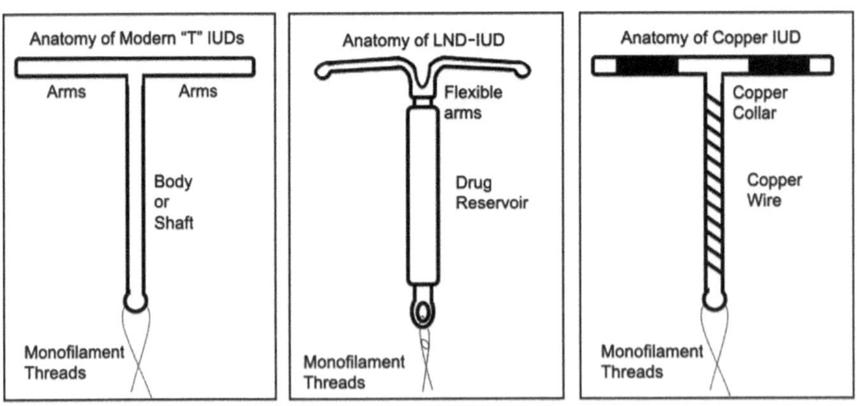


**Fig. 1.** Anatomy of modern "T"-shaped IUD, LNG-IUD, and nonhormonal copper-based IUD.

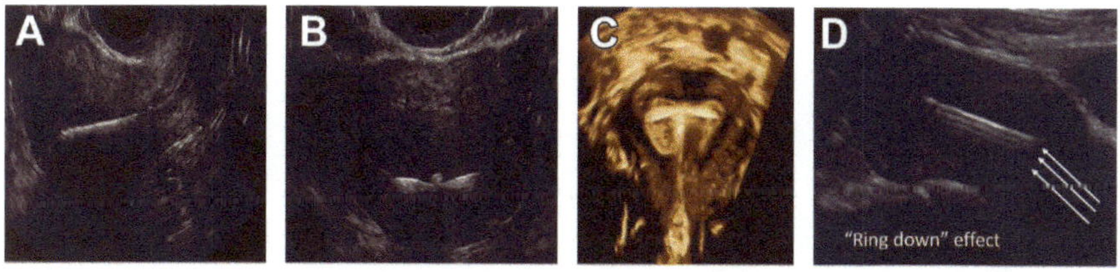


**Fig. 2.** Copper IUD seen by transvaginal imaging showing appropriate position within the endometrial cavity. Note the bright, highly echogenic appearance to the IUD from the copper. (*A*) Midsagittal position. (*B*) Transverse images of the arms appropriately within the cavity. (*C*) Coronal 3-dimentional (3D) reconstruction showing IUD completely within the cavity. (*D*) shows the "ring down" effect created by the copper bands (*arrows*).

with arms oriented slightly obliquely to the body as opposed to a true "T" shape (**Fig. 3**). Moschos quantified the difference in the imaging, demonstrating a statistically significant difference in conspicuity scores in 2-dimensional (2D) imaging between copper and LNG-IUDs in favor of the former ($P<.001$).[9]

Should a device be unable to be imaged by ultrasound, and there be a question of a "lost" IUD, radiographic imaging can be helpful, as both copper and modern LNG-IUDs are radiopaque, either from the copper or from the barium impregnated into LNG-IUDs to allow identification with radiography or intraoperative fluoroscopy (**Fig. 4**). Both copper and LNG-IUDs can also be seen on MRI and are nonferromagnetic, thereby not necessitating removal before imaging.[10]

When imaging IUDs in 2D, several key principles apply. As with all gynecologic ultrasound, transabdominal assessment with a full bladder should be performed first, followed by a transvaginal approach if more detailed imaging is needed. Although it is tempting to proceed directly with transvaginal ultrasound, depending on other uterine findings and position, important pathology or relationships between the uterus and IUD may be missed when only transvaginal imaging is used. However, transvaginal imaging is likely to provide the best imaging of IUD location, orientation, and the arm positions and therefore should be used when evaluating IUDs with concerns for placement.

When assessing an IUD in situ, the shaft/body, arms, and their relationship to each other and to the uterus must be systematically evaluated (**Box 1**). The IUD shaft must be imaged in its entirety, with care to note the relationship of the long axis to the endometrial cavity as well as whether the entire shaft is present within the endometrial cavity (**Fig. 5**). The distance from the fundal end of the endometrium to the top of the IUD

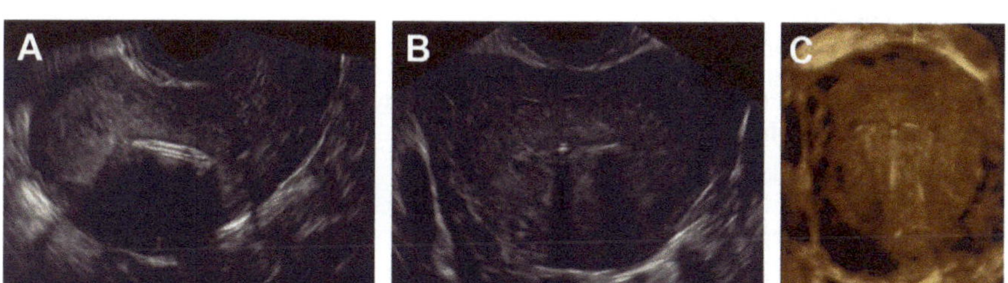


**Fig. 3.** Imaging of the body/shaft of LNG-IUD in the midsagittal position within the endometrial cavity by (*A*) midsagittal, (*B*) transverse, and (*C*) 3D coronal rendering. Note the typical "3-line" appearance of LNG-IUDs where the medication reservoir is seen to wrap the shaft.

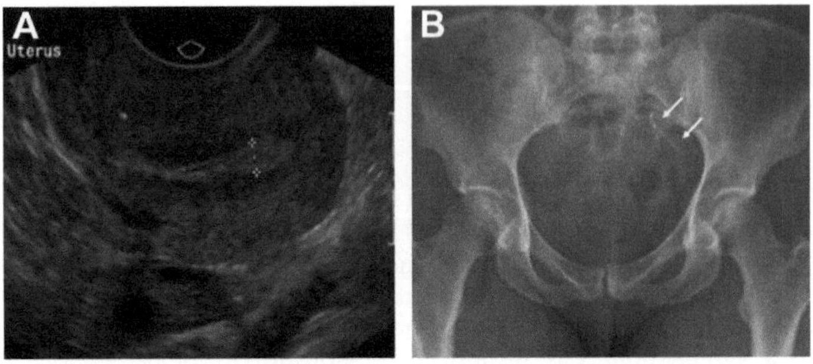


Fig. 4. "Lost" IUD evaluation by ultrasound and radiography. (*A*) The ultrasound uterine imaging shows the absence of an IUD within the cavity. (*B*) The pelvic radiograph reveals the LNG-IUD (*arrows*) in the pelvic brim on the left, which was retrieved by laparoscopy.

should be assessed (**Fig. 6**). The arms should be imaged in relationship to the body of the device, as well as to each other (extended, neutral, flexed, etc.) and to the uterine cavity. To ascertain the true uterine position of an IUD, care must be taken to image the device itself and not the acoustic shadow of the IUD (**Fig. 7**).

If the IUD or the IUD arms are thought to be out of the proper orientation, the relationship of the body and arms to the myometrium, cervix, and endometrial cavity should be thoroughly evaluated. Potential erroneous locations for an IUD include cervical canal, broad ligament/parametrium, myometrium, or abdominal. Even if the IUD appears to be in the appropriate location superiorly/inferiorly, the relationship of the entire body to the endometrial cavity should be assessed, as it can be partially or fully embedded within the myometrium (**Fig. 8**). It should be noted if the device is partially or completely located within the cervical canal (**Fig. 9**) or if there is partial abdominal placement (partially or completely through the uterine wall). If the IUD arms are not appropriately within the uterine cavity, their presence should be sought within the

**Box 1**
**Checklist for imaging position of intrauterine devices**

Images recommended:
- Midsagittal uterus and endometrium with IUD
- Long axis of IUD (if not in line w/midsagittal uterus)
- Transverse uterus with IUD body (typically in transverse)
- Transverse uterus with IUD arms
- 3D coronal reconstruction of IUD and uterus

Imaging "body" position
- Shaft length appropriate
- Orientation to long axis of uterus
- Position of ends of body in relationship to uterine cavity
- Distance from the fundus

Imaging "arm" position
- Both arms seen
- Relationship of arms to body of IUD
- Relationship of arms to uterine cavity

Other:
- Strings: are strings visible within the cervix? Uterine cavity?
- Other vaginal, uterine, tubal, and ovarian pathology evaluation

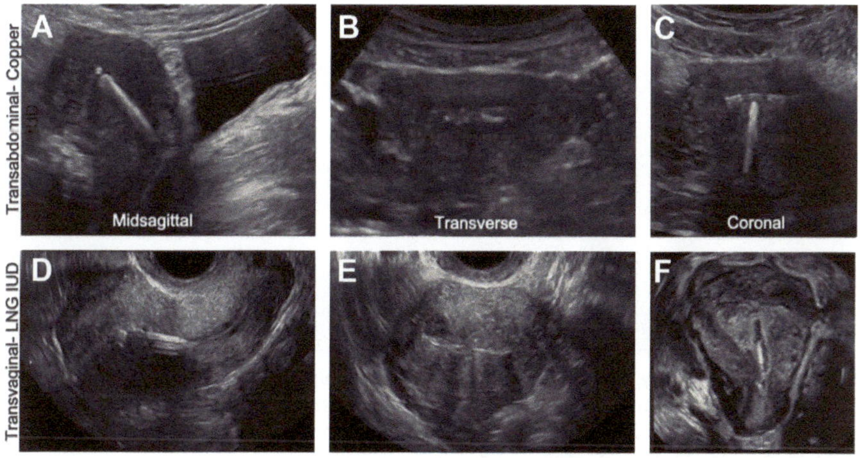


**Fig. 5.** Normally positioned IUD evaluation. (*A–C*) Transabdominal sagittal view, transverse view, and coronal view. (*D–F*) Transvaginal views. Note the relationship of body; arms to each other as well as the uterine cavity are all able to be appreciated, and the IUD is seen within to be appropriately placed completely within the uterine cavity. Also, note the difference in appearance between copper and LNG-IUDs.

uterine wall (**Fig. 10**). Their depth and location within the myometrium should be evaluated. It should be noted that IUD arms are quite thin, flexible, and may be in a variety of positions. Especially in the case of LNG-IUDs, their imaging can be quite subtle, and the operator may have to watch carefully for acoustic shadows from echogenic foci and attempt to elongate these in off-angle planes (see **Fig. 10**).

If the IUD cannot be visualized in the pelvis by ultrasound, then the first concern is typically for complete abdominal placement. A careful history should be taken to determine if device expulsion may have occurred as the cause of the device's absence. In addition, when IUDs are partially displaced or partially expelled, sideways or upside down—especially in the retroverted uterus—confirmation of the presence of the IUD within the uterus may be challenging (**Fig. 11**). In the retroverted uterus it can

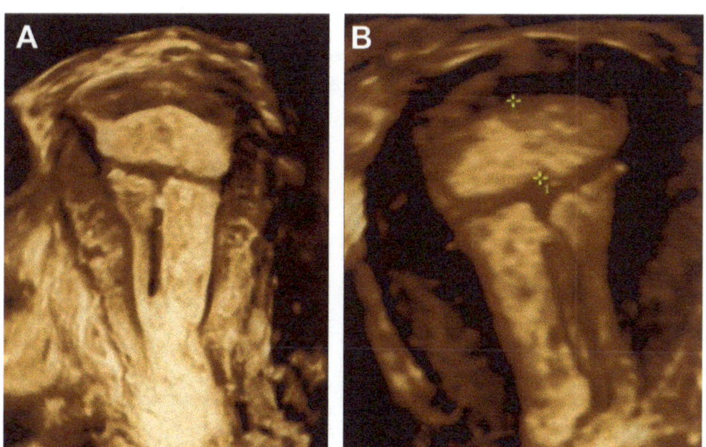


**Fig. 6.** (*A, B*) 3D coronal views of low-lying IUDs.

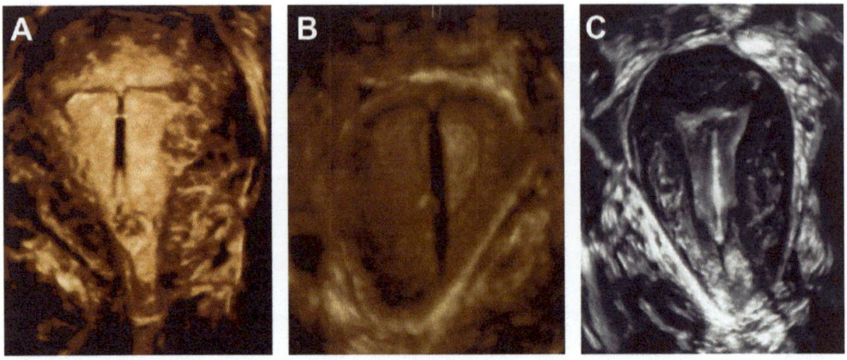


**Fig. 7.** Acoustic shadow: coronal views of LNG-IUDs. (*A, B*) The acoustic shadow, but not the IUD directly, is seen (arms, body, medication chamber, and strings are all visible). (*C*) When the IUD is brought into view, the rendering changes from black/gray (acoustic echo) to white as the barium impregnated IUD is directly visualized.

also be difficult to assess if device is within the uterus or within the posterior cul-de-sac. Coronal rendering can be very helpful in these cases to assist with device localization.

In addition to being partially or fully outside the endometrial cavity, IUDs can also be sideways (**Fig. 12**) or upside down (**Fig. 13**); in these cases the orientation may be very difficult to determine in 2D. When imaging in 2D, the inability to take a "slice" in the coronal plane limits the ability to "see" the IUD body, arms, and endometrial cavity in relationship to each other and to the endometrial cavity in a single image.

### *Three-Dimensional Ultrasonography for Imaging of Intrauterine Devices*

Given the limitations of 2D imaging, if there is a suggestion of an IUD concern, 3-dimensional (3D) imaging in the coronal plane has the ability to improve ultrasonographic imaging of the device. This requires the reconstruction of a 3D-rendered volume to create a coronal slice, which can then be used to clearly demonstrate the relationship between the uterus, endometrial cavity, and the IUD. In terms of basic 3D sonographic technique to acquire a high-quality volume, Sakhel and colleagues[11] advise incorporating the targeted pelvic anatomy at the narrowest possible angle and setting a speed that allows for maximum resolution. Furthermore, to optimize imaging in the coronal plane, Sakhel and colleagues[11] recommend "aligning the midsagittal and midtransverse planes of the uterus parallel to the horizontal plane" to automatically generate the orthogonal coronal plane.

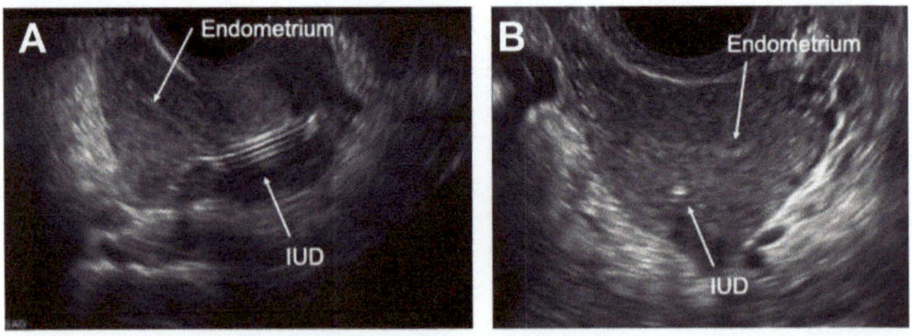


**Fig. 8.** LNG-IUD imbedded within the uterine wall. (*A*) Midsagittal view with IUD within the myometrium. (*B*) Transverse view of IUD body within the myometrium. *Arrows* on figures indicate the locations of both the IUD and the endometrium.

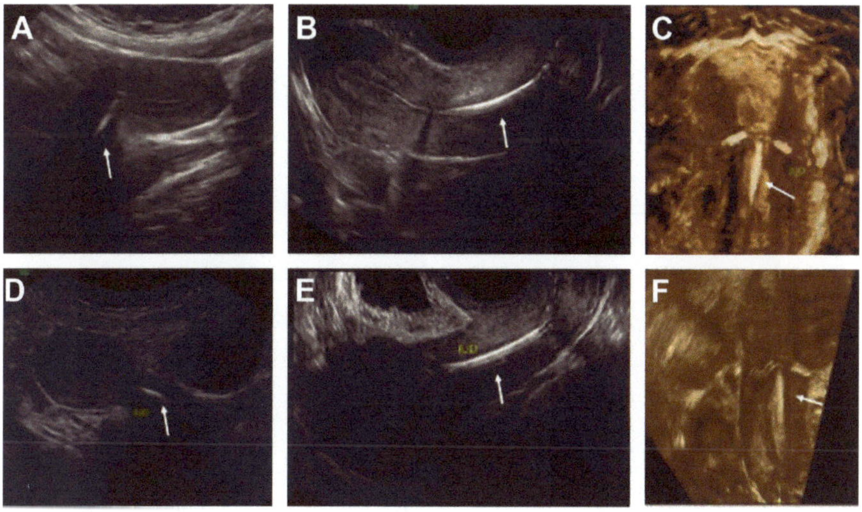


**Fig. 9.** Imaging of low-lying IUD partially within the cervix. (*A, D*) Transabdominal imaging with IUD partially within the endocervical canal. (*B, E*) Transvaginal imaging with IUD completely within the endocervical canal. (*C, F*) Coronal imaging with IUD body within the canal. (*C*) Both arms are into the lateral myometrium of the lower uterine segment; however, (*F*) the left is within the myometrium, and the right is within the canal. *Arrows* on figures indicate the locations of both the IUD and the endometrium.

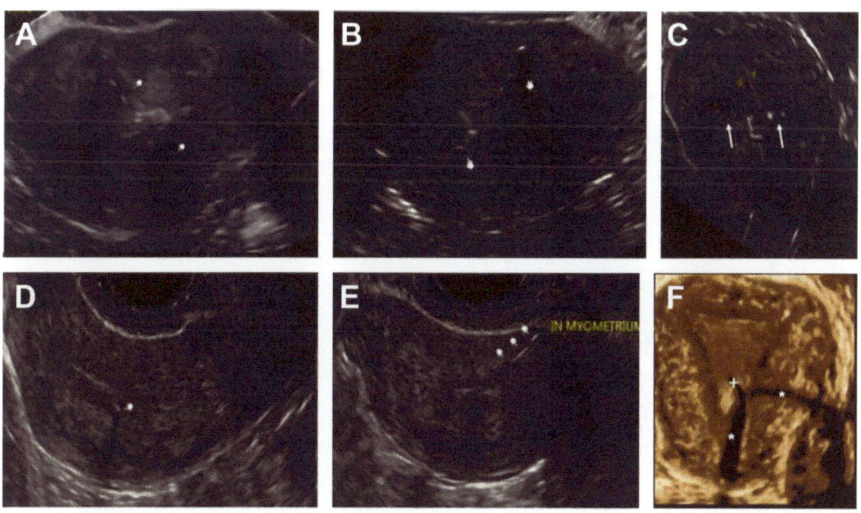


**Fig. 10.** Imaging of IUD arms. Two cases of IUD arms perforated into the myometrium. Case 1 (A, B, C)- (*A, B*) The IUD arms can be seen as linear echogenic structures in the myometrium (hands). (*C*) 3D rendering to create sagittal plane due to uterine malposition shows them outside the cavity into the anterior and posterior myometrium (*arrows*). Case 2 (D, E, F)- (*D*) The IUD arm is seen within the myometrium in oblique/transverse, creating a shadow. (*E*) The other arm is seen within the myometrium as linear density. (*F*) Coronal imaging shows the arms imbedded within the myometrium (*asterisks*). Because these are acoustic shadows, they appear elongated. Only a portion of the IUD body is seen (+), as it is partially out of plane.

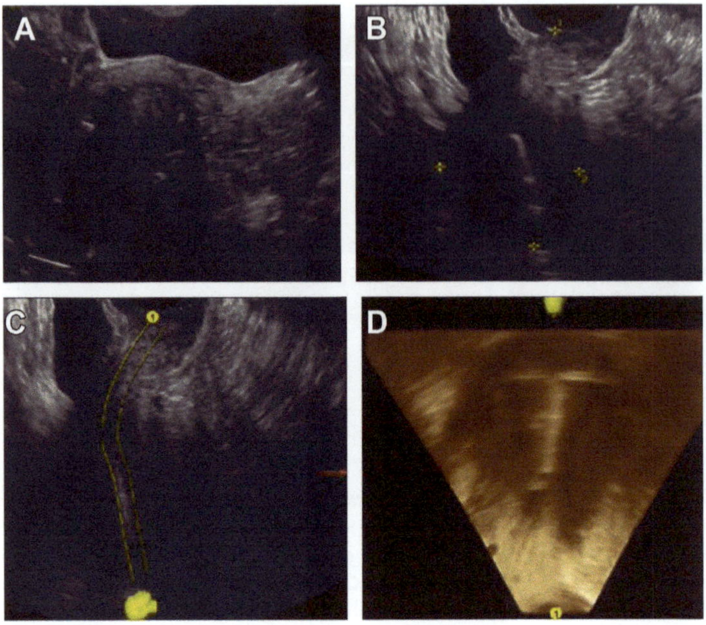

Fig. 11. IUD imaging with severely retroverted uterine positioning. On both (*A*) transabdominal and (*B*) transvaginal imaging, evaluation of the IUD position is limited. By use of omniplane (*C*) to create a coronal rendering (*D*), the IUD and uterine cavity can be recreated and position of IUD body and arms is clearly seen to be appropriately placed within the uterine cavity (*D*).

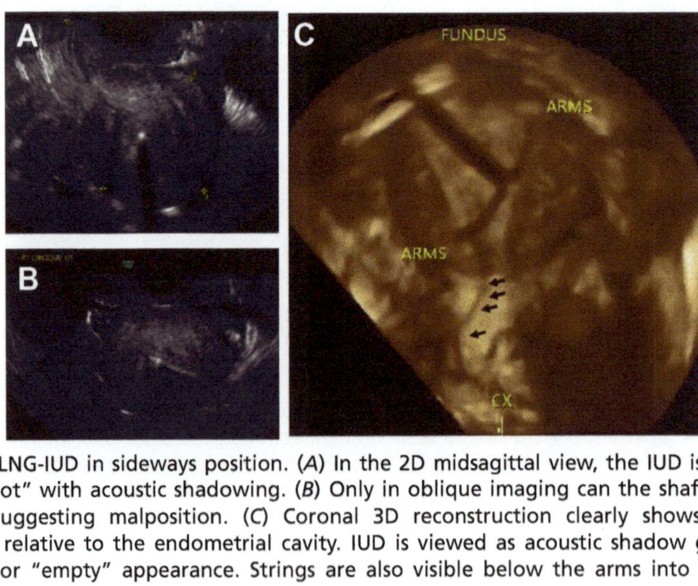


Fig. 12. LNG-IUD in sideways position. (*A*) In the 2D midsagittal view, the IUD is an echogenic "dot" with acoustic shadowing. (*B*) Only in oblique imaging can the shaft be elongated, suggesting malposition. (*C*) Coronal 3D reconstruction clearly shows the IUD position relative to the endometrial cavity. IUD is viewed as acoustic shadow giving the "black" or "empty" appearance. Strings are also visible below the arms into the cervix (*arrows*).

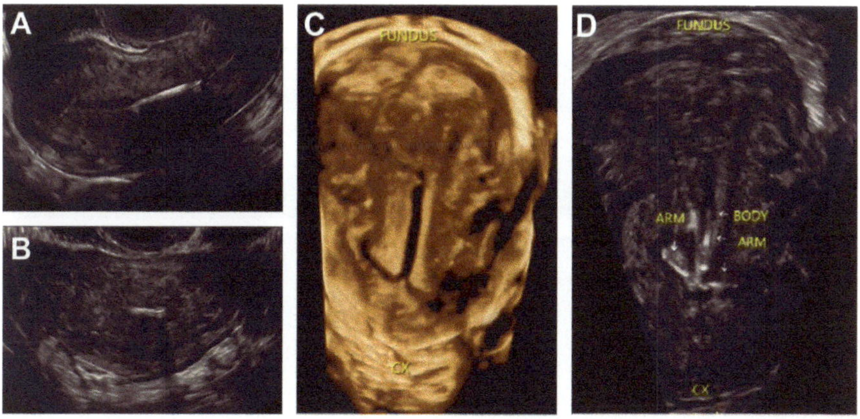


**Fig. 13.** LNG-IUD in inverted position. (*A*) In the 2D imaging, the IUD has the typical trilaminar appearance, but appears within the lower uterine segment. (*B*) The arms are seen within the cervix on transverse imaging. (*C, D*) However, on 3D coronal imaging, the position of the IUD becomes clear with the body inverted above the arms. The IUD appears as "black" or "empty space" in the reconstruction, as this is the acoustic shadow, not the IUD itself. (*D*) A second coronal reconstruction clearly shows the IUD (*white*) in position relative to the endometrial cavity.

As noted earlier, a commonly cited shortcoming of 2D sonography is the difficulty of properly visualizing the side arms of the device and their orientation with respective to uterine anatomy.[11] When an IUD is suspected to be malpositioned or imbedded, the diagnostic accuracy of 3D ultrasonography has been shown to be significantly higher than that of 2D ultrasound.[12] Three-dimensional ultrasound has also been shown to be especially helpful for IUDs with suspected malrotation (see **Figs. 12** and **13**; **Fig. 14**). However, some investigators have reported that it can be technically difficult in women with uterine scarring, retroverted uterus, or increased endometrial echogenicity/heterogeneity. In these cases, when a coronal reconstruction of the IUD itself cannot be acquired, a coronal slice of the IUD's acoustic shadow can provide evidence of intrauterine placement but cannot definitively show the true position[13] (see **Figs. 7** and **11**).

## *Evaluation of the Strings*

In some cases, but not always, the IUD strings may be visible on ultrasound. In most cases these will be subtle echogenic lines within the cervix (see **Fig. 14**). In some cases, the strings may be seen within the uterine cavity or coiled around the IUD (see **Fig. 14**). As long as they are not bothersome to the patient, and there is no bleeding or pain, their position is of no consequence unless removal is desired and they cannot be reached vaginally.

## *Evaluation of Intrauterine Device in Uterine Anomalies*

Although uterine anomalies and cavity distortions are relatively contraindications to IUD placement, they can be placed in these cases. For women with arcuate uteruses there is anecdotal discussion that expulsion rates may be higher, but the data are very limited and no prospective data exist.[14] When the IUD is imaged in these cases, the top of the IUD should be seen to abut the bottom of the septum (**Fig. 15**). For women with IUD placement in a true didelphys uterus, an IUD must be placed within each

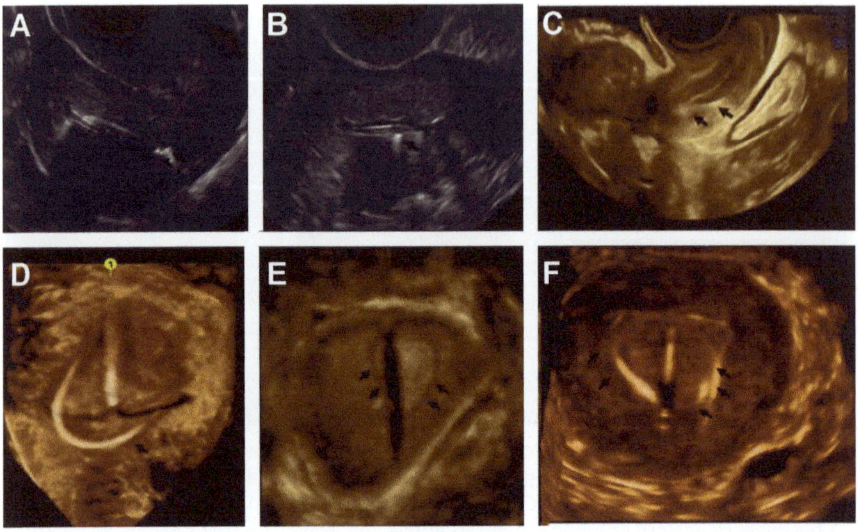


**Fig. 14.** IUD string visualization. IUD strings can be seen as subtle lines or multiple echogenic foci within the uterus or cervix in (*A*) midsagittal or (*B*) transverse imaging or (*C*) with the cervix (*arrows*). (*D–F*) On 3D coronal reconstruction, the strings can be seen wrapping around the IUD within the endometrial cavity. (*E*) The IUD in this image is also inverted. (D-body, *F*) Note the difference in appearance when visualized directly versus (D-arms, *E*) as the acoustic shadow.

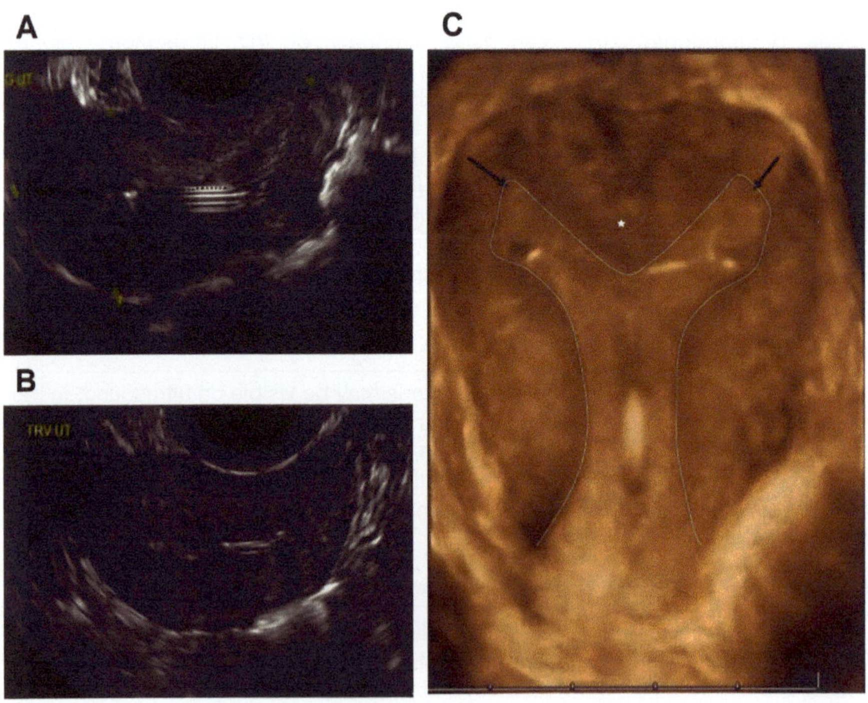


**Fig. 15.** IUD in an arcuate uterine cavity (outlined). (*A, B*) On 2D imaging, the IUD appears overall appropriately positioned. (*C*) On coronal evaluation, the IUD is seen to be positioned at the bottom of the septum (*asterisk*) with the right and left cornua extending above (*arrows*).

uterine cavity. Ultrasound guidance for placement may be helpful as the cavities may be very laterally positioned or the direction of cervical canals unclear. When assessing placement in these women, each IUD must be visualized and evaluated relative to its own cavity (**Fig. 16**).

### *Removal of Malpositioned Intrauterine Devices: When Is Ultrasound Guidance Helpful?*

In most case, the strings of an IUD will remain within the cervix and vagina even if the body or arms are partially within the walls or malpositioned, allowing for removal in the office as long as they remain visible on speculum examination. In these cases where the strings have migrated, removal with Kelly forceps or similar instrument under ultrasound guidance is generally possible.

If an IUD is deeply implanted in the myometrium or partially abdominal, the strings may longer be visible, and hysteroscopy may be necessary. If the strings have migrated, but most of the IUD remains with the uterus, it may be possible to remove the IUD vaginally if the body remains low enough to be grasped with alligator forceps, but ultrasound guidance is generally helpful. If this is unsuccessful, further evaluation with operative hysteroscopy may be needed to remove the device. If desired, another device can typically be placed after the removal.

Anytime an IUD is removed, especially when imbedded or malpositioned, the operator should inspect it to assure the entire device is removed. There are reported cases

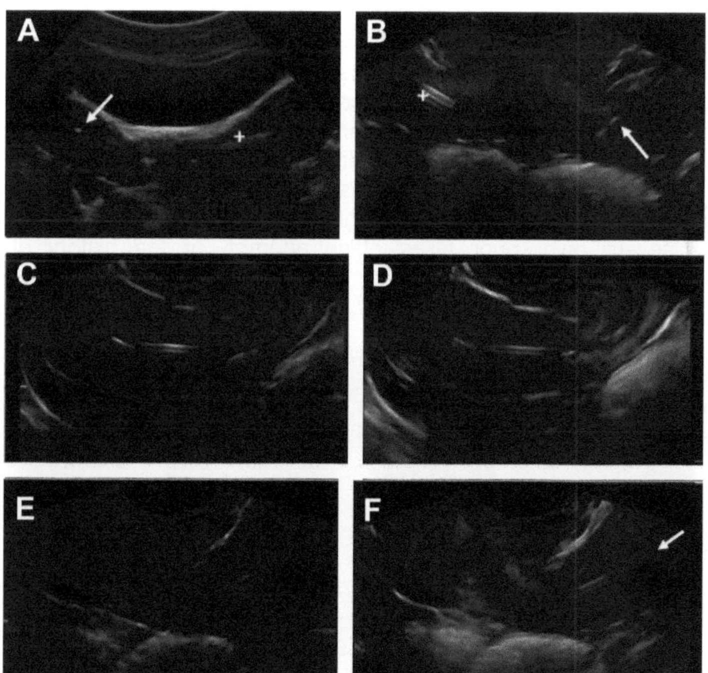


**Fig. 16.** IUD in a uterine didelphys. (*A, B*) The transverse views show 2 IUDs with one in transverse (*arrow*) when the other is in long view (+). When ultrasound is angled and each cavity viewed separately, both the (*C, D*) right and (*E, F*) left IUDs are seen to be appropriately placed with the uterine cavities. Of note, because of the extreme angle of the left horn, the superior tip of the IUD in this cavity is poorly visualized (*arrow*).

of IUD breakage and retained portions, especially with long-term retained IUDs.[15,16] In the event an IUD is removed and the entire body and arms are not identified, ultrasound may be helpful to determine the location of remaining portions, which may be able to be removed under ultrasound guidance or may require hysteroscopic removal (**Fig. 17**).

## PART III: ULTRASOUND GUIDANCE OF INTRAUTERINE DEVICE PLACEMENT

Most of the IUDs are inserted in the outpatient setting. Given barriers related to cost and access to ultrasound, it is not feasible or cost-effective for providers to place all IUDs under ultrasound guidance, and the data do not support this for uncomplicated placement. However, anecdotally it seems that there may be specific patient populations or conditions where ultrasound guidance may be helpful and/or improve safety. An exhaustive literature search yielded a relative dearth of studies exploring this question. Instead, the sources located emphasize the importance of a provider's clinical judgment regarding ultrasound as a tool to assist with technically challenging cases rather than advocating for universal use in specific circumstances.[17,18] Furthermore, multiple studies note the need for more research regarding ultrasound-guided placement in women with risk factors for IUD malposition.[19,20]

Ultrasound guidance is most commonly discussed in women with uterine structural abnormalities. Gerkowitz and colleagues[19] noted a significantly increased incidence of uterine retroflexion, and submucosal fibroids in women with malpositioned IUDs, and argued direct ultrasound visualization of IUD placement and subsequent confirmation of fundal placement may be helpful in these populations. Interestingly, this relationship, was not observed in women with retroverted uteruses or congenital uterine anomalies (CUA) such as septate or bicornuate uteruses, with the latter likely attributed to a small sample size.[19] Although the presence of a CUA was not found to be statistically significant, clinicians may find that the technical challenge posed by device placement in these women warrants ultrasound guidance. Other situations in which investigators suggest ultrasound guidance include challenging placement, nulliparity, severe pain, prior failed office attempt, or the history of an IUD expulsion.[3,17,18,21]

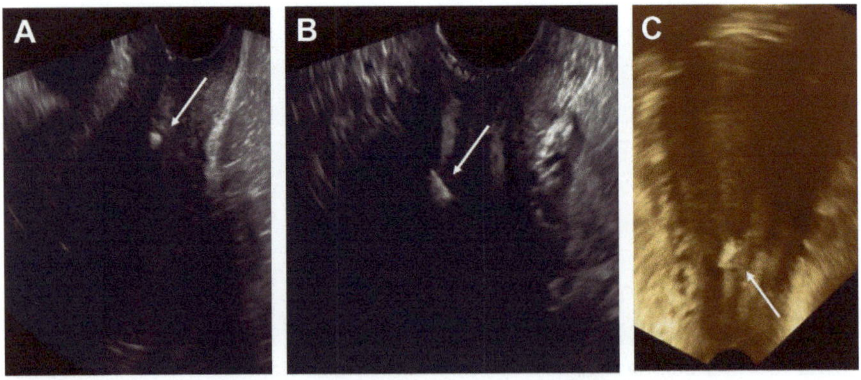


**Fig. 17.** Partial retention of IUD. After removal, an arm of the IUD was noted to be missing. Ultrasound imaging revealed the echogenic arm (*arrows*) within the lower uterine segment on both (*A*) sagittal and (*B*) transverse images. (*C*) The coronal image shows the arm (*arrow*) within the uterocervical junction and was removed under ultrasound guidance.

## OPTIMAL TECHNIQUE FOR ULTRASOUND GUIDANCE FOR INTRAUTERINE DEVICE PLACEMENT OR REMOVAL

Although there are no specific data on how to provide guidance, as with other procedures, a preprocedure "huddle" between the clinician placing the device and the scanning clinician or technician to discuss planned approach may be helpful. The patient should be imaged transabdominally, and just as when completing chorionic villous sampling (CVS), a partially (but not completely) full bladder may allow for both optimal imaging and straighten the cervical/uterine junction to improve access to the endometrial cavity.[22]

## PART IV: DETERMINING PROPER INTRAUTERINE PLACEMENT: HOW LOW IS TOO LOW?

An optimally placed IUD is located at the uterine fundus with both arms of the device extended outward toward the uterine cornua, a vertically oriented stem in the uterine body, and the IUD retrieval strings protruding approximately 2 to 3 cm from the external cervical os. Historically, "properly placed" IUDs were defined as within 3 mm of the uterine fundus, with investigators arguing that women with IUDs positioned lower than this were at increased risk for malposition, expulsion, pain, and bleeding.[18,19] However, absolute definitions of correct position have come into question as further research has examined the migration patterns of IUDs postplacement. Before addressing these arguments, it is necessary to discuss some clear differences between copper and LNG-IUDs in relation to their risk for expulsion and how malposition may affect contraceptive efficacy.

Approximately 73% of all malpositioned IUDs are located in the lower uterine segment or the cervix.[19,20,23] Copper IUDs with the vertical stem located in the cervix have been shown to have decreased contraceptive function relative to those with a fundal placement (OR = 13.93), thereby increasing the potential risk for unintended pregnancy.[24] As a result, some investigators argue in favor of immediate postinsertion ultrasound to assess positioning of a copper IUD with the recommendation of removal and replacement with a new device if malposition is noted.[20,24] The contraceptive effect of LNG-IUDs does not seem to be related to uterine or cervical positioning. A randomized controlled trial comparing pregnancy rates in women who were assigned to treatment with either LNG intracervical device or LNG-IUD did not detect a significant difference between the 2 groups.[25] Moreover, the incidence of copper IUD malposition seems to be higher than that of the LNG-IUD, which is potentially clinically significant, given the abovementioned findings.[19,26]

Although universal imaging after IUD placement may be motivated by a desire to reduce the risk of device expulsion or associated complications, routine imaging may actually cause harm to women. An early study advocated for actual replacement of a clinical office "string check" with transvaginal ultrasound within 3 months of placement, given the detection of cervically located copper IUDs, is often not evident on pelvic examination.[27] However, since then a series of studies have challenged the notion that IUDs must have a perfect fundal placement immediately after insertion. It has been demonstrated that an IUD's position in the uterine cavity is fluid, with most devices settling into a stable position by approximately 3 months after placement.[28,29] As a result, IUDs that are "malpositioned" may actually migrate into an appropriate fundal location over time.[29] A case-control study examining risk factors for IUD malpositioning found that although 66.5% of women with malpositioned IUDs had their device removed, only 30.6% received another highly effective form of contraception.[20] They subsequently concluded that women with malpositioned IUDs detected on ultrasound had a higher risk of pregnancy in the 2 years following the scan.[20] As a result, the decision regarding removal of a device if nonfundal position is noted should be a collaborative one between provider and patient.[23] Furthermore, in women without complicated IUD placement or clinical signs/symptoms of malposition (such as pain or bleeding) routine ultrasound surveillance of position 6 weeks post-placement lacked clear benefit over a pelvic examination and device string check in detecting poorly positioned devices.[30]

### *Ultrasound Guidance for Postdelivery or Postabortal Intrauterine Device Placement*

In order to reduce barriers to highly effective forms of birth control, and assist women in healthy spacing of pregnancies, IUDs can be safely placed in women immediately following placenta in both vaginal and cesarean deliveries and dilation and evacuations. It is widely accepted that postplacental IUDs should be placed within 10 minutes of completion of the third stage, as insertion beyond this is associated with higher rates of expulsion.[31–33] Thus far, the literature has not adequately explored the benefits of ultrasound-guided IUD placement or confirmed whether postplacental fundal placement reduces rates of IUD expulsion.[34] This is a particularly important area for further research, because previous studies have demonstrated a higher risk of IUD expulsion with immediate postplacental insertion relative to interval placement at 6 weeks postpartum. A randomized controlled trial by Chen and colleagues[35] noted LNG-IUD expulsion in 24% in the postplacental group relative to 4.4% of those in the delayed (6–8 weeks postpartum) placement group ($P = .008$). This statistic must be framed in a broader argument related to contraceptive access, because socioeconomic barriers to postpartum follow-up may make interval placement challenging for many patient populations. Therefore, the increased risk of expulsion should be balanced with the risk of unplanned pregnancy and this discussion should be broached as part of comprehensive antenatal contraception counseling. Overall, given the dearth of data, the Society of Family Planning states there is not enough evidence to support the routine use of ultrasound in the placement or assessment of postplacental IUDs.[34]

## PART V: INTRAUTERINE DEVICES AND PREGNANCY

Intrauterine devices are one of the most effective methods of preventing unplanned pregnancy, with an estimated contraceptive failure rate of 0.8% and 0.2% among women with typical use of copper and LNG-IUDs, respectively, within 1 year of placement.[36]

However, should pregnancy occur with an IUD in place, additional evaluation is needed (**Box 2**). First, it is important to determine whether the pregnancy is desired. In women who wish to continue with pregnancy, prompt evaluation with ultrasound is necessary to determine accurate dating, confirm an intrauterine pregnancy (IUP), and to evaluate the presence and placement of the IUD (as unreported expulsion is possible). The assessment of pregnancy location is of extreme importance in women with IUDs, because they are more likely to have an ectopic than an IUP.[23,37] As a result, if a definitive IUP is not seen, a thorough examination of the adnexa should be performed and correlated with a patient's clinical presentation and β-hCG level to determine treatment or surveillance recommendations (**Fig. 18**). Evaluation of pregnancies of unknown location is covered in detail in Drs Emily Scibetta and Christina S. Han's article, "Ultrasound in Early Pregnancy: Viability, Unknown Locations, and Ectopic Pregnancies," in this issue.

**Box 2**
**Assessment of early pregnancy in the setting of intrauterine device**

- Assess by ultrasound for intrauterine pregnancy (IUP) versus ectopic
  - If ectopic: treat as appropriate. IUD can remain in place
  - If IUD cannot be located: consider abdominal radiographic assessment after pregnancy resolution
  - For IUP with IUD in cavity: discussion of patient's desire for ongoing pregnancy
- For IUP with concurrent IUD:
  - Assess IUD location relative to the gestational sac
  - Assess for the presence of strings on pelvic examination
  - Discuss removal for IUDs low in the uterus or below the sac
  - For low IUD without visible strings, consider removal using grasper using ultrasound guidance
- Other uterine and ovarian pathology evaluation

As part of comprehensive pregnancy options, counseling, a nonbiased, nonjudgmental, and evidence-based approach, should be undertaken. Women who desire to terminate the pregnancy should be referred to an appropriate provider. In these patients, the IUD can typically be removed at the time of the abortion. Patients who are unsure of their decision or who desire to continue the pregnancy should be counseled regarding a slightly increased risk of adverse fetal outcomes whether or not the IUD is removed.[38,39] When comparing patients who conceive with an IUD in place, women who remove the device in the first trimester have a lower incidence of spontaneous abortion and are more likely to deliver at term than those who leave the device in situ.[40] A study by Ganer and colleagues[39] explored this finding in greater detail, including a group of pregnant non-IUD users as a control group. The study noted a statistically significant linear-by-linear increase in rates of adverse pregnancy outcomes—such as preterm delivery, premature rupture of membranes, and chorioamnionitis—among women who never had an IUD in place, women who had their IUD removed early in pregnancy, and those who kept an IUD in place throughout pregnancy. As a result, it seems that although removal of an IUD reduces the rate of some poor maternal/fetal outcomes, it does not revert to the level of women who conceive without an IUD.[39]

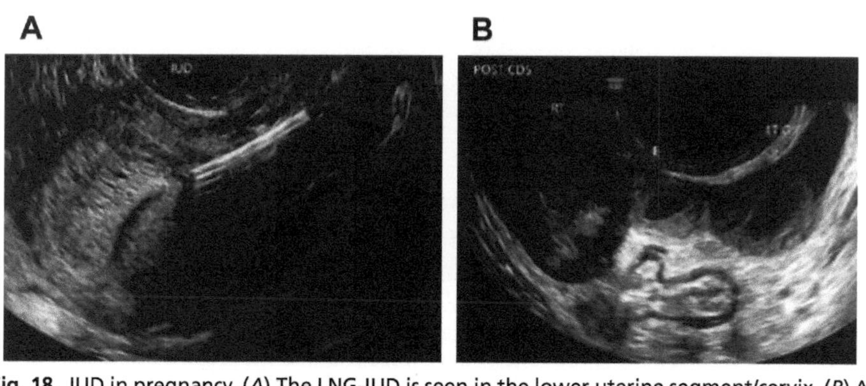


**Fig. 18.** IUD in pregnancy. (*A*) The LNG-IUD is seen in the lower uterine segment/cervix. (*B*) A concurrent left corpus luteum and ectopic pregnancy are seen in the cul-de-sac with a small amount of associated free fluid.

In desired pregnancies, during the ultrasound evaluation the position of the IUD in relationship to the gestational sac should be noted (**Fig. 19**). In pregnancies of an advanced gestational age it may be difficult to accurately assess or identify the IUD. When counseling patients, the risks of a retained IUD in pregnancy as well as the risk of possible miscarriage or vaginal bleeding with IUD removal should be reviewed. If the IUD is easily accessible and the decision is made to remove the IUD, a physical examination should be performed to assess whether the strings are visible at the cervical os (if this has not already been done). In most cases, the strings of an IUD will remain within the cervix and vagina even if the body or arms are partially imbedded in the uterine wall or malpositioned. If strings are visible, gentle traction should be applied and the device removed[23,41] (**Fig. 20**). If the strings are absent, most studies and case reports recommend an attempt be made at removal of the IUD under direct ultrasound guidance with an instrument such as alligator forceps.[18] A study by Schiesser and colleagues[42] examined the risk of miscarriage associated with ultrasound-guided removal of an IUD in pregnant patients. In terms of technique, the study used the use of transabdominal ultrasound to monitor advancement of the instrument, with the clinician attempting to grab the stem of the IUD at its most inferior point possible. The vast majority (93%) of these procedures occurred during the first trimester with a total miscarriage rate of 22.1%, with 83.2% of these within 17 days.[42]

## IMAGING LESS TYPICAL FORMS OF INTRAUTERINE DEVICES

Most women in the United States will have the traditional "T" IUD; however, the practitioner should have some familiarity with at least a few other types of IUDs that may be encountered in patients in whom the device was placed several years

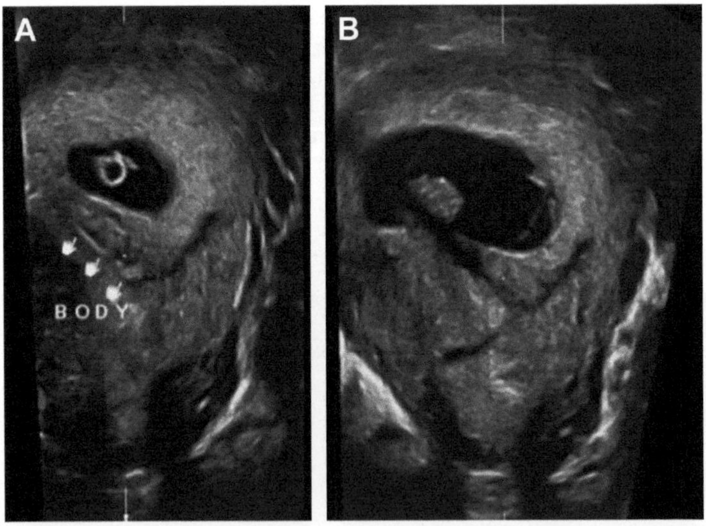


**Fig. 19.** IUD in pregnancy. (*A, B*) In both cases, the LNG-IUD is seen in the lower uterine segment, partial inverted/oblique low with arms in the lower uterine segment. A concurrent pregnancy is seen above the IUD: one with yolk sac and one with fetal pole visible. (*B*) The body of the IUD appears to partially intrude/press into the gestational sac. In both cases, the IUD was able to be removed with ultrasound guidance and the pregnancies were successfully carried to term.

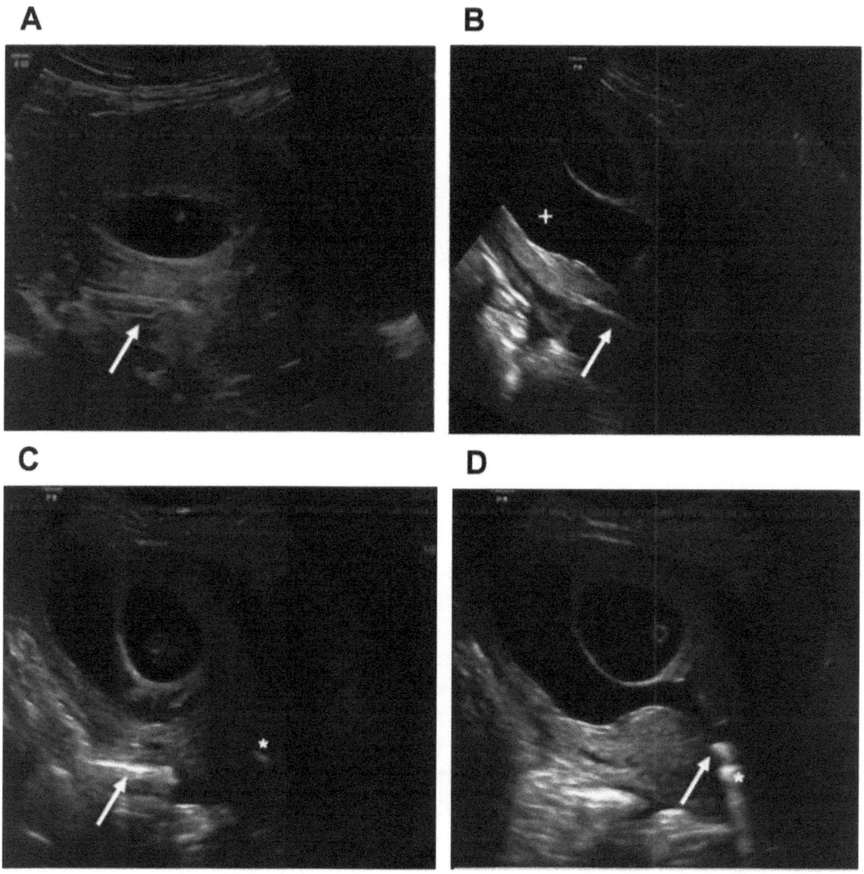


**Fig. 20.** Removal of IUD (*arrow*) under ultrasound guidance during early pregnancy. (*A*) An IUD is seen just below the gestational sac. (*B*) On return for removal, a large posterior subchorionic hemorrhage is seen (+). Under ultrasound guidance with a partially full bladder to allow visualization, alligator forceps (*asterisk*) are used to (*C*) grasp the more inferior portion of the IUD and (*D*) remove it.

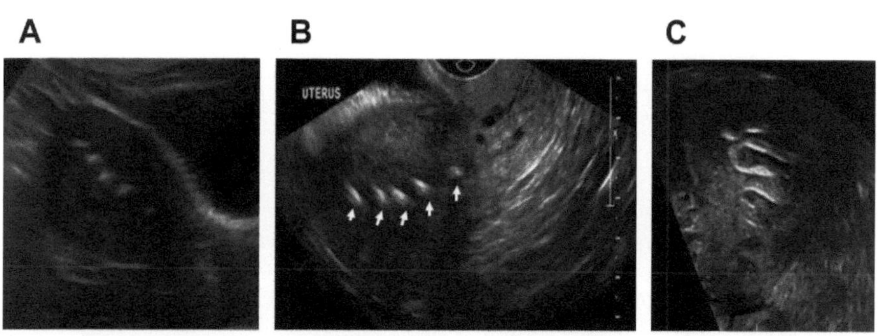


**Fig. 21.** Ultrasound images of Lippes Loop IUD in sagittal and coronal imaging. (*A, B*) On 2D sagittal imaging, this IUD appears as an evenly spaced line of echogenic points (*arrows*). (*C*) On coronal imaging, the "snake" or "double S" coil shape is apparent.

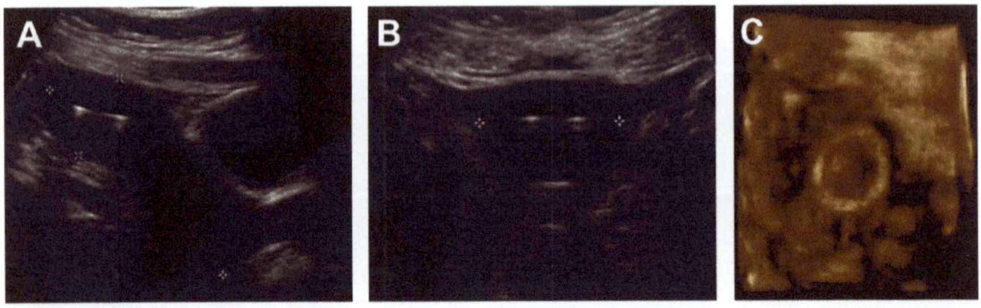


**Fig. 22.** Ultrasound images of ring IUD in (*A*) sagittal, (*B*) transverse, and (*C*) coronal imaging.

ago or in another country. One type of older medical IUDs that is seen is the Lippes Loop, which appears as a "double S" on ultrasound (**Fig. 21**). The same principle of imaging discussed earlier applies with the key difference that there are no separate arms to image. Rings are commonly used in other parts of the world, some with strings (for removal and return to fertility) and others without strings as a form of permanent contraception (**Fig. 22**). The ring should be within the endometrial cavity but can move freely. As a result, the distance between the device, the fundus, and the cervix is unimportant. Given the ring design, there are no separate arms to image.

There are reports of patients using "homemade" IUDs, which may or may not be able to be visualized well on ultrasound depending on the radiolucency of the material used. Rocks as well as a variety of other items have been described. At their unit the authors imaged an IUD made of fishing line on a postmenopausal patient that had been placed several years earlier in Puerto Rico. This unusual type of IUD appeared as multiple focal punctuations within the endometrium due to coiling and was removed hysteroscopically (**Fig. 23**).

In conclusion, the ultrasound imaging of IUDs requires the systematic assessment of the parts of the IUD relative to each other as well as each of their locations relative to the uterine cavity and walls. Both 2D imaging as well as and 3D coronal rendering are valuable in the assessment. There are limited data on routine ultrasound for IUD assessment for the asymptomatic patient or for uncomplicated placement, but for those with concurrent pregnancy or pain, loss of IUD strings, and with more complicated concerns, ultrasound assessment is the imaging modality of choice.

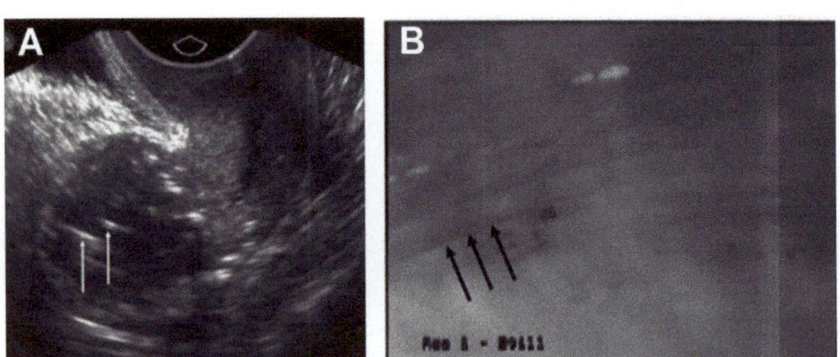


**Fig. 23.** (*A, B*) Ultrasound image of nylon string "IUD" shown on midsagittal ultrasound images as multiple focal punctuations as well as hysteroscopic image of string in situ (*arrows*).

## REFERENCES


1. Lippes J. The making of the first loop. Am J Obstet Gynecol 2018;219(2):203–6.
2. Committee on A. Contraception for adolescents. Pediatrics 2014;134(4): e1244–56.
3. Teal SB, Romer SE, Goldthwaite LM, et al. Insertion characteristics of intrauterine devices in adolescents and young women: success, ancillary measures, and complications. Am J Obstet Gynecol 2015;213(4):515.e1-5.
4. Orbo A, Arnes M, Hancke C, et al. Treatment results of endometrial hyperplasia after prospective D-score classification: a follow-up study comparing effect of LNG-IUD and oral progestins versus observation only. Gynecol Oncol 2008; 111(1):68–73.
5. Kavanaugh ML, Jerman J. Contraceptive method use in the United States: trends and characteristics between 2008, 2012 and 2014. Contraception 2018;97(1): 14–21.
6. Benacerraf BR, Abuhamad AZ, Bromley B, et al. Consider ultrasound first for imaging the female pelvis. Am J Obstet Gynecol 2015;212(4):450–5.
7. Bennett G. Evaluation of pelvic pain in the reproductive age patient. In: Norton M, Scoutt L, Feldstein V, editors. Callen's ultrasonography in obstetrics and gynecology. 6 edition. Philadelphia: Elsevier; 2017. p. 906.
8. Peri N, Graham D, Levine D. Imaging of intrauterine contraceptive devices. J Ultrasound Med 2007;26(10):1389–401.
9. Moschos E, Twickler DM. Does the type of intrauterine device affect conspicuity on 2D and 3D ultrasound? AJR Am J Roentgenol 2011;196(6):1439–43.
10. Cooper Surgical Inc.. Prescribing Information ParaGard® T 380A intrauterine copper contraceptive secondary Prescribing Information ParaGard® T 380A intrauterine copper contraceptive. 2018. Available at: https://www.paragard.com/pdf/PARAGARD-PI.pdf.
11. Sakhel K, Benson CB, Platt LD, et al. Begin with the basics: role of 3-dimensional sonography as a first-line imaging technique in the cost-effective evaluation of gynecologic pelvic disease. J Ultrasound Med 2013;32(3):381–8.
12. Chen XY, Guo QY, Wang W, et al. Three-dimensional ultrasonography versus two-dimensional ultrasonography for the diagnosis of intrauterine device malposition. Int J Gynaecol Obstet 2015;128(2):157–9.
13. Valsky DV, Cohen SM, Hochner-Celnikier D, et al. The shadow of the intrauterine device. J Ultrasound Med 2006;25(5):613–6.
14. Tepper NK, Zapata LB, Jamieson DJ, et al. Use of intrauterine devices in women with uterine anatomic abnormalities. Int J Gynaecol Obstet 2010;109(1):52–4.
15. Sinha M, Rani R, Gupta R, et al. Lippes loop inserted 45 years back: the dilemma to remove it or leave it in situ. A case report with review of literature. J Clin Diagn Res 2015;9(4):QE01–5.
16. Mohanty K. Breakage of arm of Multiload intrauterine device during removal. Int J STD AIDS 2009;20(7):512–4.
17. American College of Obstetricians and Gynecologists. Coding for the Contraceptive Implant and IUDs. Secondary Coding for the contraceptive implant and IUDs. 2018. Available at: https://www.acog.org/-/media/Departments/LARC/Coding-Guide-2018FINAL.ashx.
18. Boortz HE, Margolis DJ, Ragavendra N, et al. Migration of intrauterine devices: radiologic findings and implications for patient care. Radiographics 2012;32(2): 335–52.

19. Gerkowicz SA, Fiorentino DG, Kovacs AP, et al. Uterine structural abnormality and intrauterine device malposition: analysis of ultrasonographic and demographic variables of 517 patients. Am J Obstet Gynecol 2019;220(2):183.e1-8.
20. Braaten KP, Benson CB, Maurer R, et al. Malpositioned intrauterine contraceptive devices: risk factors, outcomes, and future pregnancies. Obstet Gynecol 2011; 118(5):1014–20.
21. Balica AC, Kim CS, Egan S, et al. Sonographically guided insertion of intrauterine device: Indications and results. J Clin Ultrasound 2018;46(2):132–5.
22. Thornburg L. Training for ultrasound procedures. Ultrasound Clin 2012;8(1): 89–103.
23. American College of Obstetricians and Gynecologists' Committee on Gynecologic Practice, Long-Acting Reversible Contraceptive Expert Work Group. Committee opinion no 672: clinical challenges of long-acting reversible contraceptive methods. Obstet Gynecol 2016;128(3):e69–77.
24. Anteby E, Revel A, Ben-Chetrit A, et al. Intrauterine device failure: relation to its location within the uterine cavity. Obstet Gynecol 1993;81(1):112–4.
25. Pakarinen P, Luukkainen T. Five years' experience with a small intracervical/intrauterine levonorgestrel-releasing device. Contraception 2005;72(5):342–5.
26. Merki-Feld GS, Schwarz D, Imthurn B, et al. Partial and complete expulsion of the Multiload 375 IUD and the levonorgestrel-releasing IUD after correct insertion. Eur J Obstet Gynecol Reprod Biol 2008;137(1):92–6.
27. Granberg S, Bundsen P, Bourne TH, et al. The use of transvaginal ultrasonography compared to routine gynecological examination to check the location of an intrauterine contraceptive device. Ultrasound Obstet Gynecol 1994;4(4):316–9.
28. Morales-Rosello J. Spontaneous upward movement of lowly placed T-shaped IUDs. Contraception 2005;72(6):430–1.
29. Faundes D, Perdigao A, Faundes A, et al. T-shaped IUDs accommodate in their position during the first 3 months after insertion. Contraception 2000;62(4):165–8.
30. de Kroon CD, van Houwelingen JC, Trimbos JB, et al. The value of transvaginal ultrasound to monitor the position of an intrauterine device after insertion. A technology assessment study. Hum Reprod 2003;18(11):2323–7.
31. Dias T, Abeykoon S, Kumarasiri S, et al. Use of ultrasound in predicting success of intrauterine contraceptive device insertion immediately after delivery. Ultrasound Obstet Gynecol 2015;46(1):104–8.
32. American College of Obstetricians and Gynecologists' Committee on Obstetric Practice. Committee Opinion No. 670: immediate postpartum long-acting reversible contraception. Obstet Gynecol 2016;128(2):e32–7.
33. Kapp N, Curtis KM. Intrauterine device insertion during the postpartum period: a systematic review. Contraception 2009;80(4):327–36.
34. Whitaker AK, Chen BA. Society of Family Planning Guidelines: Postplacental insertion of intrauterine devices. Contraception 2018;97(1):2–13.
35. Chen BA, Reeves MF, Hayes JL, et al. Postplacental or delayed insertion of the levonorgestrel intrauterine device after vaginal delivery: a randomized controlled trial. Obstet Gynecol 2010;116(5):1079–87.
36. Trussell J. Contraceptive failure in the United States. Contraception 2011;83(5): 397–404.
37. Xiong X, Buekens P, Wollast E. IUD use and the risk of ectopic pregnancy: a meta-analysis of case-control studies. Contraception 1995;52(1):23–34.
38. Brahmi D, Steenland MW, Renner RM, et al. Pregnancy outcomes with an IUD in situ: a systematic review. Contraception 2012;85(2):131–9.

39. Ganer H, Levy A, Ohel I, et al. Pregnancy outcome in women with an intrauterine contraceptive device. Am J Obstet Gynecol 2009;201(4):381.e1-5.
40. Ozgu-Erdinc AS, Tasdemir UG, Uygur D, et al. Outcome of intrauterine pregnancies with intrauterine device in place and effects of device location on prognosis. Contraception 2014;89(5):426–30.
41. Division of Reproductive Health, National Center for Chronic Disease Prevention and Health Promotion, Centers for Disease Control and Prevention (CDC). Selected Practice Recommendations for Contraceptive Use, 2013: adapted from the World Health Organization selected practice recommendations for contraceptive use, 2nd edition. MMWR Recomm Rep 2013;62(RR-05):1–60.
42. Schiesser M, Lapaire O, Tercanli S, et al. Lost intrauterine devices during pregnancy: maternal and fetal outcome after ultrasound-guided extraction. An analysis of 82 cases. Ultrasound Obstet Gynecol 2004;23(5):486–9.

# Ultrasound Evaluation in Female Infertility

## Part 1, the Ovary and the Follicle

Stuart Campbell, DSc(Lon), FRCPE, FROG

**KEYWORDS**

• Ultrasound evaluation • Female infertility • Assisted conception • Ovarian reserve
• Follicular growth • Polycystic ovarian syndrome (PCOS) • Ovarian cysts
• Oocyte collection

**KEY POINTS**

- Ultrasound is an essential component of the modern investigation of female infertility and the management of Assisted Conception.
- Ultrasound in the baseline investigation is used to assess ovarian reserve, identify polycystic ovarian syndrome.
- Ultrasound in monitoring fertility treatment is used to track follicular growth and determine the timing of the ovulation trigger injection.
- Advanced Doppler ultrasound and 3D imaging refine our understanding of ovarian function.

## INTRODUCTION

Infertility is a disease defined by the failure to achieve a successful pregnancy after 12 months or more of appropriate, timed unprotected intercourse or therapeutic donor insemination. Earlier evaluation and treatment may be justified based on medical history and physical findings and is warranted after 6 months for women over age 35 years.[1]

Ultrasound has now become an essential component of the modern investigation of female infertility and the management of assisted conception. The fertility scan not only requires a different skillset to other indications for a gynecologic scan, but also a fundamental knowledge of basic reproductive physiology, the causes of infertility and how ultrasound can aid in the investigation and treatment of this condition. Some of the current applications of ultrasound in fertility are shown in **Box 1**.

Create Fertility, 150 Cheapside, London EC2V 6ET, UK
*E-mail address:* Profscampbell@hotmail.com

Obstet Gynecol Clin N Am 46 (2019) 683–696
https://doi.org/10.1016/j.ogc.2019.08.001
obgyn.theclinics.com

**Box 1**
**Current applications of ultrasound examination in fertility**

Investigation

- Assess ovarian reserve through measurement of antral follicle count.
- Identify polycystic ovarian morphology as part of the diagnosis of polycystic ovary syndrome.
- Reveal endometrial and uterine problems that may inhibit implantation such as fibroids, adenomyosis, polyps, adhesions, and persistent fluid.
- Diagnose ovarian cysts that may affect ovulation and adnexal masses such as hydrosalpinx that may affect implantation.
- Determine the patency of the fallopian tubes through HyCoSy.

Monitoring Assisted Conception Treatment

- Track follicular growth.
- Determine the timing of the ovulation "trigger" by measurement of follicular size and vascularity.
- Determine the timing of embryo transfer through measurement of endometrial morphology thickness and vascularity.
- Guide the needle at egg collection and the catheter at embryo transfer.

Infertility can affect either one or both of the partners trying to conceive and although ultrasound is important in the investigation in the infertile male,[2] this article focuses on the investigation and treatment of the female partner. Scans are predominantly performed transvaginally, although in certain circumstances such as large uterine fibroids or difficult embryo transfer, expertise in transabdominal scanning is required. Part 1 of this article covers the baseline investigations of the ovary and follicular growth in health and disease and how transvaginal ultrasound examination is used to monitor treatment, particularly in vitro fertilization (IVF). The term IVF will be used to cover intracytoplasmic sperm injection for the clinical aspect of management of the cycle is the same. Stimulated treatment is also used for egg donation and egg freezing treatments where infertility is usually but not always an issue, but the ultrasound aspects of ovarian monitoring is appropriate for this group of women. Stimulation protocols are designed to use exogenous follicle-stimulating hormone (FSH) to encourage the growth of many of the selected follicles to mature. The aim of conventional IVF is to maximize the number of oocytes retrieved but recent research suggests that this may diminish quality. As a result, there is a move to reduce the stimulatory dose in mild IVF protocols or natural modified protocols, where the emphasis is on quality and not quantity of oocytes.[3]

Although high resolution 2-dimensional imaging provides most of the diagnostic information in the pelvic scan, modern ultrasound equipment includes advanced Doppler and 3-dimensional (3D) facilities that refine our understanding of ovarian function and will be discussed in this article. In particular, Doppler imaging is used to measure ovarian stromal blood flow to assess ovarian reserve and responsiveness to stimulation, to measure perifollicular blood flow in the prediction of follicular maturity. In this regard color and spectral Doppler seem to be more effective than the initially promising 3D VOCAL method that provides semiquantitative measures as vascularity and flow indices. Three-dimensional imaging, however, brings many advantages to the fertility scan, many of which are discussed in part 2 of this article. It is also useful in the instantaneous 3D measurement of follicles in IVF cycles and in the differential diagnosis of ovarian and extraovarian cystic structures in the pelvis.

### *The One-Stop Fertility Scan*

Infertility investigations conducted at the general hospital level are frequently prolonged over many months, which can only worsen the problem, especially for the older woman because time is her biggest enemy. An expert 1-stop fertility scan combined with semen analysis and an antimullerian hormone (AMH) blood test can now provide diagnostic information as to the cause of the infertility in a 1 hour visit in most cases[4,5] and thus allow expeditious treatment. The value of ultrasound examination over other diagnostic modalities is that it is (or should be) an interactive and informative experience for the couple with the practitioner discussing and demonstrating the findings as the scan progresses.

### *Ovarian Reserve*

The number of primordial follicles in the ovary represents the woman's ovarian reserve and is crucial to her chances of conceiving. Human oocytes cannot replicate so that the loss of oocytes cannot be recovered. In the woman her total number of primordial follicles is on average 600,000 at birth, although this number is substantially lower in women who have an early menopause. At the menarche, there are about 360,000 follicles and there is subsequently a loss of 1000 per month until the menopause, when fewer than 1000 remain.[6] Every day of her menstrual cycle, some dormant primordial follicles are recruited to grow over the course of 2 cycles before the ovulatory cycle when some will be selected to enter a race to ovulate. Recruitment is initially steady until the follicle size is 6 mm in diameter when cyclic recruitment begins as the follicle responds to FSH secretion from the anterior pituitary.

A crucial part of the growth of the follicle is the development of the antral cavity within the follicle lined by estrogen producing granulosa cells, which cover the maturing oocyte in one pole (called the cumulus). The number of these antral follicles has a positive correlation with the number of primordial follicles and is one of the key measures of the woman's ovarian reserve and its responsiveness to stimulation. The antral follicle count (AFC) can be easily measured by ultrasound examination and is given as the combined total from both ovaries; it and has now become a standard measurement of ovarian reserve. The other measure is the serum level of AMH, which is produced from the granulosa cells of the preantral and early antral follicles. A key advantage of these parameters is that they can be performed on any day of the cycle. The mean AFC and AMH levels have a linear trajectory with age until the age of 30 years when there is a gentle decrease to age 35 and a steep decrease thereafter[7,8] (**Fig. 1**). There is a great individual variation with age in these parameters and about 10% to 15% of women have a low reserve by the age of 30 years. For this reason, these tests of ovarian reserve should be recommended to any women who are not contemplating having a child in the foreseeable future. This will give the women choices such as self-egg freezing for future use.

AFC and AMH are now the standard for predicting ovarian response to stimulation and figures such as less than 10 AFC[9] and less than 7 pmol/mL (1 ng/mL)[10] have been quoted as predicting poor response. Cut off values have been used to calculate the appropriate ovarian stimulation protocol to elicit an effective and safe response[11] the lower reserve women being given higher stimulation. However, this concept has been recently challenged and a more natural form of IVF[3] has been demonstrated to be as—successful in low-reserve patients. For these women a lower limit of less than 4 pmol/L for AMH and 4 or less for AFC is more appropriate.[3] Other parameters that predict ovarian reserve are stromal blood flow using spectral Doppler (both

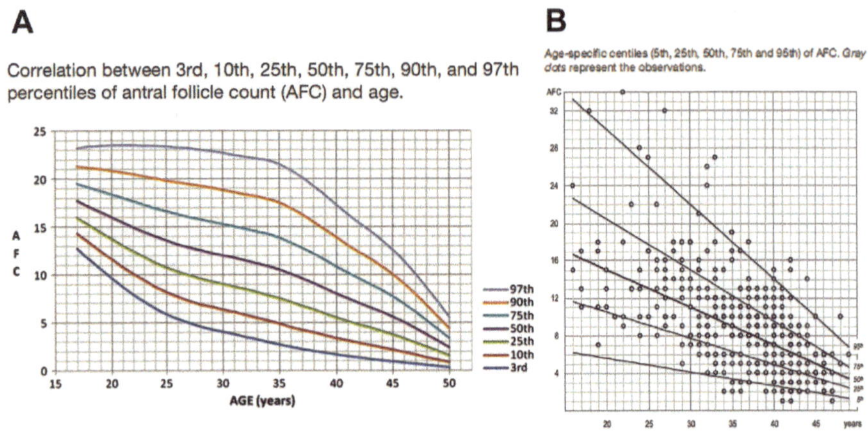


**Fig. 1.** (*A*) Relationship of AMH to age (years) (1 ng/mL = 7.14 pmol/L). (*B*) Relationship of AFC (both ovaries) to age (years). (*From* Almog B, Shehata F, Shalom-Paz E, et al. Age-related normogram for antral follicle count: McGill reference guide. Reprinted by permission from the American Society for Reproductive Medicine 2011;95(2):664; with permission.)

pulsatility index [PI] and peak systolic velocity [PSV])[12,13] and ovarian volume.[14] The mean baseline ovarian stromal PSV for a normal response is 10 cm/s while a poor or high response is associated with a the mean PSV of 5 cm/s and 15 cm/s, respectively. These parameters will give confirmatory information about ovarian reserve and response to stimulation.

Real-time 2-dimensional ultrasound imaging is generally adequate for counting ovarian follicles in clinical practice. The established practice is to measure all follicular structures 2 to 10 mm in diameter identified when scanning from one ovarian margin to the other (**Fig. 2**). Both ovaries should be included in the count.[15]

## *Follicular Growth and Oocyte Quality*

The antral follicles develop FSH receptors when 6 mm in diameter and after that cyclical growth is under the control of FSH secreted by the anterior pituitary. Follicular growth can be examined in both natural cycles and in IVF/intracytoplasmic sperm

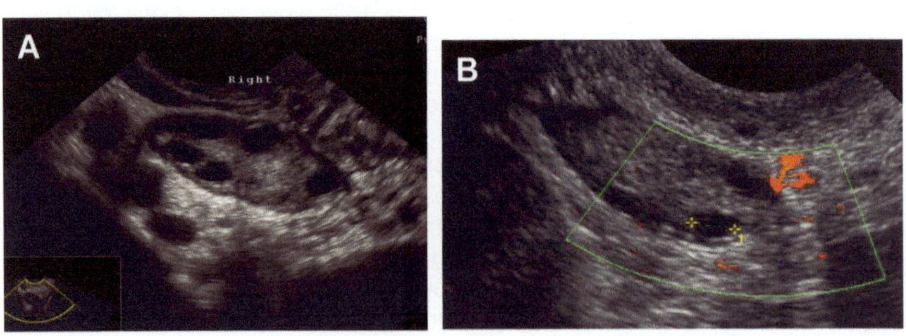


**Fig. 2.** (*A*) Normal AFC of 6 in a single maximum section of the ovary. This will underestimate the true number, which is dynamically counted by moving the transducer from one margin of the ovary to the other. (*B*) Ovary with a low AFC.

injection cycles after ovarian stimulation by exogenous FSH. Follicles are generally measured by taking the mean of 2 orthogonal diameters in one plane but after the follicles are more than 15 mm it is better to take the average of 3 diameters in 2 orthogonal planes as the follicles become more asymmetrical as they enlarge. This is especially true when there are more than 10 growing follicles in one ovary. Under these circumstances, 3D volumetry[16] is more accurate than the traditional method and takes less time (**Fig. 3**).

In a multicentre study the mean follicular diameter at the time of ovulation in a natural cycle was 20.1 mm but the range of diameters was wide and 40% of leading follicle diameters were 19 mm or less before ovulation.[17] In stimulated cycles, follicular growth is usually charted on a folliculogram every 2 days from day 5 of the cycle (day 4 of stimulation). A cut off of 17 to 18 mm at the time of trigger is generally recognized as being associated with a mature egg but this is a crude and frequently inaccurate indicator of which follicles contain the best oocytes or in choosing the best moment to trigger ovulation.[18]

Blood flow in the theca interna and externa is essential for the development of a good quality oocyte and there is good evidence that measurement of perifollicular blood flow by color and spectral Doppler is a strong marker for oocyte quality. Van Blerkom and colleagues[19] demonstrated that oxygen content of the follicle is correlated with perifollicular velocities and good oocyte quality; Nargund and colleagues[20] found that perifollicular PSV of greater than 10 cm/s at the time of the human chorionic gonadotropin trigger were associated with optimal fertilization and embryo quality. Measurement of perifollicular blood flow is especially important during mild or natural IVF cycles because there are fewer follicles and timing of the human chorionic gonadotropin trigger is crucial (**Fig. 4**). Some clinicians prefer to eyeball the completeness of the perifollicular ring of vascularity as demonstrated on power Doppler, with a more complete ring being associated with better pregnancy rates.[21] Zoomed 3D surface rendered images of the follicular wall show a ripple effect suggestive of capillaries, which are not present in dysfunctional follicles (**Fig. 5**). Although attempts have been made to visualize the cumulus, this is not consistent enough to be clinically valuable.

### *The Corpus Luteum*

Rupture of the follicle and ovulation is rarely observed on ultrasound imaging in clinical practice, but research studies have shown a sequence of events resulting in

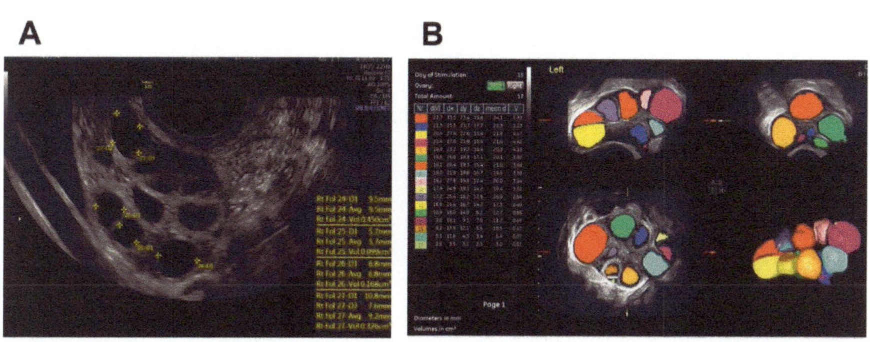

**Fig. 3.** (*A*) Measuring large numbers of follicles can be a laborious business during treatment scans and is time consuming. (*B*) The automated 3D technique; it is more efficient and accurate.

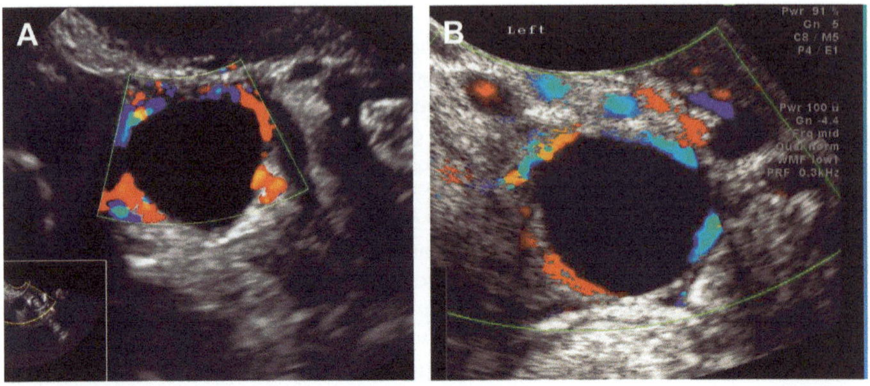


**Fig. 4.** (*A*) Good perifollicular flow in a natural IVF cycle. The mean follicular diameter is 14 mm and the PSV is 6 cm/s. The ovulation trigger injection will be given the following day. (*B*) Good perifollicular flow on day 9 of a natural modified IVF cycle. Although the mean follicular diameter is 15 mm, the PSV is 12.3 cm/s indicating follicular maturity and the optimal time for the ovulation trigger injection.

either immediate or stepwise follicular collapse over several hours. The invasion of the follicle cavity by thecal angiogenic vessels is a rapid process and high corpus luteum vascularity can be demonstrated within a few hours of rupture. Blood flow in the corpus luteum has been described as the highest per gram of any tissue in the human body.[22] The typical ultrasound appearance of the corpus luteum compared with the follicle is that of a thickened corrugated wall surrounding a blood clot which in turn is surrounded by a pronounced wreath of thecal capillaries and small arterioles and venules (**Fig. 6**). A cystic corpus luteum is common and reflects hemorrhage into the follicular cavity but occasionally it is a sign that the follicle has not ruptured and has become only partially luteinized (luteinized unruptured follicle). The blood velocities are much lower in a luteinized unruptured follicle than a

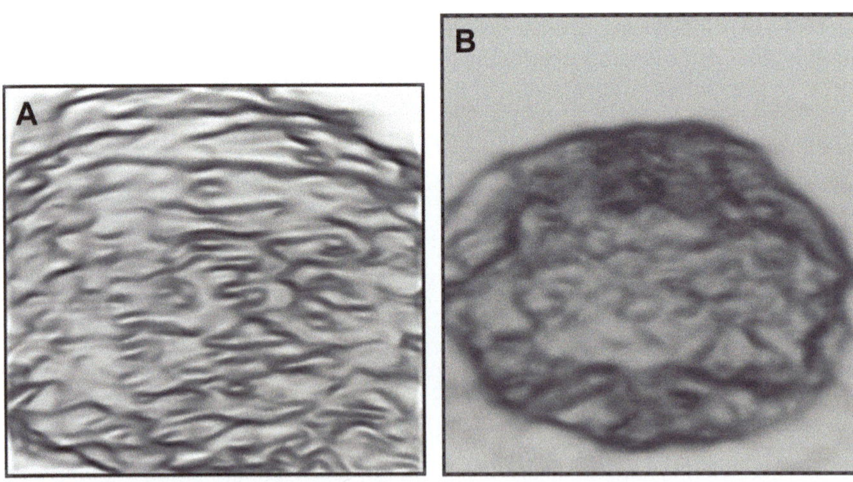


**Fig. 5.** (*A*) Normal follicle showing ripple effect on surface rendering (zoomed). (*B*) Dysfunctional follicle wall showing disrupted follicle wall ripples.

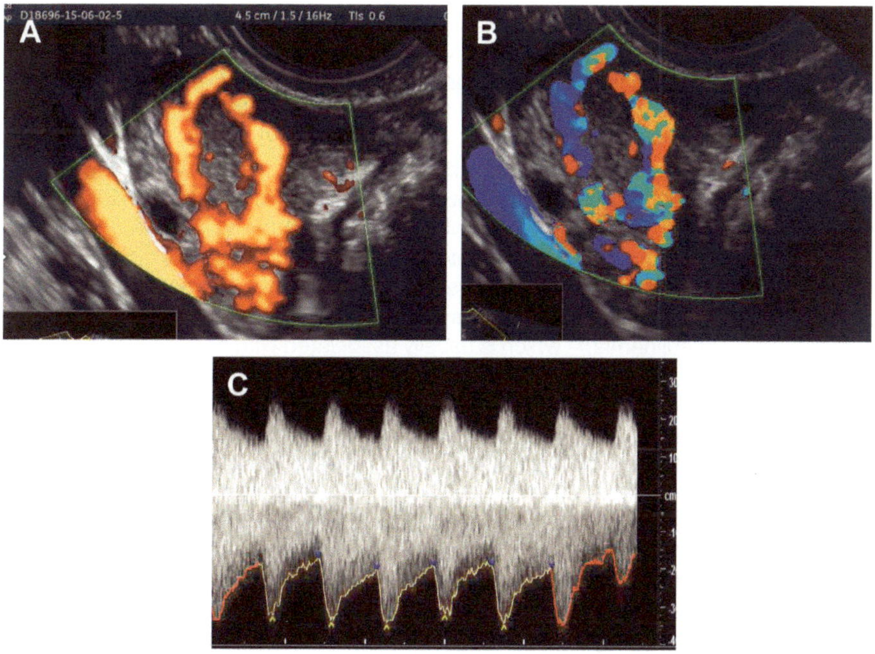


Fig. 6. Formation of the corpus luteum is associated with a large increase in angiogenesis shown here in (*A*) power Doppler, (*B*) color Doppler, and (*C*) spectral Doppler showing a massive increase in blood velocities to 35 cm/s.

healthy cystic corpus luteum so color Doppler can usually make the differential diagnosis.

The main role of the corpus luteum is to produce progesterone and estradiol to support placentation. There have been few adequate clinical studies evaluating corpus luteum function either by corpus luteum volume or vascularity but gross differences can be observed. The corpus luteum should have a lifespan of 10 days before apoptosis and autolysis begins. In women with low ovarian reserve there is often persistent corpus luteum activity which delays recruitment of follicles and gives a slow start to the cycle (**Fig. 7**).

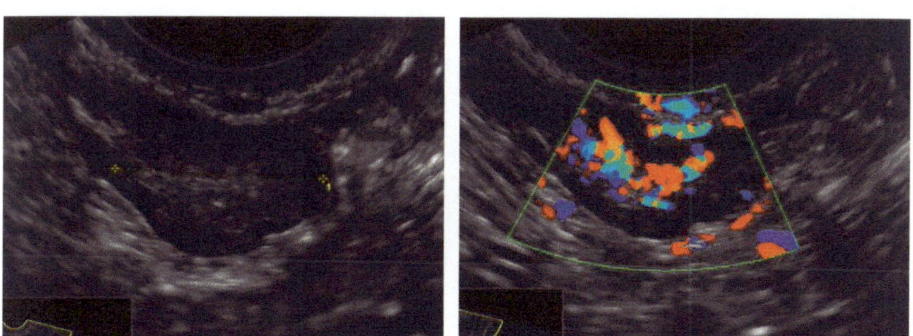

Fig. 7. Day 4 of a treatment cycle. Poor cyclical recruitment of follicles is sometimes associated with a small persistent corpus luteum.

### Polycystic Ovarian Syndrome

Polycystic ovarian syndrome (PCOS) is a major cause of anovulatory cycles and female infertility. The clinical manifestations of this important condition are hotly disputed. Some authorities believe that ovaries with polycystic morphology (PCOM) are not essential for the diagnosis and an alternative name should be given to the condition.[23] This is understandable because it is a multiorgan condition with a wide variety of endocrine and metabolic effects. However there is a growing consensus that the etiology of PCOS is primarily ovarian which is initiated by an imbalance between FSH and luteinizing hormone from the anterior pituitary in favor of luteinizing hormone causing ovarian hyperthecosis, an increase in ovarian volume and increased secretion of androgens. The hyperandrogenemia is exacerbated in 50% of cases by the development of hyperinsulinemia,[24] which is usually associated with obesity. There is also a huge increase in AMH production from the ovarian follicles and an increase in the secretion of angiogenic factors, especially vascular endothelial growth factor in the ovarian stroma. AMH decreases follicular responsiveness to FSH so the increase of AMH in the follicle causes follicular growth to stall at between 2 and 6 mm. This results in a rapid increase in the number of small antral follicles in the ovary.

The ultrasound diagnosis of altered morphology (PCOM) is therefore based on an increase in ovarian volume and stroma and the number of small antral follicles. PCOM does not imply that the woman has PCOS and it requires the addition of the clinical features and/or biochemical features of anovulation and hyperandrogenism to make the diagnosis. The term follicle number per ovary (FNPO) has supplanted AFC in the assessment of PCOM in a single ovary,[25] but this is an unsatisfactory term unless the follicular size is indicated eg, FNPO (2-10mm). Another term FNPS indicates the number of antral follicles in a single maximal cross section plane of the ovary, which was introduced to increase reproducibility to the ultrasound assessment but this has been shown to have a reduced sensitivity for PCOS.[26] The follicles are usually but not always arranged in the cortex like a necklace of pearls (**Fig. 8**). The definition of PCOM is conventionally based on the criteria set by the Rotterdam Consensus Conference,[27] that is, an ovarian volume of greater than 10 mL and AFC (2–10 mm) of greater than 12 per ovary. This definition is now disputed in view of the improvements in ultrasound technology which means that more small follicles can now be identified. In 1 paper,[28] it was found that more than 60% of women aged 25 to 30 attending a community-based clinic had polycystic morphology

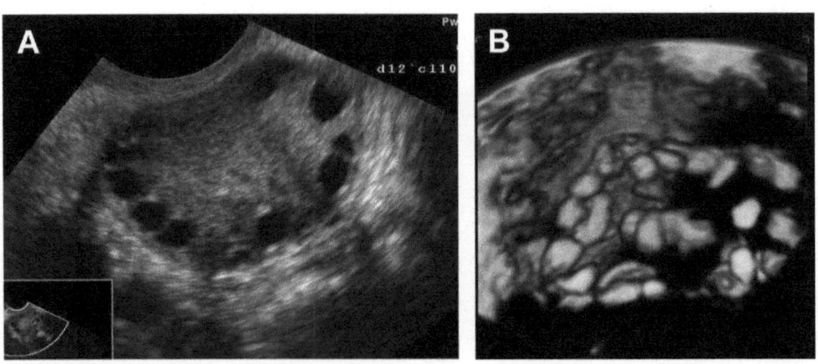


**Fig. 8.** (*A*) PCOM with 12 follicles arranged in the typical pearl necklace around increased stroma. The AFC will be higher when a count is made by continuously scanning across the ovary. (*B*) The 3D inversion mode is another method, which will permit the counting of all small follicles without the need for continuous scanning.

according to the Rotterdam criteria. For this reason there are several amended ultrasound definitions of PCOM[15,29] ranging from 19 to 25 follicles per ovary. None of these modifications challenge the acceptance of the definition of 2 to 10 mm as a small antral follicle. There are many reasons to change this definition as AFC 6 to 10 mm has not been shown to correlate with PCOS.[30] In my practice, I use the definition of 2 to 6 mm for the assessment of AFC and continue to use the original Rotterdam definition of follicle number and ovarian volume, which is well-established in clinical practice. Dewailly and colleagues[29] also recommend incorporating a serum AMH level greater than 35 pmol/L in the definition of PCOS, which is a logical step because PCOS is markedly increased at these levels.

The massive increase in angiogenic factors such as vascular endothelial growth factor in the ovarian stroma is of great significance especially when ovarian stimulation is given in IVF cycles. High stromal velocities even before stimulation are predictive of PCOS risk and have been shown to correlate with serum vascular endothelial growth factor levels[31] and the risk of ovarian hyperstimulation syndrome. If found at the baseline scan, this indicates the need to decrease the dose of stimulation and institute close monitoring of stromal velocities and estradiol during the cycle (**Fig. 9**). Sudden changes in stromal velocities during the cycle will frequently anticipate ovarian overstimulation even before the increase in estradiol is evident and in these circumstances prophylactic measures to prevent ovarian hyperstimulation syndrome such as buserelin trigger and freezing of embryos should be instituted (**Fig. 10**).

### *Ovarian Cysts*

Ovarian cysts are a common ultrasound finding in premenopausal women and can frequently cause unnecessary delay in fertility treatment. The majority of these cysts are functional and associated with an unruptured follicle or cystic corpus luteum. They frequently contain blood clot and are likely to have strong pericyst flow on Doppler examination (**Fig. 11**). The main aim is to determine whether the cyst is producing increased levels of estradiol or progesterone. If so or if the cyst is associated with menstrual irregularity, treatment should be postponed. Otherwise there is no need to interrupt treatment. Endometriotic cysts or endometriomas of the ovary are also common and can be found in the absence of endometriosis elsewhere. They contain the typical low level "ground glass" echoes of uncoagulated viscous blood and usually have a thickened wall (**Fig. 12**). The internal echoes of a hemorrhagic

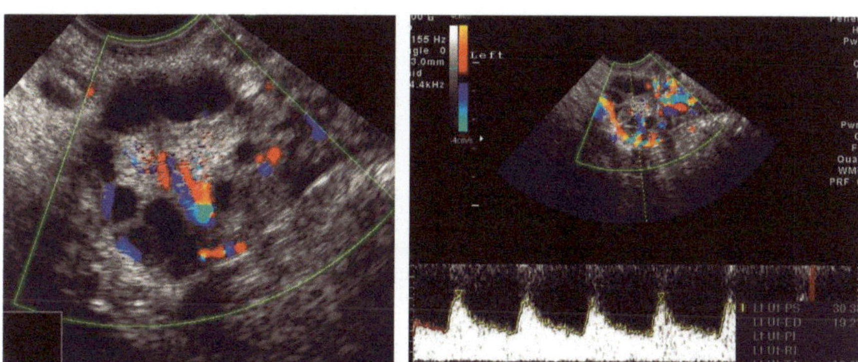


**Fig. 9.** Typical PCOS ovary with increased number of peripheral small follicles, increased stromal volume and stromal blood flow velocities of 30 cm/s on day 4 of an unstimulated cycle.

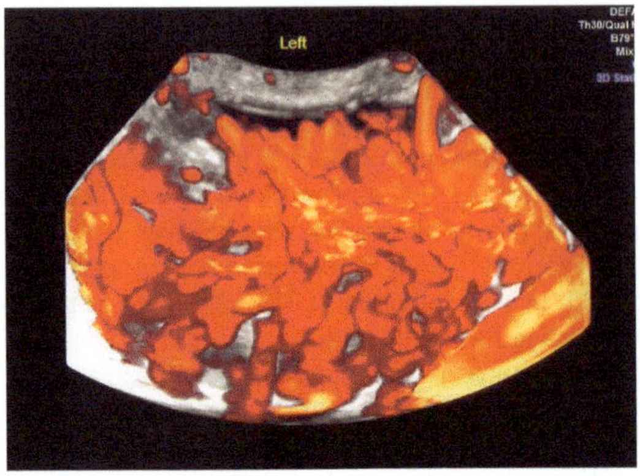


**Fig. 10.** PCOS, Massive increase in stromal flow on day 10 of a low stimulation cycle in a PCOS patient which preceded a sudden increase in serum estradiol levels.

cyst can sometimes be confused with an endometrioma but the thickened wall, the absence of blood flow and the raised serum CA125 associated with endometriomas are usually diagnostic. Endometriotic cysts providing they are not associated with widespread or deep infiltrating endometriosis do not affect the success of IVF.[32,33] It is prudent not to puncture them during egg collection because this can cause infection, but providing they do not interfere with oocyte collection their presence should not interrupt treatment. In fact there is evidence that surgical excision of endometriomas will decrease the patient's ovarian reserve.[34] Neoplastic cysts vary from simple serous to more complex cysts, of which the cystic teratoma is the most common. When identified it is important to exclude malignancy especially if there are solid internal echoes and the patient is in her 40s and a detailed Doppler examination of the solid parts should be undertaken (**Fig. 13**). There will rarely be confusion on ultrasound examination between an endometrioma and a dermoid, but occasionally an CA125 test will be helpful. It should be remembered that complex cysts such as dermoids are usually small in the premenopausal woman so the normal IOTA classification system may not apply. Neither CA125 nor Doppler is helpful in the diagnosis of borderline tumors (**Fig. 14**), which are more prevalent in premenopausal women and are diagnosed

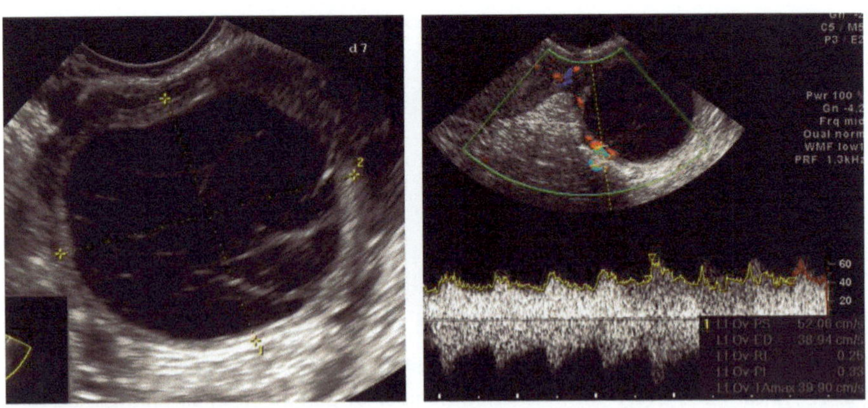

**Fig. 11.** Typical thin walled hemorrhagic cyst associated with increased peri-cyst flow typical of luteinized unruptured follicle.

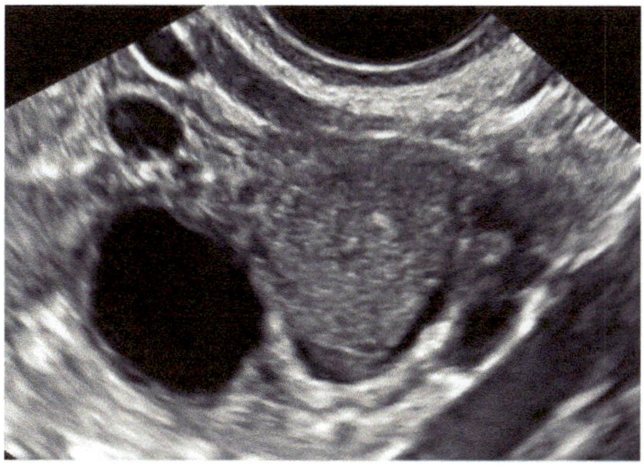

**Fig. 12.** Typical thick walled endometriotic cyst lateral to dominant follicle. The endometrioma is characteristically avascular.

primarily by their typical morphology on transvaginal ultrasound examination.[35] If the assessment of the cyst is reassuring, then treatment can proceed, although continued monitoring of the dimensions of the cyst should continue.

### *Oocyte Collection*

Oocyte retrieval is carried out 35 to 37 hours after the ovulation trigger injection. The technique of oocyte collection has evolved over many years from the laparoscopic approach first described by Steptoe to the now generally accepted ultrasound directed transvaginal aspiration method.[36] The procedure is usually carried out in dedicated surgical suite under aseptic conditions. Conscious sedation is usually given in the form of a combination of propofol, fentanyl, and midazolam. A needle guide is fixed to the transvaginal probe and after identification of the follicles a needle is inserted through the vaginal skin of each lateral fornix and aspiration of the oocytes from both ovaries accomplished with low pressure suction. Any follicle over 14 mm mean diameter should be aspirated. Care should be taken to avoid vessels because puncture of these can cause intraperitoneal bleeding. In most cases the follicles will be close to the vaginal wall but where there is any distance, Color Doppler should be used to identify any vessels that may be situated between the probe and the follicle.

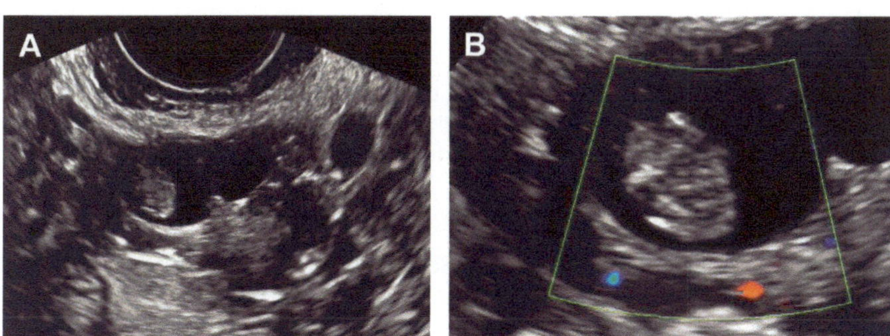


**Fig. 13.** (*A*) Small dermoid cyst noted in left ovary during a treatment scan. (*B*) The solid area was zoomed and Doppler studies performed at low PRF. No blood flow signals were detected. A CA125 was normal. The treatment cycle was continued. PRF, pulse repetition frequency.

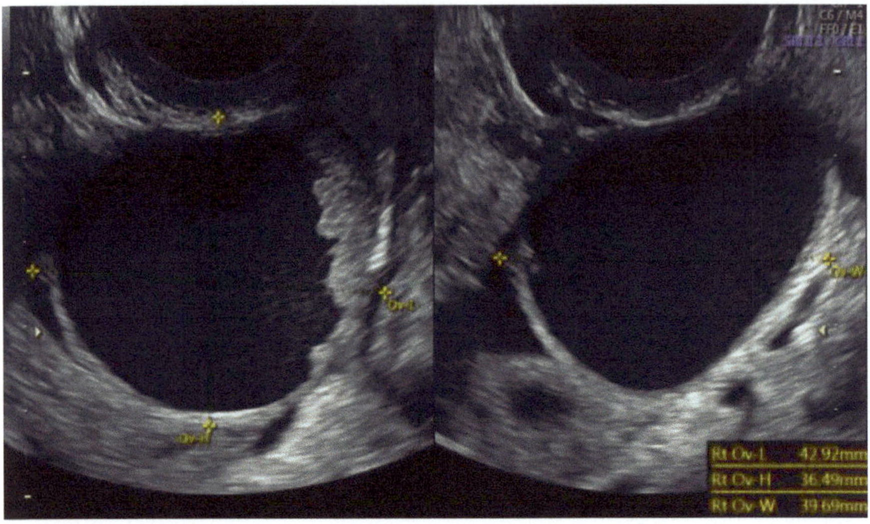


**Fig. 14.** Borderline epithelial tumor in 40 year old woman undergoing a 1-stop fertility scan. High-grade serous cancers are rarely found during a woman's reproductive years but borderline tumors are more common. Ultrasound provides the highest detection rate (sensitivity 91% in the UK Collaborative Trial of Ovarian Cancer Screening trial) and are suspected by their typical morphologic appearance of low flat papillae and minimal vascularity.

Puncture of an endometriotic cyst is the principal cause of infection and ultrasound expertise is required to avoid this. Where possible after aspiration of a follicle, the needle is directed to the next follicle without removal and reinsertion. When no oocyte is found in the aspirate it is usual to carry out a flushing of the follicle with 5 mL of culture medium. A limit on the number of flushes should be observed as excessive flushing can damage the formation of the corpus luteum. Some studies have demonstrated that flushing brings no benefit but in women with few follicles 2 or 3 flushes will sometimes produce a mature egg. Antibiotic cover for the procedure is usually given. The procedure usually takes 20 to 30 minutes and patient recovery time is about 1 hour. The procedure has a low incidence of complications; a recent large study[37] reported the overall complication rate to be 0.4% of procedures with intraperitoneal bleeding, infection, and anesthetic complications being the main reasons.

## ACKNOWLEDGMENTS

The work described in this chapter uses the latest ultrasound equipment provided for research purposes by Create Fertility. I thank Professor Nargund, Medical Director of Create Fertility for her constant support for this work.

## REFERENCES

1. Practice Committee of the American Society for Reproductive Medicine. Definitions of infertility and recurrent pregnancy loss: a committee opinion. Fertil Steril 2013;99(1):63.
2. Lotti F, Maggi M. Ultrasound of the male genital tract in relation to male reproductive health. Human Reproduction Update 2015;21(1):56–86.
3. Nargund G, Datta AK, Fauser BCJM. Mild stimulation for in vitro fertilization. Fertil Steril 2017;108(4):558–67.

4. Kelly SM, Sladevicius P, Campbell S, et al. Investigation of the infertile couple: a one-stop ultrasound based approach. Human Reproduction 2001;16(1):2481–4.
5. Benacerraf BR, Abuhamad AZ, Bromley B, et al. Consider ultrasound first for imaging the female pelvis. Am J Obstet Gynecol 2015;212(4):450–5.
6. Wallace WH, Kelsey TW. Human ovarian reserve from conception to the menopause. PLoS One 2010;5(1):e8772.
7. La Marca A, Spada E, Sighinolfi G, et al. Age-specific nomogram for the decline in antral follicle count throughout the reproductive period. Fertil Steril 2011;95(2):684–8.
8. Almog B, Shehata F, Suissa S, et al. Age-related normograms of serum antimüllerian hormone levels in a population of infertile women: a multicenter study. Fertil Steril 2011;95(7):2359–63, 2363.e1.
9. Jayaprakasan K, Chan YY, Islam R, et al. Prediction of in vitro fertilization outcome at different antral follicle count thresholds in a prospective cohort of 1,012 women. Fertil Steril 2012;98(3):657–63.
10. Ficicioglu C, Cenksoy OP, Yildirim G, et al. Which cut-off value of serum anti-Mullerian hormone level can predict poor ovarian reserve, poor ovarian response to stimulation and in vitro fertilization success? A prospective data analysis. Gynecol Endocrinol 2014;30(5):372–6.
11. La Marca A, Sunkara SK. Individualization of controlled ovarian stimulation in IVF using ovarian reserve markers: from theory to practice. Hum Reprod Update 2014;20(1):124–40.
12. Zaidi J, Barber J, Kyei-mensah A, et al. Relationship of ovarian stromal blood flow at the baseline ultrasound scan to subsequent follicular response in an in vitro fertilization program. Obstet Gynecol 1996;88:779–84.
13. Engmann L, Sladkevicius P, Agrawal R, et al. Value of ovarian stromal blood flow velocity measurement after pituitary suppression in the prediction of ovarian responsiveness and outcome of in vitro fertilization treatment. Fertil Steril 1999;71(1):22–9.
14. Syrop CH, Willhoite A, Van Voorhis BJ. Ovarian volume: a novel outcome predictor for assisted reproduction. Fertil Steril 1995;64:1167–71.
15. Coelho Neto MA, Ludwin A, Borrell A, et al. Counting ovarian antral follicles by ultrasound: a practical guide. Ultrasound Obstet Gynecol 2018;51(1):10–20.
16. Raine-Fenning N, Jayaprakasan K, Clewes J, et al. SonoAVC: a novel method of automatic volume calculation. Ultrasound Obstet Gynecol 2008;31(6):691–6.
17. Mikolajczyk RT, Stanford JB, Ecochard R. Multilevel model to assess sources of variation in follicular growth close to the time of ovulation in women with normal fertility: a multicenter observational study. Reprod Biol Endocrinol 2008;6:61.
18. Revelli A, Martiny G, Delle Piane L, et al. A critical review of bi-dimensional and three-dimensional ultrasound techniques to monitor follicle growth: do they help improving IVF outcome? Reprod Biol Endocrinol 2014;12:107.
19. Van Blerkom J, Antczak M, Schrader R. The developmental potential of the human oocyte is related to the dissolved oxygen content of follicular fluid: association with vascular endothelial growth factor levels and perifollicular blood flow characteristics. Hum Reprod 1997;12(5):1047–55.
20. Nargund G, Bourne T, Doyle P, et al. Associations between ultrasound indices of follicular blood flow, oocyte recovery and preimplantation embryo quality. Hum Reprod 1996;11(I):109–13.
21. Robson SJ, Barry M, Norman RJ. Power Doppler assessment of follicle vascularity at the time of oocyte retrieval in in vitro fertilization cycles. Fertil Steril 2008;90(6):2179–82.

22. Parsons AK. Imaging the human corpus luteum. J Ultrasound Med 2001;20: 811–9.
23. Conway G, Dewailly D, Diamanti-Kandarakis E, et al, ESE PCOS Special Interest Group. The polycystic ovary syndrome: a position statement from the European Society of Endocrinology. Eur J Endocrinol 2014;171(4):P1–29.
24. Rosenfield RL, Ehrmann DA. The pathogenesis of polycystic ovary syndrome (PCOS): the hypothesis of PCOS as functional ovarian hyperandrogenism revisited. Endocr Rev 2016;37(5):467–520.
25. Dewailly D, Lujan ME, Carmina E, et al. Definition and significance of polycystic ovarian morphology: a taskforce report from the Androgen Excess and Polycystic Ovary Syndrome Society. Hum Reprod Update 2014;20:334–52.
26. Christ JP, Willis AD, Brooks ED, et al. Follicle number, not assessments of the ovarian stroma, represents the best ultrasonographic marker of polycystic ovary syndrome. Fertil Steril 2014;101(1):280–7.e1.
27. Rotterdam ESHRE/ASRM-Sponsored PCOS Consensus Workshop Group. Revised 2003 consensus on diagnostic criteria and long-term health risks related to polycystic ovary syndrome. Fertil Steril 2004;81:19–25.
28. Johnstone EB, Rosen MP, Neril R, et al. The polycystic ovary post-Rotterdam: a common, age-dependent finding in ovulatory women without metabolic significance. J Clin Endocrinol Metab 2010;95(11):4965–72.
29. Dewailly D, Gronier H, Poncelet E, et al. Diagnosis of polycystic ovary syndrome (PCOS): revisiting the threshold values of follicle count on ultrasound and of the serum AMH level for the definition of polycystic ovaries. Hum Reprod 2011; 26(11):3123–9.
30. Jonard S, Robert Y, Cortet-Rudelli C, et al. Ultrasound examination of polycystic ovaries: is it worth counting the follicles? Hum Reprod 2003;18(3):598–603.
31. Agrawal R, Sladkevicius P, Engmann L, et al. Serum vascular endothelial growth factor concentrations and ovarian stromal blood flow are increased in women with polycystic ovaries. Hum Reprod 1998;13:651–5.
32. Jayaprakasan K, Becker C, Mittal M, on behalf of the Royal College of Obstetricians and Gynaecologists. The effect of surgery for endometriomas on fertility. Scientific impact paper No. 55. BJOG 2018;125(6):e19–28.
33. Barnhart K, Dunsmoor-Su R, Coutifaris C. Effect of endometriosis on in vitro fertilization. Fertil Steril 2002;77:1148–55.
34. Somigliana E, Berlanda N, Benaglia L, et al. Surgical excision of endometriomas and ovarian reserve: a systematic review on serum antimullerian hormone level modifications. Fertil Steril 2012;98:1531–8.
35. Campbell S, Gentry-Maharaj A. The role of transvaginal ultrasound in screening for ovarian cancer. Climacteric 2018;21(3):221–6.
36. Healy MW, Hill MJ, Levens ED. Optimal oocyte retrieval and embryo transfer techniques: where we are and how we got here. Semin Reprod Med 2015;33:83–91.
37. Levi-Setti PE, Cirillo F, Scolaro V, et al. Appraisal of clinical complications after 23,827 oocyte retrievals in a large assisted reproductive technology program. Fertil Steril 2018;109(6):1038–43.e1.

# Ultrasound Evaluation in Female Infertility

## Part 2, the Uterus and Implantation of the Embryo

Stuart Campbell, DSc(Lon), FRCPE, FROG

**KEYWORDS**

- Ultrasound evaluation • Female infertility • Implantation • Endometrial polyps
- Submucous fibroids • Adenomyosis • Mullerian duct abnormalities
- Embryo Transfer • Hysterosalpingo Contrast Sonography (HyCoSy)

**KEY POINTS**

- Ultrasound now plays a pivotal role in the investigation and management of the female partner in infertile couples. There is now a need for advanced ultrasound training to take center stage in fellowship training programs in reproductive medicine.
- Although high-resolution two-dimensional imaging provides most of the diagnostic information in the pelvic scan, modern ultrasound equipment includes advanced Doppler and three-dimensional facilities that refine understanding and evaluate uterine and endometrial blood flow in the assessment of endometrial receptivity.
- Three-dimensional scanning provides surface rendered images, which are diagnostically helpful. It is principally used to define the relationship of fibroids to the endometrium and the position of endometrial polyps and other structures relative to the implantation site, to diagnose adenomyosis, to reveal and classify congenital uterine malformations, and in the differential diagnosis of ovarian and extraovarian cystic structures in the pelvis.

## INTRODUCTION

Part 1 of this article described the role of ultrasound in identifying ovarian abnormalities, assessing ovarian reserve, measuring follicular growth, and the retrieval of oocytes in an in vitro fertilization (IVF) program. The aim of these procedures is directed toward the creation of an embryo.

Part 2 covers the role of ultrasound in assessing endometrial and uterine factors affecting the implantation of the embryo. Although high-resolution two-dimensional (2D) imaging provides most of the diagnostic information in the pelvic scan, modern ultrasound equipment includes advanced Doppler and 3D facilities that refine the evaluation of uterine and endometrial blood flow in the assessment of

Create Fertility, 150 Cheapside, London EC2V 6ET, UK
*E-mail address:* Profscampbell@hotmail.com

Obstet Gynecol Clin N Am 46 (2019) 697–713
https://doi.org/10.1016/j.ogc.2019.08.002

endometrial receptivity. 3D scanning is principally used to define the relationship of fibroids to the endometrium and the position of endometrial polyps and other structures relative to the implantation site, to diagnose adenomyosis, to reveal and classify congenital uterine malformations, and in the differential diagnosis of ovarian and extra-ovarian cystic structures in the pelvis.

## ENDOMETRIAL FACTORS

Successful implantation in the normal uterus is the culmination of a complex interaction between many factors, and ultrasonography can give important information on many of these. The endometrium thickens and undergoes morphologic changes under the influence of increasing estradiol levels from the developing ovarian follicles. This process is also associated with an increased vascularity from the basal arteries with sprouting angiogenic vessels developing along the lengthening glandular crypts of the functional layer. Implantation failure can occur because of a missed implantation window, which is defined by the development of endometrial pinopods at luteinizing hormone peak +9 days (range, 6–12 days). Vascular development and angiogenesis during implantation are mediated by numerous cell types and cell products, especially vascular endothelial growth factor, and aberrant vascularity is a likely contributor to implantation failure and early pregnancy loss.[1] These factors may influence the timing of the ovulation trigger in IVF cycles and frozen embryo transfer (FET) cycles to prevent missing the implantation window. Another factor in the maturation of the endometrium is the development of waves of contractions in the junctional zone (JZ) of the subendometrial myometrium. These contractions increase under the influence of estradiol, which promotes waves principally from cervix to fundus in the estradiol-only phase of the cycle and vanish immediately or reverse after the administration of progesterone. They seem to have an important physiologic role in implantation and are clearly visible on the scan but are difficult to quantify and have not been found to be useful in clinical practice.

Ultrasound monitoring of the endometrium in a natural or stimulated transfer cycle usually involves measuring the endometrial thickness (ET) and studying changes in morphology up to the time of ovulation. ET is measured in the midsagittal plane of the uterus as the maximum distance between the 2 interfaces of the endometrial-myometrial junction. Endometrial morphology is classified as pattern A (triple layer: characterized by a hypoechoic endometrium with a central line; **Fig. 1**A); pattern B

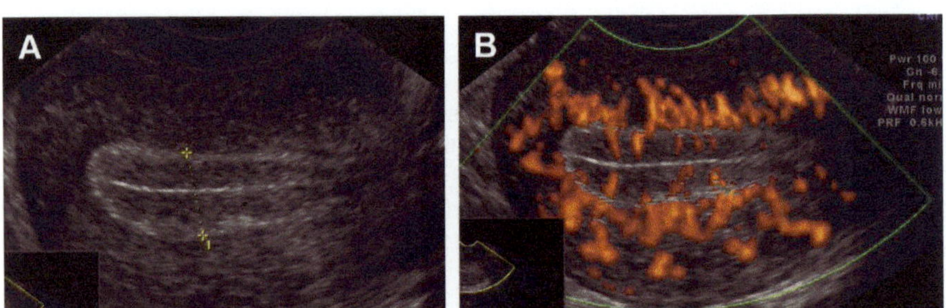


**Fig. 1.** (*A*) Typical triple-layer endometrium in the late follicular phase of the cycle. This pattern together with an ET greater than 7 mm is strongly associated with implantation. (*B*) Grade 3 endometrial flow with spiral arteries observed penetrating the functional layer of the endometrium. Optimal vascularization at the implantation site is associated with implantation.

(isoechoic endometrium with poorly defined outer walls and central echogenic line), and pattern C (homogeneous hyperechoic morphology).[2] Various studies have reported that the mean ET at the time of ovulation in natural cycles is between 10 and 12.5 mm.[3,4] Raine-Fenning and colleagues[3] found that both ET and volume increased significantly during the follicular phase, reaching a peak at the time of ovulation, and that both thickness and endometrial volume remained stable throughout the luteal phase. Bakos and colleagues[4] found triple-layer morphology at 5 to 6 days before ovulation, which continued to the day of ovulation. Studies relating ET and morphology to successful implantation are confounded by difficulties in controlling for embryo quality, which is the most important factor[5] for successful implantation. However, most large studies[6,7] undertaken in IVF cycles show that both ET and triple-layer endometrium have a positive relationship with the clinical pregnancy rate, although there is no universal agreement.[8] Other studies have identified a lower ET threshold below which clinical pregnancy was significantly reduced; this can vary between 6 and 8 mm.[9,10] Zhang and colleagues[11] in a large retrospective study of embryo transfers in women with morphologically good blastocysts found that ET on oocyte retrieval day was associated with improved live birth rate but live births were achieved in one-third of women who had an ET less than 6 mm.

Endometrial vascularity is usually assessed by visually assessing power Doppler images of endometrial vascularity before the ovulation trigger injection. Vascular penetration of the endometrium is usually graded as grade 1, no subendometrial blood flow detected; grade 2, subendometrial blood flow detected; and grade 3, both endometrial and subendometrial blood flow detected[12] (**Fig. 1**B). Most studies show that grade 3 flow is associated with significantly higher clinical pregnancy rates,[13,14] although there are some dissenting studies.[8] Examining subendometrial flow requires careful attention to certain details. The endometrial triple or double layer in the region of the implantation site should occupy at least 50% of the screen, the power Doppler color box should be made as small as possible (to increase the frame rate), and a few seconds should be allowed for the flow signals to appear as flow is reduced during endometrial contractions. In the author's experience, grade 3 flow is a good predictor of implantation even in the presence of persistently thin endometrium (**Fig. 2**).

Measurement of uterine artery blood flow gives a global assessment of uterine perfusion and is very useful in identifying a small subgroup with average pulsatility index greater than 3.5 before the trigger injection.[15,16] Reverse flow in the uterine artery

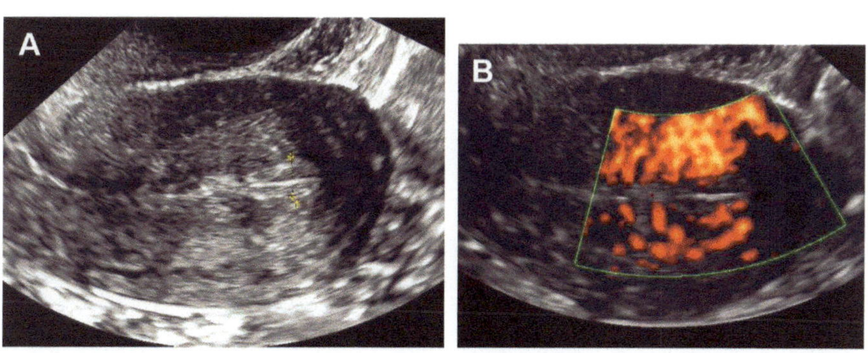


**Fig. 2.** (*A*) Persistently thin endometrium (5.8 mm) in patient having a medicated FET cycle with high doses of estradiol. Triple-layer morphology is visible at the fundus. (*B*) Transfer was performed because of strong grade 2 endometrial flow resulting in implantation and successful pregnancy.

is associated with such low implantation rates that the embryos should be frozen. In these circumstances, the uterine circulation and implantation can be improved in a subsequent medicated cycle with oral and subcutaneous estrogen, and aspirin.

### Endometrial polyps

Endometrial polyps are small, discrete, localized, hyperplastic overgrowths of endometrium that contain both endometrial glands and stroma and are usually benign in premenopausal women. They are either sessile or (more commonly) pedunculated and have feeder vessels that sustain their growth. They can vary in number, size, and position in the uterine cavity. Polyps are easily diagnosed by 2D ultrasound, especially in the proliferative phase of the cycle around the 6th to 14th day of the cycle when they are identified by their bright edge and increased echogenicity (**Fig. 3**A). The feeder vessel can also be identified by Doppler (**Fig. 3**B). 3D ultrasound both in the coronal (**Fig. 4**A) and sagittal planes (**Fig. 4**B) is especially helpful in identifying the position of the polyp. Occasionally, particularly during IVF-stimulated cycles, false-positive diagnoses can be made by misinterpreting folds in the endometrial epithelium for a polyp, and saline sonohysterography may be required to clarify the situation. Hysteroscopic removal is a simple procedure and should be performed for all polyps 5 mm or greater close to the implantation area. Hysteroscopy plus polyp removal has been shown to have higher live-birth rates than diagnostic hysteroscopy alone.[17]

### Endometrial fluid

The presence of persistent fluid in the endometrium at the time of ovulation can inhibit implantation. There is generally a consensus that when excessive fluid is noted in the uterine cavity embryo implantation will fail. The 4 most common causes for persistent fluid are endometrial adhesions, hydrosalpinges, dehiscent cesarean scar, and subclinical intrauterine infection.

Endometrial adhesions are usually associated with Asherman syndrome in which overenthusiastic curettage has removed the basal layer of the endometrium, resulting in synechiae between the anterior and posterior walls. Fluid becomes trapped between the synechiae giving a typical 2D appearance. The finding of small fluid collections in a thin endometrium is frequently the first indication of the condition. The diagnosis is usually made by 2D scanning, although 3D can give information of the extent of the lesions (**Fig. 5**). The confirmatory diagnosis is by hysteroscopy and treatment is by hysteroscopic surgery. This surgery is usually successful, although in a

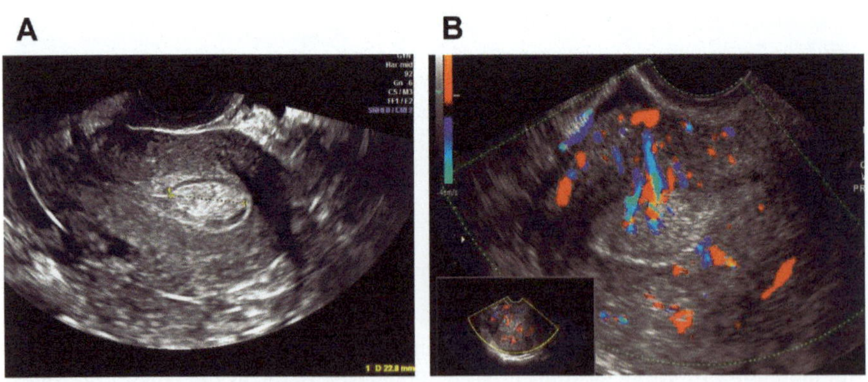


**Fig. 3.** (*A*) Typical appearance on 2D of polyp with its bright edge. (*B*) The feeder vessel of the endometrial polyp is diagnostic.

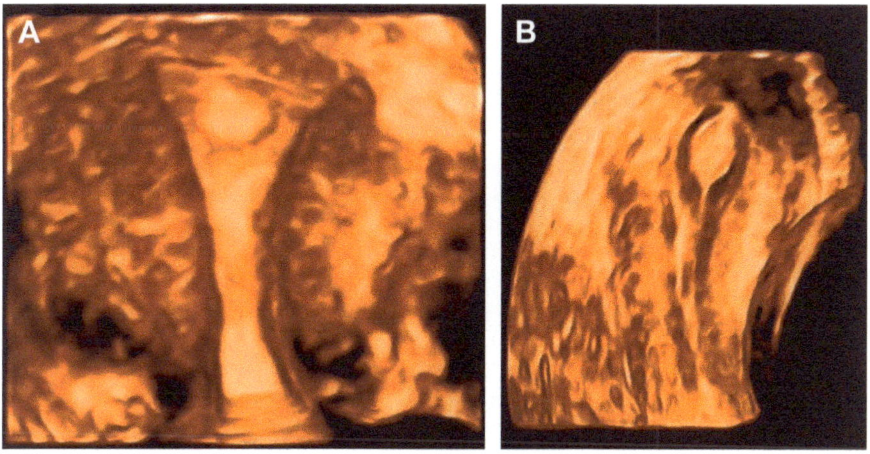


**Fig. 4.** (*A*) The position of the polyp in relation to the implantation site can best be shown in the 3D coronal view of the uterine cavity. (*B*) Rotating the image plane to a sagittal section often improves visualization of the polyp and its pedicle.

significant number of cases endometrial damage is so extensive that receptivity cannot be restored.

The presence of hydrosalpinges during IVF treatment, especially if they are bilateral, is associated with a significant reduction of live-birth rates by 30%, and early miscarriage rates are also high but only when the hydrosalpinges are visible by ultrasound.[18,19] The cause is the reflux of tubal fluid into the endometrium, which is toxic to the embryo and endometrium. The endometrial fluid is easily identified and, when seen, should prompt a search for the hydrosalpinges. The typical adnexal appearance is of multiple elongated irregular "cysts" in the adnexal region, which frequently have incomplete septae. The appearances can vary widely and single or double cysts may be the only presentation (**Fig. 6**A,B). 3D ultrasound helps to confirm the diagnosis by linking the separate loops (**Fig. 6**C) into 1 tubal mass. Surgical removal of the dilated tubes or proximal tubal clipping restores implantation rates to normal.[20]

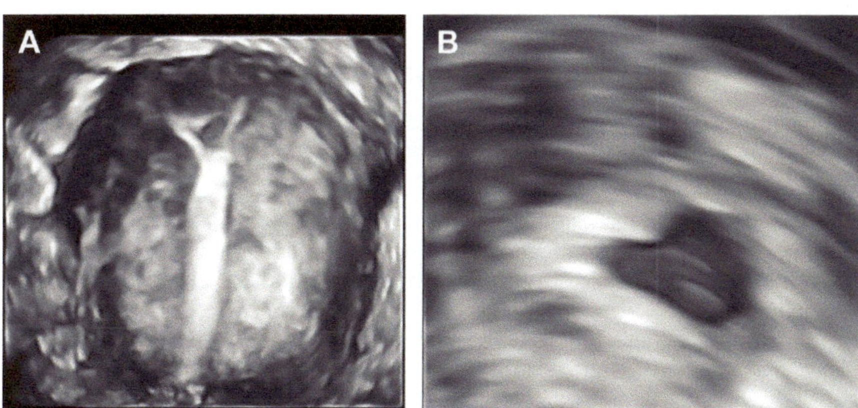


**Fig. 5.** (*A*) Thin endometrium and trapped fluid at the implantation site caused by intracavitary adhesions. (*B*) Zoomed image of the fluid suggesting adhesions.

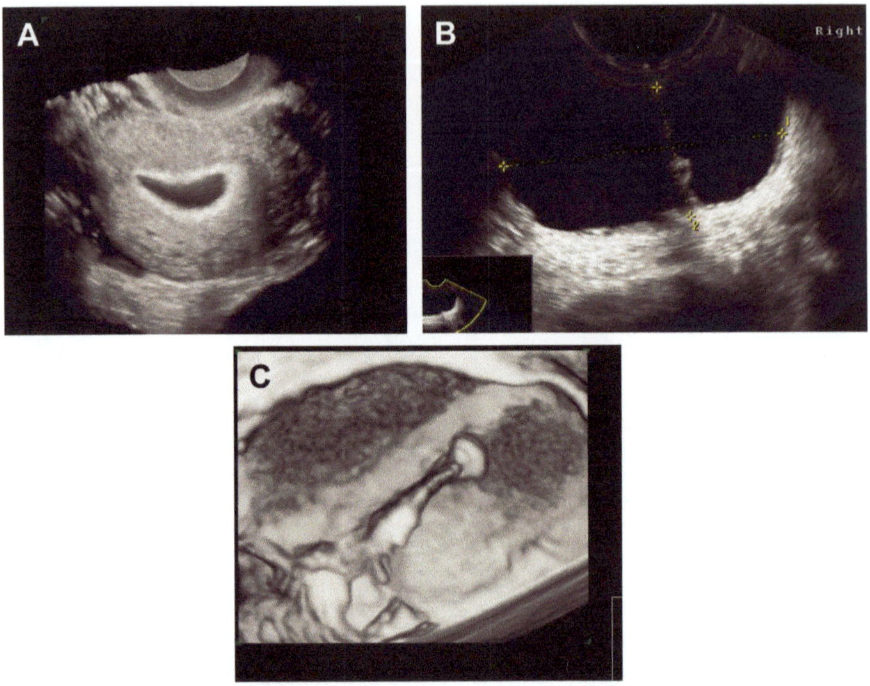


**Fig. 6.** (*A*) Transverse section of the uterus with significant amount of endometrial fluid. Associated with cystic adnexal mass. (*B*) Atypical appearance of hydrosalpinx, although the nodular appearance of the septum suggests this diagnosis. (*C*) 3D image of adnexal cyst in **Fig. 6**B confirming the diagnosis of hydrosalpinx with incomplete septum.

Endometrial fluid emanating from a fully dehiscent cesarean section (CS) scar has not been described before but the author has observed this on many occasions (**Fig. 7**). The fluid may pass from the peritoneum through the scar and reach the fundus by peristalsis. The treatment is resuture of the CS scar. Endometrial infections are rare during a woman's reproductive years but endometrial fluid has been reported in association with chlamydia and cervical bacterial infections. Antibiotic therapy is indicated. Aspiration of the fluid before embryo transfer has been reported to be successful.[21]

## UTERINE FACTORS AFFECTING IMPLANTATION

The uterine size should be a standard ultrasound measurement in the pelvic examination because uterine abnormalities are usually associated with deviations from the normal. Standard measurements should be:

1. Uterine length from the external cervix to the fundus in the sagittal plane with the cervix and uterine corpus measured separately and added if they are angulated.
2. Maximal anteroposterior (AP) diameter in the sagittal plane perpendicular to the endometrial line.
3. Uterine width from each side of the uterine corpus in the transverse plane at its maximal diameter.

The uterus declines slightly in length throughout the reproductive years and becomes rounder, but approximate sizes are longitudinal, 68 to 75 mm; AP, 34 to 41 mm; and width, 44 to 50 mm.[22] The myometrium should be studied for its

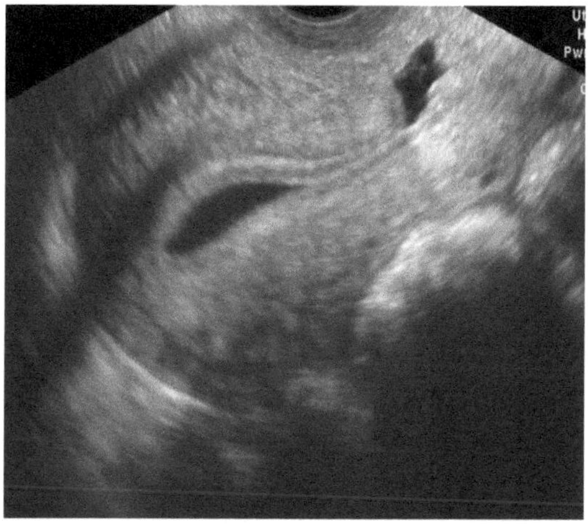

**Fig. 7.** Endometrial fluid caused by a full-thickness separation of a CS scar. Pregnancy occurred after repair of the dehiscence.

morphology and the 3 layers identified (ie, external longitudinal, middle spiral, and inner junctional). This morphology is best shown on a 3D scan, which should be performed in the coronal view from the cervix to the fundus to show the junctional layer or JZ, which should be less than 8 mm in diameter (**Fig. 8**).

The following abnormalities are associated with reduced implantation.

### *Submucous fibroids*

Uterine fibromyomas (fibroids) are common benign tumors of the smooth muscle of the uterus. Prevalence is higher than was originally thought, and there is ultrasound evidence to suggest that fibroids occur in more than 50% of premenopausal women.[23] Fibroids are classified into subserous (ie, projecting from the serosal surface),

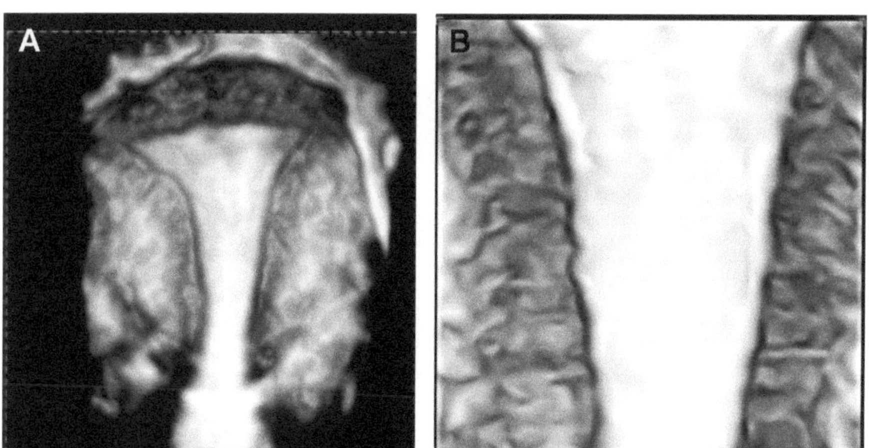


**Fig. 8.** (*A*) 3D coronal view of endometrium showing the JZ layer and middle spiral and outer longitudinal layers. (*B*) Zoomed view of normal JZ (gradient light algorithm) showing radial arteries crossing to the endometrium.

intramural (contained entirely within the myometrium), and submucous, which are situated partially or completely within the endometrial cavity. Submucous fibroids are subdivided into type 0, a polyp fibroid; type1, in which less than 50% of the fibroid is contained within the myometrium; and type 2, greater than 50% of the fibroid is contained within the myometrium.[24] It is generally considered that subserous fibroids have no effect on implantation and that submucous fibroids do reduce implantation rates and live-birth rates depending on their size and site.[25] The removal of submucous fibroids by hysteroscopic surgery is associated with improved clinical pregnancy and live-birth rates, which are proof of their adverse effect on implantation.[26] The effect of intramural fibroids on live-birth rates is more controversial, with proponents either way, but Sunkara and colleagues,[27] in a detailed systematic review of 6087 well-documented observational IVF cycles, found that the presence of non–cavity-distorting intramural fibroids on average reduces the live birth rate by 21% and the clinical pregnancy rate by 15% per IVF cycle compared with no fibroids. This reduction is small compared with the 70% reduction associated with submucous fibroids reported by Somigliana and colleagues[28] in their meta-analysis.

It seems that the current focus of ultrasound should be on the diagnosis of submucous and endometrial distorting fibroids because of their proven effect on reducing live-birth rates. The role of myomectomy with non–cavity-distorting intramural fibroids is less certain, although removal of very large fibroids makes visualization of the ovaries and oocyte collection easier.

Unlike large intramural fibroids, submucous fibroids are usually capable of being accurately assessed in terms of site and size by transvaginal (TV) scanning. This technique allows a better evaluation of the relationship of the fibroid to the endometrial cavity, especially if 3D imaging is used (**Fig. 9**A). Surgery is has risks and not all need to be removed if it is judged that the fibroid will not significantly affect implantation (**Fig. 9**B). It should be recognized that knowing when not to operate is as important as when to operate, because inappropriate surgery can worsen uterine receptivity. Doppler ultrasound of the fibroid must be performed to assess its vascularity because it indicates the propensity of the fibroid to grow and disrupt the normal endometrial blood flow.

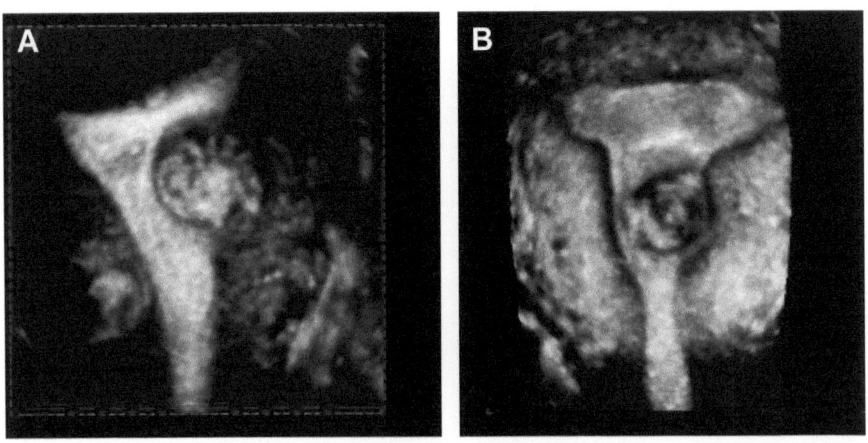


**Fig. 9.** (*A*) 3D image of type 1 submucous fibroid affecting the implantation area; this fibroid should be removed by hysteroscopic surgery. (*B*) 3D image of type 1 submucous fibroid situated below the implantation area. Surgery in this case may not be necessary.

### Adenomyosis

Adenomyosis is caused by encroachment of endometrial glands into the myometrium, resulting in uterine enlargement and focal and global lesions in the myometrium. The principal differential diagnosis is with uterine fibroids.

The ultrasound characteristics of adenomyosis compared with fibroids are:

- Poorly defined borders
- Minimal distortion of endometrium
- Lack of calcification
- Lack of edge shadowing
- Myometrial cysts and small echogenic nodules distributed throughout the lesion
- Linear striations from endometrium into the myometrium
- No capsular flow on power Doppler but presence of palisading veins through the lesion

Until recently, adenomyosis was under-recognized in infertile women because the 2D images could sometimes be subjective and the definitive histologic diagnosis could only be made after hysterectomy. MRI imaging identified diagnostic features such as expanded JZ greater than 12 mm, lower signal strength compared with the surrounding myometrium, and bright discrete foci throughout the lesion as diagnostic features.[29] However, MRI is an expensive investigation and is not often now used for this diagnosis. The development of 3D ultrasound permitted study of the JZ and the spread of the adenomyotic tissue into the myometrium (**Fig. 10**). This technique has revealed the true prevalence of adenomyosis in women of reproductive age. In a study of 72 premenopausal women who had 2D/3D ultrasound before hysterectomy, the incidence of adenomyosis was 44.5%; 2D features were myometrial cysts and heterogeneous myometrium, and 3D features were JZ widening greater than or equal to 4 mm and myometrial infiltration.[30] In a meta-analysis of 8 studies on the likelihood of clinical pregnancy in infertile women with or without adenomyosis undergoing IVF/intracytoplasmic sperm injection,[31] there was a significantly reduced clinical pregnancy rate by more than 40% and increase in miscarriage rate by more than 40% in the adenomyosis arm. Treatment of severe generalized adenomyosis is difficult, but successful pregnancies have been obtained following gonadotropin-releasing hormone agonist therapy for several months. Localized adenomyosis close to the endometrium can be successfully resected with good results.[32]

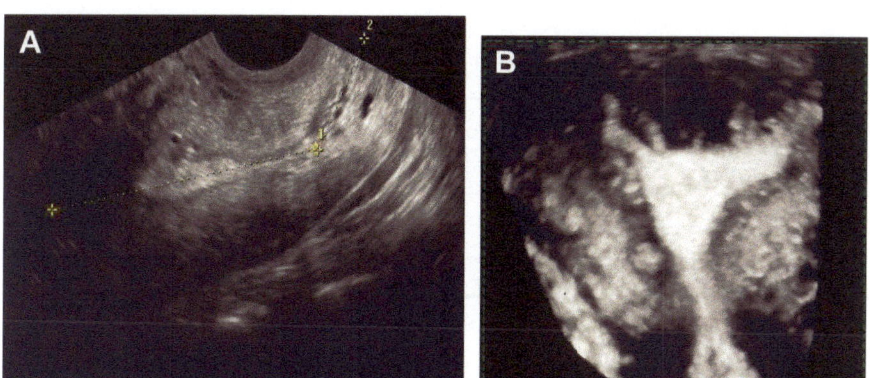


**Fig. 10.** (*A*) 2D image of uterus with (apparently) mild adenomyotic changes. (*B*) The 3D image shows marked adenomyosis with endometrium observed streaming into the junctional layer and myometrium.

### *Müllerian duct abnormalities*

The müllerian ducts differentiate in the fetus to form the fallopian tubes, uterus, the uterine cervix, and the superior aspect of the vagina. Normal development depends on the completion of 3 phases: organogenesis, fusion, and septal resorption.

The most commonly reported müllerian duct anomalies (MDAs) are septate, arcuate, didelphys, unicornuate, or hypoplastic uteri. Using the latest diagnostic techniques, the prevalence of MDAs is about 6.7% of the general population, 7.3% of the infertile population, and 16.7% of women with a history of recurrent miscarriage.[33] In the past, these anomalies were diagnosed by a combination of hysteroscopy or x-ray contrast hysterography to delineate cavity defects and laparoscopy to visualize any corporeal abnormalities of the uterine fundus. The diagnostic landscape has recently completely changed and it is generally accepted that MRI and 3D ultrasound are the optimal techniques because both, in a single examination, allow classification of both the cavity and corporeal defects. Both techniques have been compared and found to correlate closely in the diagnosis of cavity and corpus MDAs with a high degree of accuracy.[34] Because 3D ultrasound is part of the ultrasound investigation and is less expensive and more interactive, it is currently the method of choice, and MRI is reserved for when there are difficulties in the ultrasound examination. Any suspected diagnosis should be followed by investigation of the renal tract because the relationship of fusion defects and renal abnormalities is well documented, especially in women with unicornuate uterus.

The American Society for Reproductive Medicine (ASRM) classification[35] of MDAs is the one most widely used and may not be superseded by the European Society of Human Reproduction and Embryology (ESHRE)/European Society for Gynaecological Endoscopy (ESGE) classification,[36] which does away with the traditional terminology used by most gynecologists.

Essentially, the task of MRI and 3D ultrasound is to determine whether there is a serious dysmorphic defect, and to define the extent of the cavity defect in cases of resorption failure and the degree of separation of the uterine fundi in cases of fusion defects of the corpus. A meta-analysis on the impact of the most common defects on fertility and reproduction[37] is summarized in **Table 1**. Essentially, early miscarriage

**Table 1**
**Meta-analysis of effects of common müllerian abnormalities on reproduction: 9 studies involving 3805 women**

| Defect | Conception | First Trimester Misc | Second Trimester Misc | Preterm Birth | Malpresentation at Delivery |
|---|---|---|---|---|---|
| Arcuate | NS | NS | ** | NS | *** |
| Subseptate | NS | *** | NS | * | ** |
| Septate | NS | *** | ** | *** | *** |
| Bicornuate | NS | * | * | *** | *** |
| Didelphys | NS | NS | NS | *** | *** |
| Unicornuate | NS | * | NS | *** | ** |

*Abbreviations:* Misc, miscellaneous; NS, not significant.
* Some effect (*P*<.05).
** Moderate effect (*P*<.01).
*** Significant effect (*P*<.001).

*Adapted from* Chan YY, Jayaprakasan K, Tan A, et al. Reproductive outcomes in women with congenital uterine anomalies: a systematic review. Ultrasound Obstet Gynecol 2011;38(4):376; with permission.

is strongly related to septal defects, whereas the bicornuate uterus has a greater impact on preterm birth and malpresentation at delivery. Most interestingly, neither group of defects seems to be a cause of infertility. Fertility specialists should therefore focus on the prevention of miscarriage. Numerous studies have attested to the effectiveness of ultrasonography-guided hysteroscopic resection of the septum, but all are based on nonrandomized and mainly retrospective cohort trials with a high risk of bias. However, it is widely accepted that the procedure is indicated for women with a history of miscarriage and a septal defect.

A key diagnostic task is to distinguish a septal from a corporeal defect (ie, septate from bicornuate uterus), which makes a major difference in determining any approach to surgery. The ASRM defines the bicornuate uterus as having a fundal notch of greater than 1 cm[38]; other suggested criteria are a distance between the horns of more than 4 cm and an angulation between the horns of greater than 105°.[39] The significance of the septum can be determined by obtaining a coronal view showing both tubal ostia and drawing a line between them. If the distance from a vertical line from the interostial line to the fundus is less than that of the line to the lower part of the septum (ie, the septum exceeds 50% of the uterine wall thickness), then it is likely to be significant and differentiates it from the arcuate uterus, in which the ratio is reversed. The definition favored by the ASRM defines a septum as being greater than 1.5 cm from the interostial line and an angle of indentation at the apex of the septum of less than 90%.[38] Some authorities regard the arcuate uterus as a variation of normal and this diagnosis does not even feature in the ESHRE/ESGE classification, but it is worth noting these features because there could be some impact in the second and third trimesters of pregnancy, as shown in **Table 1**. Some examples of MDAs are given in **Figs. 11–13**.

## HYSTEROSALPINGO CONTRAST SONOGRAPHY

Determining the patency of the fallopian tubes is a fundamental examination in the fertility work-up. The investigation is performed unnecessarily in many patients in whom IVF is the preferred option; for example, in women who are more than 40 years

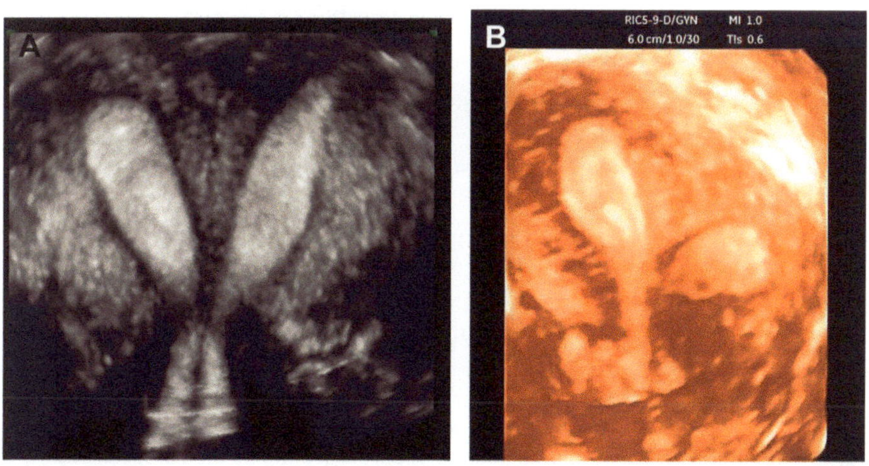


**Fig. 11.** (*A*) Complete septate uterus and cervix. Note the narrow angle of separation of the 2 cavities. (*B*) Partial bicornuate uterus. Note the wide angle of separation of the uterine horns.

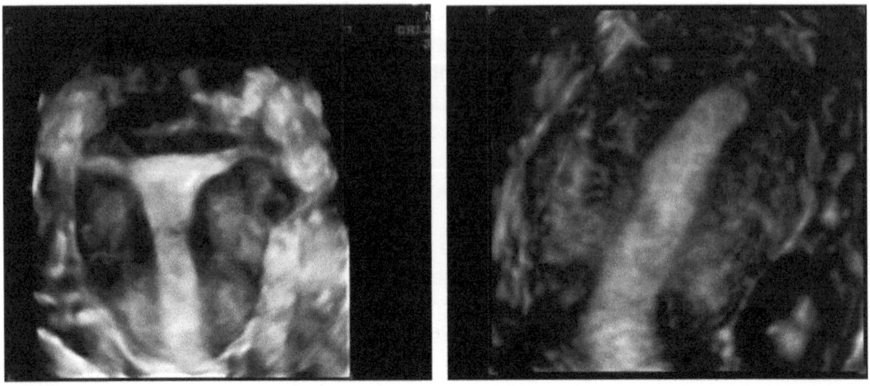

**Fig. 12.** T-shaped uterus classified as a dysmorphic anomaly associated with a high risk of miscarriage. Unicornuate uterus. There is a strong association of this defect with renal anomalies.

old or have low ovarian reserve. It is essential for couples who are not contemplating immediate treatment and for single women and same-sex couples who are having in utero insemination treatment.

In the past, the investigation was performed by x-ray hysterosalpingography (XHSG), but this test has been gradually overtaken by the ultrasonography-based hysterosalpingo contrast sonography (HyCoSy) test, which is usually performed by the familiar fertility team in the reproductive medicine department and avoids the problem of exposure to ionizing radiation. The optimal time for the test is in the proliferative phase of the cycle after day 7 to avoid the possibility of menstrual bleeding and of disturbing an early pregnancy. The TV procedure is usually performed in a sterile room or theater. A small balloon catheter (1–2 mL) is frequently inserted into the uterus to prevent leakage of contrast. Because positive contrast medium is not suitable for examining the uterine cavity, HyCoSy is usually

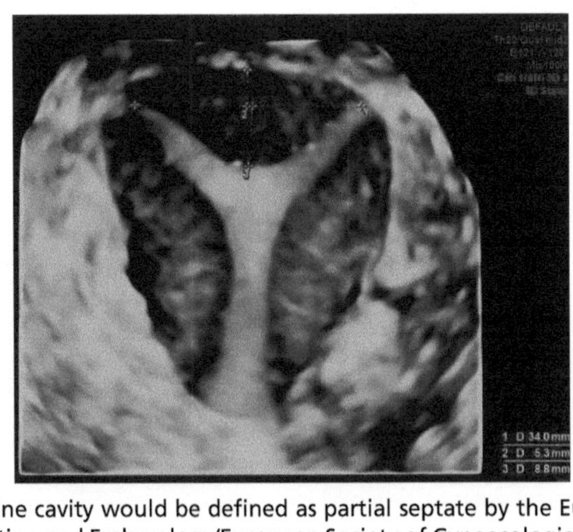

**Fig. 13.** This uterine cavity would be defined as partial septate by the European Society of Human Reproduction and Embryology/European Society of Gynaecological Oncology definition but arcuate by the ASRM definition. Note the narrow cavity angles at the ostia. A history of miscarriages would be required before surgery was recommended.

preceded by injection of a negative contrast such as saline, which helps to define cavity defects. It is then customary to inject a positive contrast medium of some kind. These media are based on the reflectivity of microbubbles held in suspension in a milky fluid so that that visual intratubal flow can be traced from the tubal ostia to the fimbrial end and also to show the spill of fluid in the peritoneum (**Fig. 14**). These contrast media can be expensive and merely shaking a saline solution in air provides enough bubbles to provide a diagnosis in most cases, although the contrast will be visible for a shorter time. The operator should be careful not to inject the contrast too quickly because this can induce a vasovagal attack in the patient, and small boluses of 2 mL usually suffice if the tubes are patent. In general, each side is visualized separately following a separate bolus. Because of the tortuosity of the tubes, it is rare to visualize the whole length of the tube, and much depends on the visualization of spill of contrast from the fimbrial end into the peritoneum. Even these echoes can sometimes be confused with bowel echoes. These problems can be minimized by the technique of automated 3D coded contrast HyCoSy,[40] which permits simultaneous visualization of both tubes throughout their lengths (**Fig. 15**). The technique requires expensive ultrasound equipment and software and the true strength of HyCoSy is that it is a quick, simple technique that rapidly confirms tubal patency and allows treatment to commence without delay. In this regard, it has high concordance with XHSG in showing tubal patency. However, there is a 10% false-positive rate for obstruction, so failure to identify patency should be followed up by laparoscopy and dye perturbation.[41] The procedure is well tolerated; severe pain can occur in about 15% of cases and is usually associated with tubal obstruction.

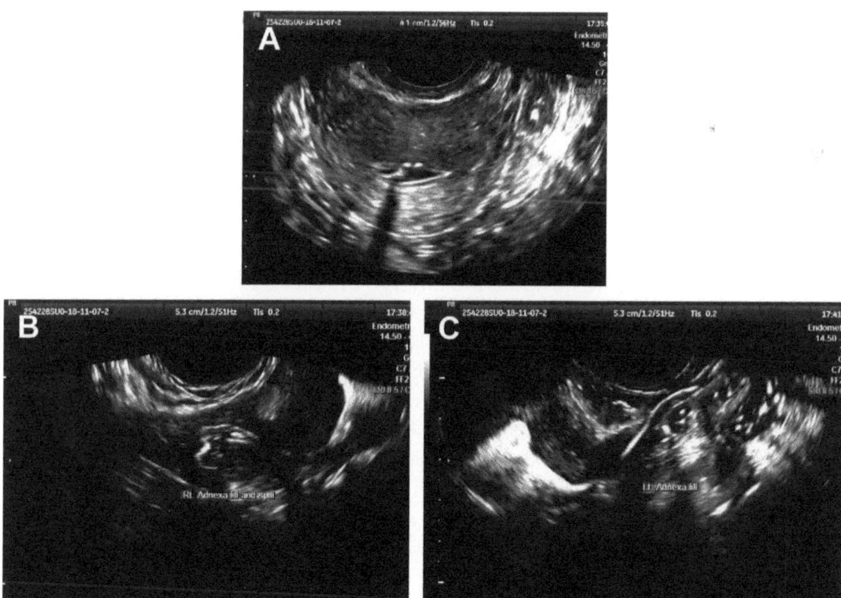


**Fig. 14.** HyCoSy procedure. (*A*) Cross section of the uterus with the catheter and negative contrast. (*B*) Right fallopian tube: the positive contrast can be seen outlining the tube with peritoneal spill visible. (*C*) Left fallopian tube: contrast can be seen outlining about half of the length of the tube. Peritoneal spill can be assumed by the presence of bubbles in the peritoneal cavity.

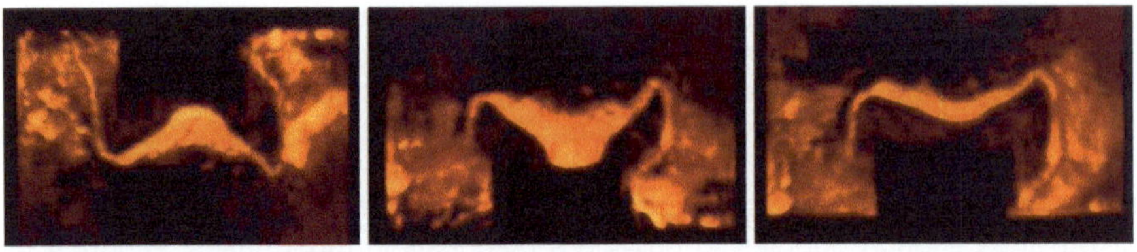

**Fig. 15.** Automated 3D coded contrast HyCoSy technique overcomes many of the problems associated with the conventional HyCoSy because it provides simultaneous improved imaging of both fallopian tubes and spill. (*From* Exacoustos C, Di Giovanni A, Szabolcs B, et al. Automated three-dimensional coded contrast imaging hysterosalpingo-contrast sonography: feasibility in office tubal patency testing. Ultrasound Obstet Gynecol 2013;41(3):330; with permission.)

### *Embryo Transfer*

The embryo transfer procedure is the culmination of IVF treatment and is a crucial step that can affect success or failure. Many centers restrict embryo transfers to a select few people with demonstrably "green fingers." For fresh transfers, the procedure is usually performed in an operating theater 3 to 6 days after the egg collection, the timing being influenced by whether the embryo is transferred at cleavage or blastocyst stage. FETs are now increasingly performed and for these it is usual to administer oral estrogen until the ET on ultrasound has reached 7 to 8 mm and then to add vaginal progesterone for the number of days proportional to the stage of development of the embryo being transferred.

The procedure is usually performed with only mild oral sedation and takes on average 15 to 20 minutes. The cardinal rules of the procedure are[42]:

- Avoid disruption of the endometrium by the catheter
- Minimize induction of the uterine contractions
- Protect the embryos
- Deposit the embryos in an optimal position within the uterine cavity

Ultrasound guidance of the catheter is usually performed transabdominally because it is difficult to perform the procedure transvaginally while a speculum is in the vagina. Therefore, the patient's bladder should be moderately full, which improves ultrasound visualization and helps to "straighten" the anteverted uterus. Transabdominal ultrasound helps the operator to navigate the embryo transfer catheter through the internal cervical os, especially in patients with acutely anteverted or retroverted uteri or a long cervical canal. The operator can use this information to mold the tip of the embryo catheter to match that of the patient's uterocervical angle and decrease difficult or bloody entries and transfers.[43] It also allows direct visualization of the catheter tip during the entire passage to avoid disruption of the endometrium. Embryo transfers performed using abdominal ultrasound guidance have been shown to increase pregnancy rates by 4% to 8% compared with the clinical touch method[44] and to reduce the number of difficult transfers.

## SUMMARY

Ultrasound now plays a pivotal role in the investigation and management of the female partner in infertile couples. The development of high-resolution ultrasound equipment with 3D imaging and color Doppler has meant that ultrasound can now give important information on ovarian function and has supplanted other imaging techniques such as MRI and radiology as the first-line investigative technique for uterine and tubal abnormalities. There is now a need for advanced ultrasound training to take center stage in fellowship training programs in reproductive medicine.

**ACKNOWLEDGMENTS**

I would like to thank Professor Geeta Nargund for her inspirational support and Create Fertility for providing the equipment for this work.

**REFERENCES**

1. Torry DS, Leavenworth J, Chang M, et al. Angiogenesis in implantation. J Assist Reprod Genet 2007;24:303–15.
2. Chen SL, Wu FR, Luo C, et al. Combined analysis of endometrial thickness and pattern in predicting outcome of in vitro fertilization and embryo transfer: a retrospective cohort study. Reprod Biol Endocrinol 2010;8:30.
3. Raine-Fenning NJ, Campbell BK, Clewes JS, et al. Defining endometrial growth during the menstrual cycle with three-dimensional ultrasound. BJOG 2004;111: 944–9.
4. Bakos O, Lundkvist O, Wide L, et al. Ultrasonographical and hormonal description of the normal ovulatory menstrual cycle. Acta Obstet Gynecol Scand 1994; 73(10):790–6.
5. Laasch C, Puscheck E. Cumulative embryo score, not endometrial thickness, is best for pregnancy prediction in IVF. J Assist Reprod Genet 2004;21:47–50.
6. Richter KS, Bugge KR, Bromer JG, et al. Relationship between endometrial thickness and embryo implantation, based on 1,294 cycles of in vitro fertilization with transfer of two blastocyst-stage embryos. Fertil Steril 2007;87(1):53–9.
7. Zhao J, Zhang Q, Li Y. The effect of endometrial thickness and pattern measured by ultrasonography on pregnancy outcomes during IVF-ET cycles. Reprod Biol Endocrinol 2012;10:100.
8. Schild RL, Knobloch C, Dorn C, et al. Endometrial receptivity in an in vitro fertilization program as assessed by spiral artery blood flow, endometrial thickness, endometrial volume, and uterine artery blood flow. Fertil Steril 2001;75:361–6.
9. Wu Y, Gao X, Lu X, et al. Endometrial thickness affects the outcome of in vitro fertilization and embryo transfer in normal responders after GnRH antagonist administration. Reprod Biol Endocrinol 2014;12:96.
10. Traub ML, Van Arsdale A, Pal L, et al. Endometrial thickness, Caucasian ethnicity, and age predict clinical pregnancy following fresh blastocyst embryo transfer: a retrospective cohort. Reprod Biol Endocrinol 2009;7:33.
11. Zhang T, Li Z, Ren X, et al. Endometrial thickness as a predictor of the reproductive outcomes in fresh and frozen embryo transfer cycles: A retrospective cohort study of 1512 IVF cycles with morphologically good-quality blastocyst. Medicine (Baltimore) 2018;97(4):e9689.
12. Chien LW, Au HK, Chen PL, et al. Assessment of uterine receptivity by the endometrial-subendometrial blood flow distribution pattern in women undergoing in vitro fertilization-embryo transfer. Fertil Steril 2002;78(2):245–51.
13. Wang L, Qiao J, Li R, et al. Role of endometrial blood flow assessment with color Doppler energy in predicting pregnancy outcome of IVF-ET cycles. Reprod Biol Endocrinol 2010;8:122.
14. Zaidi J, Campbell S, Pittrof R, et al. Endometrial thickness, morphology, vascular penetration and velocimetry in predicting implantation in an in vitro fertilization program. Ultrasound Obstet Gynecol 1995;6(3):191–8.

15. Levi-Setti PE, Rognoni G, Bozzo M, et al. Color-Doppler velocimetry of uterine arteries in pregnant and nonpregnant patients during multiovulation induction for IVF. J Assist Reprod Genet 1995;12(7):413–7.
16. Steer CV, Campbell S, Tan SL, et al. The use of transvaginal color flow imaging after in vitro fertilization to identify optimum uterine conditions before embryo transfer. Fertil Steril 1992;57:372–6.
17. Bosteels J, van Wessel S, Weyers S, et al. Hysteroscopy for treating subfertility associated with suspected major uterine cavity abnormalities. Cochrane Database Syst Rev 2018;12:CD009461.
18. de Wit W, Gowrising CJ, Kuik DJ, et al. Only hydrosalpinges visible on ultrasound are associated with reduced implantation and pregnancy rates after in-vitro fertilization. Hum Reprod 1998;13(6):1696–701.
19. Cohen MC, Lindheim SR, Sauer MV. Hydrosalpinges adversely affect implantation in donor oocyte cycles. Hum Reprod 1999;14(4):1087–9.
20. Tsiami A, Chaimani A, Mavridis D, et al. Surgical treatment for hydrosalpinx prior to in-vitro fertilization embryo transfer: a network meta-analysis. Ultrasound Obstet Gynecol 2016;48:434–45.
21. Griffiths AN, Watermeyer SR, Klentzeris LD. Fluid within the endometrial cavity in an IVF cycle—a novel approach to its management. J Assist Reprod Genet 2002; 19(6):298–301.
22. Verguts T, Amaye L, Bourne T, et al. Normative data for uterine size according to age and gravidity and possible role of the classical golden ratio. Ultrasound Obstet Gynecol 2013;42:713–7.
23. Ahrendt HJ, Tylkoski H, Rabe T, et al. Prevalence of uterine myomas in women in Germany: data of an epidemiological study. Arch Gynecol Obstet 2016;293(6): 1243–53.
24. Brady PC, Stanic AK, Styra AK. Uterine fibroids and subfertility: an update on the role of myomectomy. Curr Opin Obstet Gynecol 2013;25:255–9.
25. Bajekal N, Li TC. Fibroids, infertility and pregnancy wastage. Hum Reprod Update 2000;6:614–22.
26. Casini ML, Rossi F, Agostini R, et al. Effects of the position of fibroids on fertility. Gynecol Endocrinol 2006;22:106–9.
27. Sunkara SK, Khairy M, El-Toukhy T, et al. The effect of intramural fibroids without uterine cavity involvement on the outcome of IVF treatment: a systematic review and meta-analysis. Hum Reprod 2010;25:418–29.
28. Somigliana E, Vercellini P, Daguati R, et al. Fibroids and female reproduction: a critical analysis of the evidence. Hum Reprod Update 2007;13:465–76.
29. Novellas S, Chassang M, Delotte J, et al. MRI characteristics of the uterine junctional zone: from normal to the diagnosis of adenomyosis. AJR Am J Roentgenol 2011;196(5):1206–13.
30. Exacoustos C, Brienza L, Di Giovanni A, et al. Adenomyosis: three-dimensional sonographic findings of the junctional zone and correlation with histology. Ultrasound Obstet Gynecol 2011;37(4):471–9.
31. Vercellini P, Consonni D, Dridi D, et al. Uterine adenomyosis and in vitro fertilization outcome: a systematic review and meta-analysis. Hum Reprod 2014;29(5): 964–77.
32. Gordts S, Campo R, Brosens I. Hysteroscopic diagnosis and excision of myometrial cystic adenomyosis. Gynecol Surg 2014;11(4):273–8.
33. Saravelos SH, Cocksedge KA, Li T-C. Prevalence and diagnosis of congenital uterine anomalies in women with reproductive failure: a critical appraisal. Hum Reprod Update 2008;14:415–29.

34. Graupera P, Pascual MA, Hereter L, et al. Accuracy of three-dimensional ultrasound compared with magnetic resonance imaging in diagnosis of Mullerian duct anomalies using ESHRE–ESGE consensus on the classification of congenital anomalies of the female genital tract. Ultrasound Obstet Gynecol 2015;46: 616–22.
35. The American Fertility Society classifications of adnexal adhesions, distal tubal occlusion, tubal occlusion secondary to tubal ligation, tubal pregnancies, mullerian anomalies and intrauterine adhesions. Fertil Steril 1988;49(6):944–55.
36. Grimbizis GF, Gordts F, Sardo ADS, et al. The ESHRE–ESGE consensus on the classification of female genital tract congenital anomalies. Hum Reprod 2013; 28:2032–44.
37. Chan YY, Jayaprakasan K, Tan A, et al. Reproductive outcomes in women with congenital uterine anomalies: a systematic review. Ultrasound Obstet Gynecol 2011;38:371–82.
38. Practice Committee of the American Society for Reproductive Medicine. Uterine septum: a guideline. Fertil Steril 2016;106(3):530–40.
39. Spanish Infertility SWOT Group (SISG), Checa MA, Bellver J, Bosch E, et al. Hysteroscopic septum resection and reproductive medicine: A SWOT analysis. Reprod Biomed Online 2018;37(6):709–15.
40. Exacoustos C, Di Giovanni A, Szabolcs B, et al. Automated three-dimensional coded contrast hysterosalpingo-contrast-sonography: feasibility in office tubal patency testing. Ultrasound Obstet Gynecol 2013;41:328–35.
41. Campbell S, Bourne T, Tan SL, et al. Hysterosalpingo contrast sonography (hyCoSy) and its future role within in the investigation of infertility in Europe. Ultrasound Obstet Gynecol 1994;4:25–253.
42. Tıras B, Cenksoy PO. Practice of embryo transfer: recommendations during and after. Semin Reprod Med 2014;32:291–6.
43. Sallam HN, Agameya AE, Rahman AF, et al. Ultrasound measurement of the uterocervical angle before embryo transfer: a prospective controlled study. Hum Reprod 2002;17:1767–72.
44. Sallam HN, Sadek SS. Ultrasound-guided embryo transfer: a meta-analysis of randomized controlled trials. Fertil Steril 2003;80(4):1042–6.

# Ultrasonography in Pelvic Floor Dysfunction

Hadas Allouche Kam, MD[a], Simcha Yagel, MD[b,c,*], Vered H. Eisenberg, MD, MHA[d,e]

**KEYWORDS**

- Transperineal ultrasonography • Pelvic floor imaging • OASI • Levator trauma
- Avulsion defect

**KEY POINTS**

- Obstetric anal sphincter injury (OASI) and levator ani muscle (LAM) trauma are common disorders in parous women.
- Ultrasonography enables an anatomic and functional assessment of the pelvic floor with dynamic and static imaging.
- Four sonographic signs can be detected in OASI: external and/or internal anal sphincter discontinuity; thickening of the external anal sphincter (EAS) at the area of repair; thinning of the internal anal sphincter (IAS) in the area of rupture in conjunction with thickening opposite the rupture site ("half-moon" sign); and abnormality of the mucous folds ("mucosal star" sign).
- Levator ani trauma can be asymptomatic; abnormality may arise years later with levator hiatus enlargement.
- Discontinuity of the levator ani muscle, levator avulsion, is the main sonographic sign, along with increased hiatal area, called hiatal ballooning in severe cases.

## INTRODUCTION TO TRANSPERINEAL ULTRASONOGRAPHY

### *Indications for Transperineal Ultrasonography*

Ultrasonography enables an anatomic and functional assessment of the pelvic floor with dynamic as well as static imaging. The common reasons for referrals for pelvic floor ultrasonography are evaluation of the anal sphincter after obstetric anal sphincter

Disclosure Statement: The authors have nothing to disclose.
[a] Department of Obstetrics and Gynecology, Hadassah Mount Scopus – Hebrew University Medical Center Jerusalem, PO Box 24035, Mt Scopus, Jerusalem 91240, Israel; [b] Department of Obstetrics and Gynecology, Hadassah – Hebrew University Medical Centers, PO Box 24035, Mt Scopus, Jerusalem 91240, Israel; [c] Obstetrics and Gynecology Ultrasound Unit, Jerusalem, Israel; [d] Department of Obstetrics and Gynecology, Sheba Medical Center, Tel Hashomer 5265601, Israel; [e] Sackler Faculty of Medicine, Tel Aviv University, Tel Aviv, Israel
* Corresponding author. Department of Obstetrics and Gynecology, Hadassah-Hebrew University Medical Centers, PO Box 24035, Mt Scopus, Jerusalem 91240, Israel.
*E-mail address:* simcha.yagel@gmail.com

Obstet Gynecol Clin N Am 46 (2019) 715–732
https://doi.org/10.1016/j.ogc.2019.07.006 obgyn.theclinics.com

injury (OASI) or evaluation of the levator ani in women with a history of OASI, or those complaining of cystocele, rectocele, or uterine prolapse. Pelvic floor imaging is currently preformed in specialized urogynecology centers, and few sonographers are familiar with the technique in comparison with obstetric sonography.

## *Technical Overview*

### *Machine type and requirements*

A 2-dimensional ultrasound examination may be performed with any machine of good resolution, preferably a B-mode ultrasound machine equipped with cine-loop function, convex transducers of 3 to 6 MHz, and a field of view of at least 70°. The area is scanned in the transverse and sagittal planes. When the probe is appropriately placed in the midsagittal plane, the pelvic floor will be fully visualized.

The transvaginal and transabdominal probes each have advantages and disadvantages, and their use depends mostly on operator preference. The transvaginal probe provides better resolution and higher-quality imaging, but its drawback is decreased visualization at the 12 o'clock position. In addition, the transvaginal probe requires pressure on the fourchette to prevent the probe from sliding backward, which may cause patient discomfort and may disrupt full visualization of the distal part of the sphincter. The transabdominal probe allows better visualization at the 12 o'clock position as well as a thorough examination of the pelvic floor, simply by tilting the transducer.

### *Preparation of the probes*

One should cover the transducer with a nonpowdered glove, condom, or thin plastic wrap to maintain asepsis. The powder in gloves can produce reverberations that impair image quality and are therefore to be avoided. In compliance with multiple ultrasound societies, disinfection of internal transducers with high-level disinfectants is necessary between patients.[1]

### *Preparation of the patient*

The patient must void before the examination, although bowel emptying is not mandatory. The patient reclines in the dorsal lithotomy position with the hips flexed and slightly abducted. Bringing the heels closer to the buttocks can assist by improving the pelvic tilt. Imaging is performed at rest, during maximal Valsalva maneuver, and during maximal pelvic floor muscle contraction (PFMC).

## *Basic Pelvic Ultrasonography*

### *Two-dimensional ultrasonography assessment*

Although obesity usually does not interfere with imaging, scar tissue or mesh implants may impair visibility. A standard midsagittal image can be obtained by placing the transducer on the perineum to reveal, from anterior to posterior: the symphysis pubis, bladder and urethra, vagina, distal part of the rectum with the anorectal junction, and proximal part of the anal canal (**Figs. 1–3**). The hyperechoic structure visualized further posterior to the anorectal junction is the puborectalis sling.[2]

Parasagittal or transverse views can provide additional information, such as visualization of the urethra, puborectalis muscle attachment, and depiction of mesh implants. Vaginal prolapse, the pubic bone, or rectocele may cause artifacts and acoustic shadowing, which can obscure the posterior compartment or the vaginal apex.

### *Three-dimensional ultrasonography assessment*

Three-dimensional ultrasonography (3DUS) is currently the standard of care for pelvic floor imaging. Among its modalities, 3DUS provides tomographic multislice imaging in

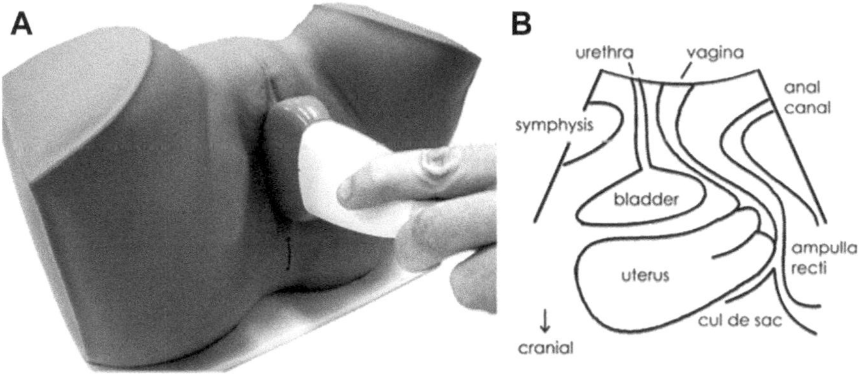


**Fig. 1.** (*A*) Transducer placement and (*B*) field of view in the midsagittal plane when using a curved array transducer designed for abdominal or obstetric applications. (*From* Dietz HP. Pelvic floor ultrasound: a review. Am J Obstet Gynecol 2010;202(4):322; with permission.)

a chosen plane, which produces a picture resembling computed tomography scanning, called tomographic ultrasound imaging (TUI). TUI enables extensive assessment of the entire puborectalis muscle and its attachment to the pubic rami, measurement of the diameter and area of the levator hiatus, and determination of the degree of hiatal

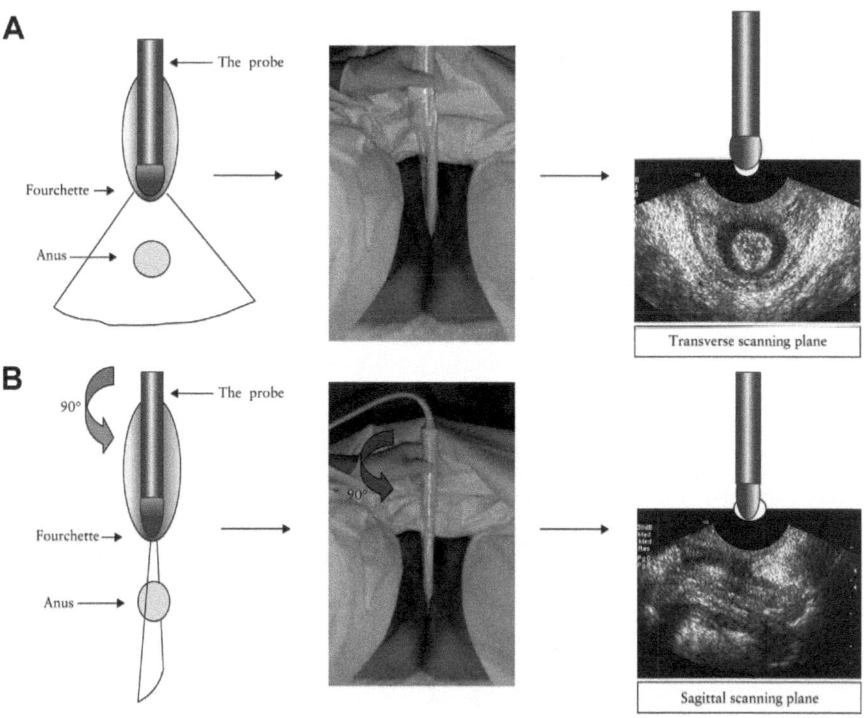


**Fig. 2.** The technique of the anal sphincter ultrasound examination. (*A*) The vaginal ultrasound probe is placed in the fourchette of the vaginal introitus to obtain the transverse section of the anal sphincter. (*B*) Turning the vaginal ultrasound probe 90°, the sagittal section is obtained. (*From* Timor-Tritsch IE, Monteagudo A, Smilen SW, et al. Simple ultrasound evaluation of the anal sphincter in female patients using a transvaginal transducer. Ultrasound Obstet Gynecol 2005;25(2):178; with permission.)

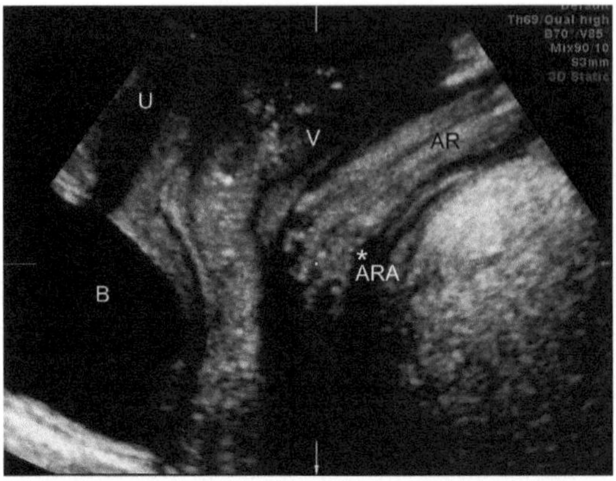


Fig. 3. Sagittal plane of the pelvic floor. The optimal plane shows the urinary bladder (B), urethra (U), and vagina (V) along their entire lengths, and the anorectal angle (ARA). The anorectum (AR) is visualized to its maximum length. (*From* Valsky DV, Yagel S. Three-dimensional transperineal ultrasonography of the pelvic floor. J Ultrasound Med 2007;26:1375; with permission.)

distension on Valsalva maneuver.[3] This technique enables volume ultrasound storage and assessment without the patient being present, which can shorten examination time for the patient and allow for second opinion consultation when necessary.

## OBSTETRIC ANAL SPHINCTER INJURY ASSESSMENT

### *Background*

The anal sphincter complex consists of the external and internal anal sphincters (EAS and IAS, respectively) separated by a longitudinal smooth muscle (LSM) and the puborectalis part of the levator ani muscle (LAM)[4] (**Fig. 4**). The IAS, a continuation of the circular smooth muscle of the bowel, ends at the junction of the superficial and subcutaneous part of the EAS.[5] Sympathetic innervation is via L5 and parasympathetic innervation via S2 to S4. The IAS accounts for 50% to 85% of the resting

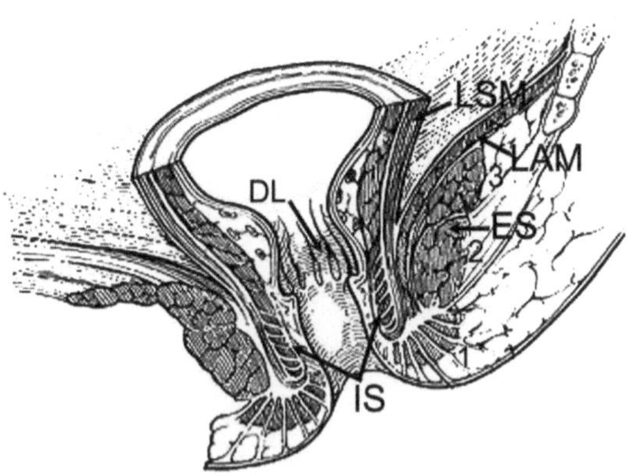


Fig. 4. Schematic diagram of the anal sphincter complex. DL, dentate line; LAM, levator ani muscle; LSM, longitudinal smooth muscle. Portions of the external sphincter (ES): 1, subcutaneous; 2, superficial; 3, deep. (*From* Valsky DV, Yagel S. Three-dimensional transperineal ultrasonography of the pelvic floor. J Ultrasound Med 2007;26:1380; with permission.)

pressure and the EAS is innervated by the inferior rectal branch of the pudendal nerve, and contributes 15% to 30% of the resting anal pressure and 70% of the squeeze anal pressure.[5]

***Definition (classification of obstetric anal sphincter injury assessment)***

OASIs are classified into 4 degrees of injury, as depicted in **Fig. 5**.

First- and second-degree lacerations include those involving skin and perineal muscles but not the anal sphincter. Third-degree lacerations are further subdivided into 3 subcategories. The 3A and 3B subtypes involve the EAS (to an extent lesser or greater than 50%, respectively), whereas the 3C subtype involves the IAS. A fourth-degree tear resembles a 3C subtype, combined with disruption of the anal mucosa.

***Risk factors, clinical significance, and prevalence of obstetric anal sphincter injury assessment***

In cases of a suspected third-degree anal tear, a digital examination is performed for assessment of the anal muscles. The 1998 to 2010 US Nationwide Inpatient Sample reported a third-degree laceration rate of 3.3% and fourth-degree laceration rate of 1.1% for women who had vaginal deliveries.[6] Clinically, anal sphincter tears are detected in 0.36% to 8.4% of all deliveries.[7,8] Unrecognized or occult sphincter damage is far more common, estimated at 11.5% to 35.4% among primiparous women.[9–11]

Known risk factors for OASI are primiparity, birth weight greater than 4 kg, occipitoposterior position at delivery, and instrumental delivery.[12] Forceps delivery was associated with a 4- to 10-fold increased risk of OASI, and vacuum extraction with up to a 2-fold increased risk, compared with noninstrumental deliveries.[13,14] The

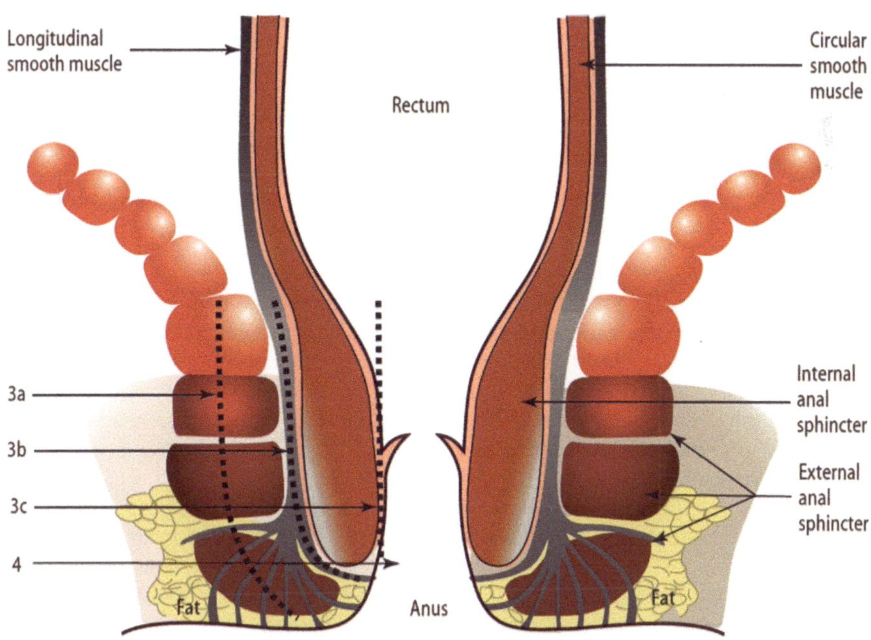


**Fig. 5.** Schematic representation of obstetric anal sphincter injuries. (*From* Sultan AH, Kettle C. Diagnosis of perineal trauma. In: Sultan AH, Thakar R, Fenner DE, editors. Perineal and anal sphincter trauma. London: Springer London; 2009; with permission.)

use of a mediolateral episiotomy during both vacuum delivery and forceps delivery is associated with a 5- to 10-fold reduction in the rate of OASI in primiparous and multiparous women but not in noninstrumental delivery.[15]

The long-term complications of OASI include anal incontinence (AI), rectovaginal fistula, and pain. The true prevalence of AI related to OASI may be underestimated. The reported rates of AI following the primary repair of OASI range between 15% and 61%, with a mean of 39%.[16] A prospective follow-up of 125 women with OASI reported a significantly increased incidence of anal incontinence (*P*<.001) in women who had 3B to fourth-degree tears, in comparison with women having 3A tears.[17] The risk of a third- or fourth-degree tear in a subsequent delivery is 3% to 7%. All women should be counseled regarding the mode of delivery, and an elective cesarean section may be considered with a history of a prior fourth-degree tear.[6,18–20] Early recognition and surgical repair of OASI will substantially reduce AI.[21]

## *Ultrasonographic Approach*

In the past decade, transperineal ultrasonography (TPUS) has emerged as an effective modality to evaluate anal sphincter injuries. Previously these images were usually evaluated by endoanal ultrasonography (EAUS), but EAUS requires specialized equipment. Its high cost and relative invasiveness prompted clinicians to explore alternative imaging techniques, such as TPUS. Further research comparing these modalities is needed.[22–24] The current understanding is that TPUS is comparable with EAUS, especially for IAS assessment. Although EAUS is considered the gold standard among gastroenterologists and colorectal surgeons, the painless, noninvasive nature of TPUS, its acceptability among patients, and its clinical applicability make it a feasible alternative to EAUS. Another advantage of TPUS is that contrary to the endoanal approach, which by the insertion of the transducer may distort the anal canal, the transperineal approach, using either a vaginal or an abdominal probe, does not cause distortion by the transducer and enables evaluation of the anal sphincter and mucosa in the resting position.

## *Practical Issues*

### *Timing of examination*

To allow the edema commonly present in the immediate postpartum to subside, the examination is best performed at least 10 to 12 weeks postpartum.

### *Methodology of anal sphincter assessment*

Using either a vaginal or an abdominal probe, the examination begins with placement of the transducer on the fourchette and perineal body. In a midsagittal scan, the anorectum will be fully visualized, with the anal verge on one side of the screen and the anorectal angle on the other (**Fig. 6**). Image directions can be reversed as long as consistency is maintained. Rendering is initiated with the 2D transverse view positioned 1.5 cm from the distal margin of the anus, where the characteristic star shape of the anal mucosa can be visualized.

The anterior and posterior aspects of the IAS are seen as 2 well-defined, almost parallel hypoechoic structures, approximately 2 to 4 mm in width and approximately 4 cm in length.[25]

Postprocessing is best performed with the transverse plane in the A frame of the multiplanar projection screen. The image is adjusted with the x-, y-, and z-axis sliders to display the (A) transverse, (B) sagittal, and (C) coronal planes for optimal evaluation of sphincter integrity (**Fig. 7**). The navigation dot is placed in the middle of the anal mucosa. The EAS and IAS widths can be measured in the A plane, 1.5 cm from the distal

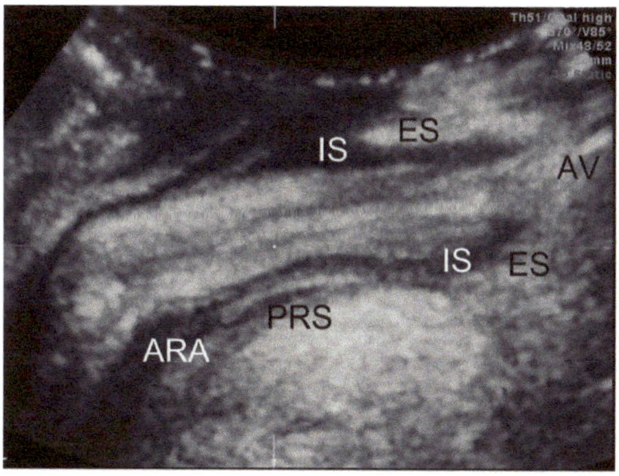


**Fig. 6.** Normal midsagittal scanning plane of the anal sphincter complex. The internal sphincter (IS) is visualized as a hypoechoic line on the sagittal scan; the external sphincter (ES) is depicted as an area of mixed echogenicity surrounding the IS. Note that the ES begins before the IS, and the superior portion of the ES is shorter than the inferior portion, which continues into the puborectal sling (PRS). ARA, anorectal angle; AV, anal verge. (*From* Valsky DV, Yagel S. Three-dimensional transperineal ultrasonography of the pelvic floor. J Ultrasound Med 2007;26:1381; with permission.)

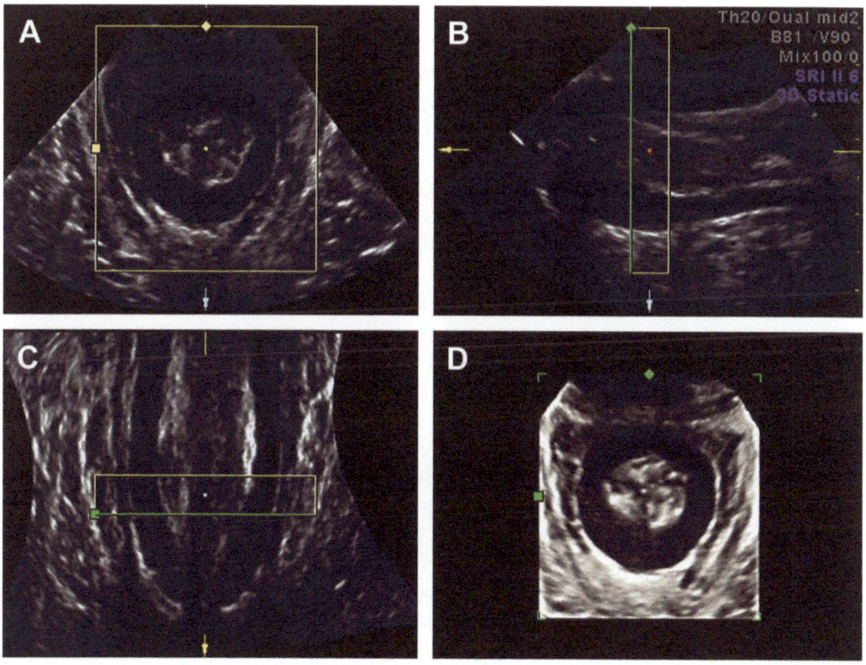


**Fig. 7.** Multiplanar reconstruction of a 3D TPUS scan of the normal posterior compartment. The volume is acquired in the transverse plane (shown in the A plane of the multiplanar reformatting [MPR] screen). The images in the B and C planes are adjusted along the x, y, and z axes to optimize the orthogonal sagittal plane for anal sphincter complex assessment. To obtain the optimal rendered image (*D* plane), the bounding box is placed tightly around the region of interest in the B plane, with the active side (green) set from anterior to posterior. The slice thickness is set to the thinnest feasible to avoid missing small findings. (*From* Valsky DV, Yagel S. Three-dimensional transperineal ultrasonography of the pelvic floor. J Ultrasound Med 2007;26:1382; with permission.)

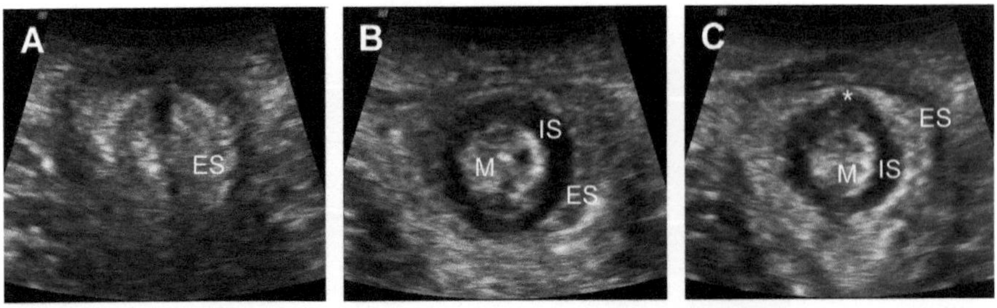


**Fig. 8.** (*A, B*) Normal transverse scanning planes of the anal sphincter complex (*A*) at the anal verge and the external sphincter (ES) (*B*) at the midpoint of the anal canal, where measurements are usually taken. M indicates mucous folds. (*C*) In the most proximal area to the anorectal junction, normal anatomic thinning of the ES (*asterisk*) should not be misconstrued as a defect. IS, internal sphincter. (*From* Valsky DV, Yagel S. Three-dimensional transperineal ultrasonography of the pelvic floor. J Ultrasound Med 2007;26:1382; with permission.)

margin of the anus. The puborectalis muscle is visualized as a U-shaped echogenic area surrounding the EAS posteriorly near the anorectal junction, forming the anorectal angle (see **Fig. 6**; **Fig. 8**). The transverse perinei muscles (superficial and deep) can be visualized superior/cephalad to the EAS in the A plane. Other postprocessing modalities such as TUI can be applied (**Fig. 9**). Nine sequential imaging slices of the anal sphincter in the transverse plane are displayed in a $3 \times 3$ matrix. This will suffice in most cases, since the EAS anteriorly rarely exceeds a length of 3 cm; therefore, an interslice interval of 2 mm allows full view of the sphincter length as well as a thorough assessment of any sphincter defect.

### *Sonographic signs of damage to the anal sphincter*

A defect in the EAS is suspected when discontinuity in the hyperechogenic ring is observed, whether affecting the whole or only part of the EAS thickness. One must keep in mind that the anterior EAS is 0.5 to 1 cm shorter than the posterior when integrity of the EAS is assessed in the most proximal area near the anorectal junction, so that normal variant anatomy is not misconstrued as an EAS defect (**Fig. 10**). The minimal accepted requirements for diagnosis are that a defect is seen in 3 central slices of the TUI image, but assessment of all the slices of the TUI is mandatory to minimize false-positive and false-negative results. The size of the defect is measured with a generic 2-line angle from the postprocessing program menu, with the angle vertex placed in the center of the anal mucosa (**Fig. 11**). A significant residual defect is defined as $\geq 30°$ on the clock face, seen on the ultrasonogram on at least 3 slices.[26]

As the authors have previously published, 4 sonographic signs can be detected: EAS or IAS sphincter discontinuity; thickening of the EAS at the area of repair; thinning of the IAS in the area of rupture in conjunction with thickening opposite the rupture site (the "half-moon" sign); and the "mucosal star sign"[11] (**Fig. 12**). The mucosal star sign was first described by Timor-Tritsch and colleagues.[27] It is seen on transverse sections and accounts for an abnormality of the mucosal folds, which appear as an asymmetric star.

### *Reporting*

The examination report might resemble the form reported by Eisenberg and colleagues[28]: "Using an abdominal (or a vaginal) probe, the anal canal was visualized

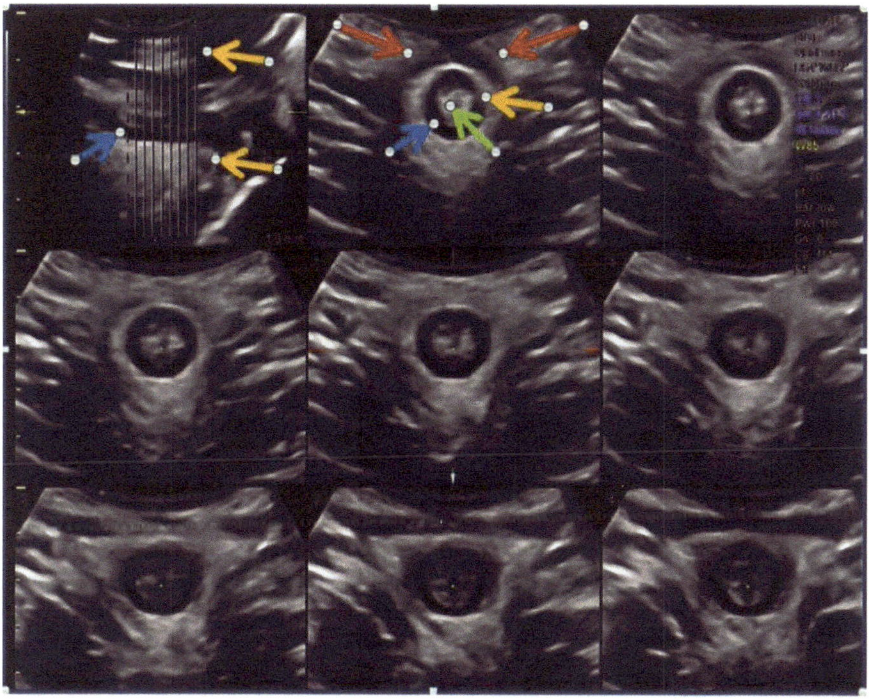

**Fig. 9.** Tomographic ultrasound imaging of external anal sphincter (EAS) using a transabdominal probe. Longitudinal plane encompassing the entire length of the EAS is used as reference frame (*upper left image*). Interslice interval is set at 2 mm, but can be adjusted further as necessary. Sphincter is normal in all transverse slices. Arrows depict: transverse perinei muscles (*red*); external anal sphincter (*yellow*); internal anal sphincter (*blue*); and anal mucosa (*green*). Moving the region of interest to the left would yield the subcutaneous part of the sphincter. (*From* Eisenberg VH, Valsky DV, Yagel S. Transperineal ultrasound assessment of the anal sphincter after obstetric anal sphincter injury (OASI). Ultrasound Obstet Gynecol 2019;53(2):158–65; with permission.)

in its entirety with transperineal 3D sonography. In the longitudinal section the length of the EAS is 10 mm. In the transverse section there is a residual full thickness defect between 10 to 14 hours in the EAS, corresponding to 120° of the clock face, which can be visualized in all sections of the TUI (2 mm interslice interval). The IAS and mucosal folds appear normal. The measurements in the 12 o'clock position are: EAS—not present, IAS 2 mm, transverse perinei muscles 5 mm."

## LEVATOR ANI ASSESSMENT

### *Background*

The pelvic floor mainly consists of a musculotendinous sheet called the LAM. The levator ani originates from the pubis and arcus tendineus anteriorly and ischial spines laterally. It inserts to the coccyx and to the midline area of the pelvic floor.[25] The LAM is subdivided into the iliococcygeus, pubococcygeus, and ischiococcygeus. The pubococcygeus, also known as the pubovisceral muscle, is further subdivided into the pubourethralis, pubovaginalis, and puborectalis, through which pass the urethra, vagina, and rectum, respectively. Therefore, the pubococcygeus muscle plays an important role in formation of the sphincters of these organs.[4]

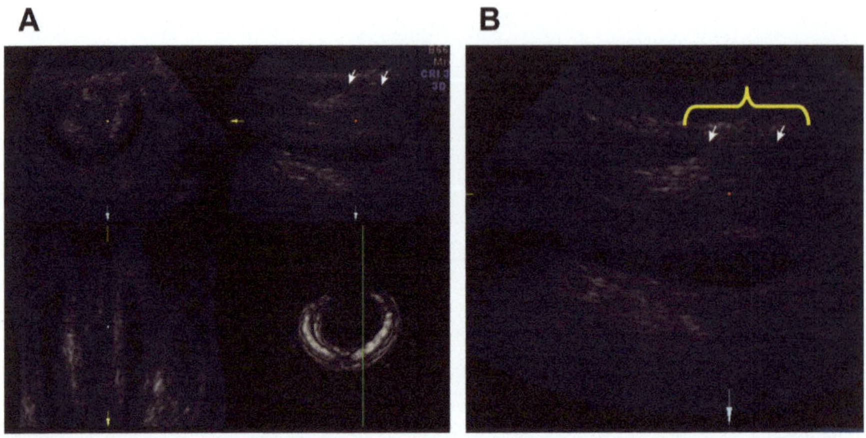


**Fig. 10.** (*A*) Multiplanar projection of a sphincter tear. Arrows mark the tear in the A plane. Compare the inversion mode–rendered image at the bottom left of the MPR image; note the disruption of the anal sphincter and the mucous fold pattern, which are distorted toward the defect. (*B*) Sagittal plane enlarged. Note the defect in the IS (bracket). Examination of this plane allows for localization and assessment of the defect. (*Adapted from* Valsky DV, Yagel S. Three-dimensional transperineal ultrasonography of the pelvic floor. J Ultrasound Med 2007;26:1383; with permission.)

The LAM has a constant tone providing support to the pelvic floor and is capable of relaxation during voiding and defecation, and contraction in cases of increased abdominal pressure such as during coughing and sneezing. During vaginal delivery the LAM stretches up to 3.3 times its initial length to enable passage of the fetus.[29,30]

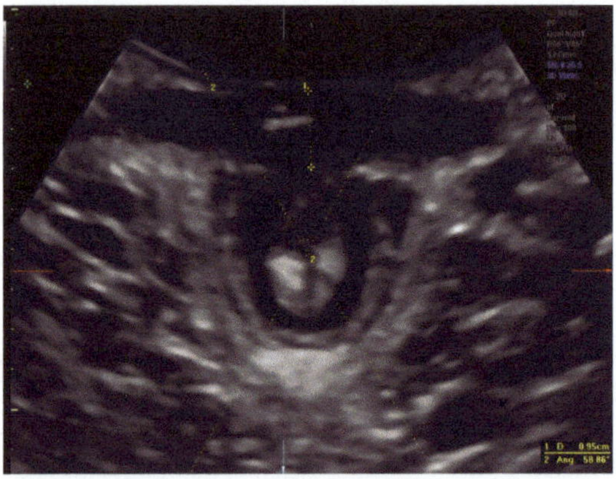

**Fig. 11.** Tomographic ultrasound imaging (TUI) applied to a 3D TPUS acquired volume (using a transabdominal probe) of the anal sphincter complex. The interslice interval is set to 2 mm. The size of the defect is measured with a generic angle from the menu using a 2-line angle with the angle vertex placed at the center of the anal mucosa, corresponding here to 59°. The EAS and IAS are missing at 12 o'clock. The transverse perinei muscles measure 9.5 mm. The transverse perinei muscles are seen here as hypoechoic rather than the usual hyperechoic characteristics, resulting from residual scar tissue following repair and resolution of edema. (*From* Eisenberg VH, Valsky DV, Yagel S. Transperineal ultrasound assessment of the anal sphincter after obstetric anal sphincter injury (OASI). Ultrasound Obstet Gynecol 2019;53(2):158–65; with permission.)

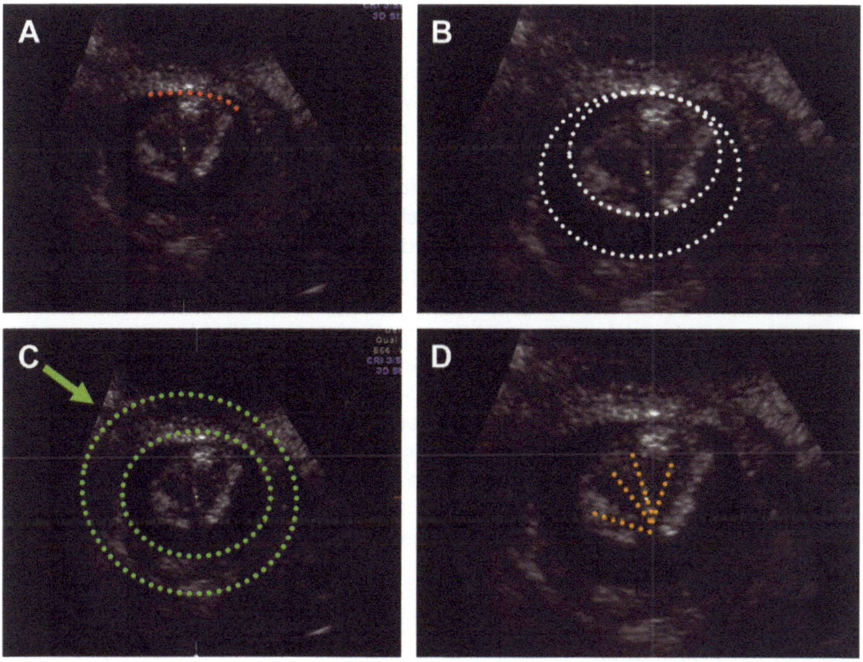


**Fig. 12.** Four sonographic signs can be detected in OASI: (*A*) external and/or internal anal sphincter discontinuity (*red dots*); (*B*) thinning of the IAS in the area of rupture in conjunction with thickening opposite the rupture site (the "half-moon" sign) (*white dots*); (*C*) asymmetry and thickening of the EAS at the area of repair (*green dots, arrow*); and (*D*) abnormality of the mucous folds (the "mucosal star sign") (*orange dots*).

The main effect of levator avulsion is an enlargement of the levator hiatus.[31] Unlike sphincter injury, which is apparent to the trained eye after delivery, LAM injury is rarely visible clinically. Most women with trauma to the levator ani are asymptomatic, and abnormality may arise years later with levator hiatus enlargement. An enlarged levator hiatus can be either congenital or the result of irreversible overdistension or avulsion injury. This may produce excessive loading of ligamentous and fascial structures, which over time may lead to connective tissue failure, the development of prolapse, and pelvic pain syndromes.[32] Correlations between clinical assessment and imaging findings of pelvic floor disorders have been widely investigated, both in the immediate postpartum and later, among women presenting to urogynecology clinics.[33] A substantial alteration of functional anatomy affecting the puborectalis component of the LAM is observed in about 13% to 36% of women after vaginal birth.[33,34]

### *Definition*

Trauma of the LAM can occur by overdistension of the muscle and by detachment of the muscle from its insertion to the pubic bone (avulsion).[30] Avulsion can be either partial or complete and can be unilateral or bilateral. The most frequent finding seems to be an avulsion injury to the anterior and inferomedial aspects of the pubovisceral muscle, that is, a detachment of this muscle from its insertion on the arcus tendinous fasciae pelvis.[35,36] Obstetric trauma is the main cause for the development of LAM avulsion.[36]

***Prevalence, risk factors, and clinical significance of levator ani injury***

The prevalence of levator avulsion defects is approximately 10% to 36% of primiparous women.[36,37] Levator ani trauma is associated with vaginal delivery, because no cases of trauma were observed in women who underwent elective cesarean delivery.[34,38] Forceps delivery was significantly associated with avulsion in primiparous women (odds ratio [OR] 3.83–11.0), with a prevalence of LAM avulsion of 35% to 71%.[34,38,39] Use of the Kristeller maneuver (fundal pressure in second stage) is associated with a higher prevalence of LAM avulsion and a larger hiatal area on maximum Valsalva maneuver.[40] Other risk factors found to be associated with LAM avulsion are fetal head circumference,[41] third- and fourth-degree OASI,[24,42,43] higher maternal age,[36] and prolonged second stage of labor.[41] Lin and colleagues[44] assessed patients with OASIs or LAM avulsion 23 years after their first delivery. LAM avulsion was diagnosed in 15.2% of women, and 12.6% had significant anal sphincter defect. An approximately one-third reduction in muscle strength is estimated when avulsion defect is identified,[45,46] and a marked alteration in anatomy may follow.[47] When assessed by TPUS, patients with a levator ani defect were 4 times more likely to suffer from uterine prolapse and 2.3 times more likely to have a significant cystocele, compared with those without.[46] In another study, prolapse was associated with levator avulsion (OR 4.17) and levator hiatus area (OR 1.52), and inversely with muscle strength (OR 0.87).[48]

## *Ultrasonographic Approach*

***Timing of the examination***

Most ultrasound examinations are performed years after childbirth, once symptoms arise. However, Valsky and colleagues[49] found that a LAM defect identified in the immediate postpartum period persists months or years after delivery and, therefore, the examination may be performed following delivery or may be delayed without affecting the result. In another study, 62% of levator avulsions assessed 3 months postpartum were no longer evident 1 year postpartum.[50] As in assessment of OASI, waiting for postpartum edema to subside is common practice.

***Methodology of levator ani assessment***

The clearest visualization of defects is achieved on maximal PFMC,[51] with TUI being particularly useful for this purpose.[52] Some patients may be unable to achieve a satisfactory PFMC.[53] Dietz and colleagues[54] assessed the accuracy of avulsion assessment when performed at rest and found it to be noninferior to that obtained during PFMC; however, the examination should be performed during PFMC if possible.

Determination of the hiatal area is best performed in the axial plane showing the minimal anteroposterior diameter. An oblique axial plane will display the "plane of minimal hiatal dimensions."[3] The plane of minimal dimensions can be used as a reference plane for the puborectalis muscle assessment on multislice or tomographic ultrasonography.[52] (**Fig. 13**). An interslice interval of 2.5 mm enables visualization of a reliable image of the entire puborectalis from its most caudal to its most cranial aspects.[32,55,56] Dimensions of the pubovisceral muscle and levator ani hiatus as calculated in nulliparous women are listed in **Table 1**.

***Sonographic signs of damage to the levator ani muscle***

To diagnose a full avulsion, an abnormal insertion must be identified in at least the 3 central slices of a tomographic series.[57] **Fig. 14** presents TUI of a unilateral avulsion visible in 4 slices.

Dietz and colleagues[58] proposed normal and pathologic dimensions of the levator hiatus according to sonographic and clinical evaluations, as well as patient

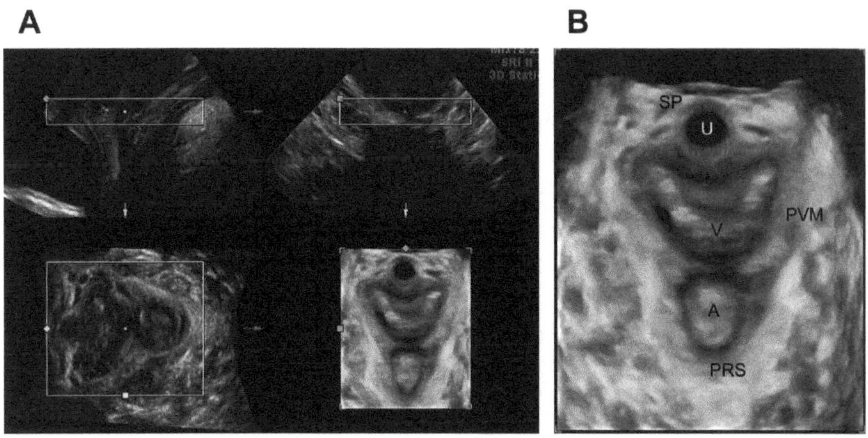


**Fig. 13.** (*A*) Multiplanar projection of a normal pelvic floor examination. The upper left A plane shows the midsagittal plane, while the C plane and rendered image (right upper image and left lower image) show the pelvic hiatus in axial plane. (*B*) The structures visualized on the rendered image are: symphysis pubis (SP), urethra (U), vagina (V), pubovisceral muscle (PVM) component of the levator ani, and puborectal sling (PRS). (*From* Valsky DV, Yagel S. Three-dimensional transperineal ultrasonography of the pelvic floor. J Ultrasound Med 2007;26:1376; with permission.)

complaints. Normal values were calculated as mean plus two standard deviations, as well as by receiver-operating characteristic curves, using symptoms attributable to the phenotypic observation in question. Both approaches yield a "normality" cutoff of 25 $cm^2$. A hiatal area on Valsalva maneuver of 25 to 29.9 $cm^2$ can be defined as "mild" enlargement, 30 to 34.9 $cm^2$ as "moderate," 35 to 39.9 $cm^2$ as "marked," and $\geq$40 $cm^2$ as "severe" ballooning. Excessive distensibility of the hiatus ("ballooning"; **Fig. 15**) whether as a result of childbirth or a congenital variant, is associated with symptoms and signs of prolapse[58] and with the complaint of vaginal laxity.[59] Marked ballooning is likely to reduce the odds of success for both pessary management and prolapse correction.[60]

**Table 1**
**Biometric indices of the pubovisceral muscle and levator hiatus determined in the axial and coronal planes**

| Parameter | Mean | SD |
|---|---|---|
| Pubovisceral muscle diameter (axial) (cm) | 0.73 | 0.16 |
| Pubovisceral muscle area (axial) ($cm^2$) | 7.59 | 1.72 |
| Levator hiatus at rest (AP) (cm) | 4.52 | 0.67 |
| Levator hiatus at rest (LR) (cm) | 3.75 | 0.50 |
| Hiatal area at rest ($cm^2$) | 11.25 | 2.70 |
| Hiatal area on Valsalva maneuver ($cm^2$) | 14.05 | 5.87 |
| Pubovisceral muscle diameter (coronal) (cm) | 1.33 | 0.55 |
| Pubovisceral muscle area (coronal) ($cm^2$) | 1.33 | 0.59 |
| Distance from perineal surface (cm) | 2.42 | 0.44 |

*Abbreviations*: AP, sagittal (anteroposterior); LR, coronal (left to right).

*From* Dietz HP, Shek C, Clarke B. Biometry of the pubovisceral muscle and levator hiatus by three-dimensional pelvic floor ultrasound. Ultrasound Obstet Gynecol 2005;25(6):583; with permission.

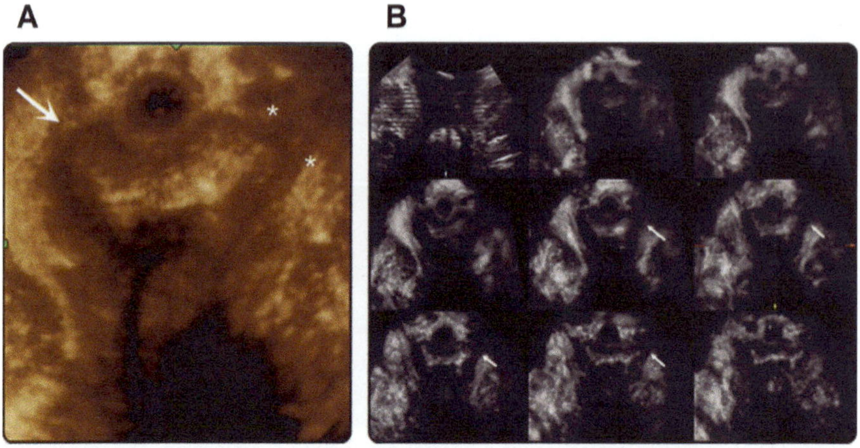


**Fig. 14.** (*A*) Rendered image from patient with unilateral levator ani muscle (LAM) injury. Discontinuity to LAM on left (*asterisks*); compare with right (*arrow*) showing continuity of muscle. (*B*) Tomographic ultrasound imaging in the same patient was used to verify results. Visualization of defect in several planes is mandatory to differentiate true injury from artifact. In this examination of the patient with right-sided unilateral LAM avulsion, frames −4 to −2 appear normal, whereas frames −1 to 2 demonstrate disturbance to the normal appearance of the vagina and fornices. (*From* Valsky DV, Lipschuetz M, Bord A, et al. Fetal head circumference and length of second stage of labor are risk factors for levator ani muscle injury, diagnosed by 3-dimensional transperineal ultrasound in primiparous women. Am J Obstet Gynecol 2009;201(1):91.e3; with permission.)

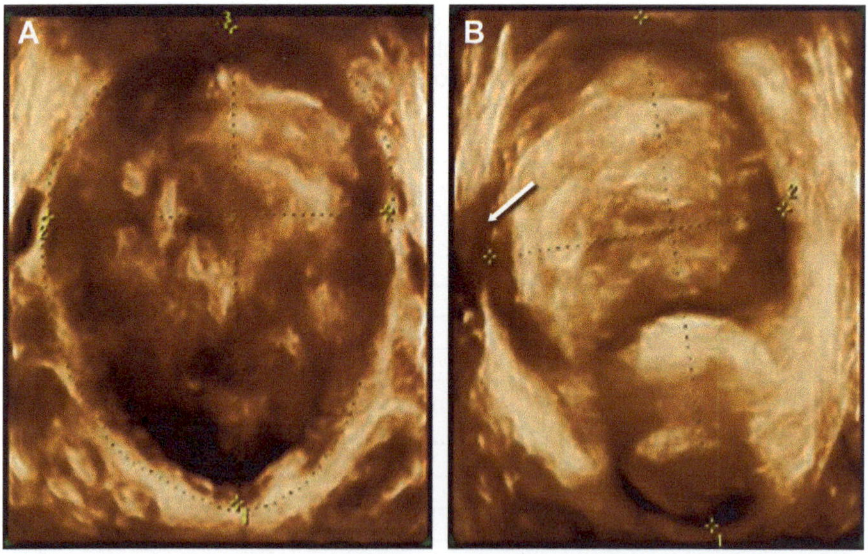


**Fig. 15.** Ballooning. (*A*) 3D rendered image of severe ballooning in a 42-year-old patient with total pelvic organ prolapse. (*B*) 3D rendered image of moderate ballooning in a 63-year-old patient with pelvic organ prolapse. Note asymmetry, which was corroborated by complete right avulsion defect in this patient (*arrow*).

***Reporting***

LAM avulsion can be reported as follows:

> *On TUI there is evidence of complete levator avulsion bilaterally on all the central slices with moderate ballooning on Valsalva maneuver (hiatal area 32 cm$^2$). There is weak contraction.*

## REFERENCES


1. American Institute of Ultrasound in Medicine. Guidelines for cleaning and preparing external- and internal-use ultrasound probes between patients, safe handling, and use of ultrasound coupling gel. 2017. Available at: https://www.aium.org/accreditation/Guidelines_Cleaning_Preparing.pdf.
2. Dietz HP. Pelvic floor ultrasound: a review. Am J Obstet Gynecol 2010;202(4):321–34.
3. Dietz HP, Shek C, Clarke B. Biometry of the pubovisceral muscle and levator hiatus by three-dimensional pelvic floor ultrasound. Ultrasound Obstet Gynecol 2005;25(6):580–5.
4. Sultan AH, Thakar R, Fenner DE, editors. Perineal and anal sphincter trauma. London: Springer London; 2007. https://doi.org/10.1007/978-1-84628-503-5.
5. Lone F, Sultan A, Thakar R. Obstetric pelvic floor and anal sphincter injuries. Obstet Gynaecol 2012;14(4):257–66.
6. American College of Obstetricians and Gynecologists' Committee on Practice Bulletins—Obstetrics. Practice Bulletin No. 165: prevention and management of obstetric lacerations at vaginal delivery. Obstet Gynecol 2016;128(1):e1–15.
7. Pirhonen JP, Grenman SE, Haadem K, et al. Frequency of anal sphincter rupture at delivery in Sweden and Finland—result of difference in manual help to the baby's head. Acta Obstet Gynecol Scand 1998;77(10):974–7.
8. Starck M, Bohe M, Valentin L. Results of endosonographic imaging of the anal sphincter 2-7 days after primary repair of third- or fourth-degree obstetric sphincter tears. Ultrasound Obstet Gynecol 2003;22(6):609–15.
9. Varma A, Gunn J, Gardiner A, et al. Obstetric anal sphincter injury: prospective evaluation of incidence. Obstet Gynecol Surv 2003;55(7):414–5.
10. Dockery DW, Pope CA III, Xu X, et al. An association between air pollution and mortality in six U.S. cities. N Engl J Med 1993;329(24):1753–9.
11. Valsky DV, Messing B, Petkova R, et al. Postpartum evaluation of the anal sphincter by transperineal three-dimensional ultrasound in primiparous women after vaginal delivery and following surgical repair of third-degree tears by the overlapping technique. Ultrasound Obstet Gynecol 2007;29(2):195–204.
12. Sultan AH, Kamm MA, Hudson CN, et al. Third degree obstetric anal sphincter tears : risk factors and outcome of primary repair. BMJ 1994;308(6933):887–91.
13. Christianson LM, Bovbjerg VE, Mcdavitt EC, et al. Risk factors for perineal injury during delivery. Am J Obstet Gynecol 2003;189(1):255–60.
14. De Leeuw JW, Struijk PC, Vierhout ME, et al. Risk factors for third degree perineal ruptures during delivery. BJOG 2001;108(4):383–7.
15. van Bavel J, Hukkelhoven CWPM, De Vries C, et al. The effectiveness of mediolateral episiotomy in preventing obstetric anal sphincter injuries during operative vaginal delivery : a ten-year analysis of a national registry. Int Urogynecol J 2018;29(3):407–13.

16. Sultan AH, Thakar R. Third and fourth degree tears. In: Sultan AH, Thakar R, Fenner DE, editors. Perineal and anal sphincter trauma. London (UK): Springer; 1999. p. 33–51.
17. De Leeuw JW, Vierhout ME, Struijk PC, et al. Anal sphincter damage after vaginal delivery : functional outcome and risk factors for fecal incontinence. Acta Obstet Gynecol Scand 2001;80(9):830–4.
18. Jangö H, Dmsc JL, Rosthøj S, et al. Mode of delivery after obstetric anal sphincter injury and the risk of long-term anal incontinence. Am J Obstet Gynecol 2016; 214(6):733.e1-13.
19. No GG. The management of third- and fourth-degree perineal tears. Green-top guideline No. 29. London (UK): Royal College of Obstetricians & Gynaecologists; 2015. Available at: https://www.rcog.org.uk/globalassets/documents/guidelines/gtg-29.pdf.
20. Jangö H, Langhoff-roos J, Rosthøj S, et al. Long-term anal incontinence after obstetric anal sphincter injury—does grade of tear matter? Am J Obstet Gynecol 2018;218(2):232.e1-10.
21. Faltin DL, Boulvain M, Floris LA, et al. Diagnosis of anal sphincter tears to prevent fecal incontinence. Obstet Gynecol 2010;106(1):6–13.
22. Ros C, Mart EI, Wozniak MM, et al. Postpartum two- and three-dimensional ultrasound evaluation of anal sphincter complex in women with obstetric anal sphincter injury. Ultrasound Obstet Gynecol 2017;49(4):508–14.
23. Cornelia L, Stephan B, Michel B, et al. Trans-perineal versus endo-anal ultrasound in the detection of anal sphincter tears. Eur J Obstet Gynecol Reprod Biol 2002;103(1):79–82.
24. Volløyhaug I, Taithongchai A, Van Gruting I, et al. Levator ani muscle morphology and function in women with obstetric anal sphincter injury. Ultrasound Obstet Gynecol 2019;53(3):410–6.
25. Valsky DV, Yagel S. Three-dimensional transperineal ultrasonography of the pelvic floor. J Ultrasound Med 2007;26:1373–87.
26. Roos AM, Thakar R, Sultan AH. Outcome of primary repair of obstetric anal sphincter injuries (OASIS): does the grade of tear matter? Ultrasound Obstet Gynecol 2010;36(3):368–74.
27. Timor-Tritsch IE, Monteagudo A, Smilen SW, et al. Simple ultrasound evaluation of the anal sphincter in female patients using a transvaginal transducer. Ultrasound Obstet Gynecol 2005;25(2):177–83.
28. Eisenberg VH, Valsky DV, Yagel S. Transperineal ultrasound assessment of the anal sphincter after obstetric anal sphincter injury (OASI). Ultrasound Obstet Gynecol 2019;53(2):158–65.
29. Hoyte L, Damaser MS, Warfield SK, et al. Quantity and distribution of levator ani stretch during simulated vaginal childbirth. Am J Obstet Gynecol 2008;199(2): 198.e1-5.
30. Lien K, Mooney B, DeLancey J, et al. Levator ani muscle stretch induced by simulated vaginal birth. Obstet Gynecol 2005;103(1):31–40.
31. Dietz HP, Franco AVM, Shek KL, et al. Avulsion injury and levator hiatal ballooning: two independent risk factors for prolapse? An observational study. Acta Obstet Gynecol Scand 2012;91(2):211–4.
32. Eisenberg VH. Female pelvic floor imaging with emphasis on the overactive pelvic floor. In: Padoa A, Rosenbaum TY, editors. The overactive pelvic floor. Cham (Switzerland): Springer International Publishing; 2016. p. 205–32. https://doi.org/10.1007/978-3-319-22150-2_13.

33. Dietz HP, Steensma AB. The prevalence of major abnormalities of the levator ani in urogynaecological patients. BJOG 2006;113(2):225–30.
34. Shek KL, Dietz HP. Intrapartum risk factors for levator trauma. BJOG 2010; 117(12):1485–92.
35. DeLancey JOL, Kearney R, Chou Q, et al. The appearance of levator ani muscle abnormalities in magnetic resonance images after vaginal delivery. Obstet Gynecol 2003;101(1):46–53.
36. Dietz HP, Lanzarone V. Levator trauma after vaginal delivery level of evidence: II-3. Obstet Gynecol 2005;106(4):707–12.
37. Shek KL, Dietz HP. OC003: the effect of vaginal childbirth on levator hiatal dimensions. Ultrasound Obstet Gynecol 2008;32(3):243–4.
38. van Delft K, Thakar R, Sultan AH, et al. Levator ani muscle avulsion during childbirth : a risk prediction model. BJOG 2014;121(9):1155–63.
39. Keane D, Herlihy CO, Delancey JOL. Levator ani injury in primiparous women with forceps delivery for fetal distress, forceps for second stage arrest, and spontaneous delivery. Int J Gynaecol Obstet 2011;111(1):19–22.
40. Youssef A, Salsi G, Cataneo I, et al. Fundal pressure in second stage of labor (Kristeller maneuver) is associated with increased risk of levator ani muscle avulsion. Ultrasound Obstet Gynecol 2019;53(1):95–100.
41. Valsky DV, Lipschuetz M, Bord A, et al. Fetal head circumference and length of second stage of labor are risk factors for levator ani muscle injury, diagnosed by 3-dimensional transperineal ultrasound in primiparous women. Am J Obstet Gynecol 2009;201(1):91.e1-7.
42. Shek KL, Green K, Hall J, et al. Perineal and vaginal tears are clinical markers for occult levator ani trauma: a retrospective observational study. Ultrasound Obstet Gynecol 2016;47(2):224–7.
43. Valsky DV, Cohen SM, Lipschuetz M, et al. Third- or fourth-degree intrapartum anal sphincter tears are associated with levator ani avulsion in primiparas. J Ultrasound Med 2016;35(4):709–15.
44. Lin S, Atan IK, Dietz HP, et al. Delivery mode, levator avulsion and obstetric anal sphincter injury: a cross-sectional study 20 years after childbirth. Aust N Z J Obstet Gynaecol 2019. https://doi.org/10.1111/ajo.12948.
45. Miller JM, Umek W, Fenner DE, et al. Comparison of levator ani muscle defects and function in women with and without pelvic organ prolapse. Obstet Gynecol 2010;109(2):295–302.
46. Dietz HP, Shek C. Levator avulsion and grading of pelvic floor muscle strength. Int Urogynecol J 2008;19(5):633–6.
47. Abdool Z, Shek KL, Dietz HP. The effect of levator avulsion on hiatal dimension and function. Am J Obstet Gynecol 2009;201(1):89.e1-5.
48. Handa VL, Roem J, Blomquist JL, et al. Pelvic organ prolapse as a function of levator ani avulsion, hiatus size, and strength. Am J Obstet Gynecol 2019;221(1): 41.e1-7.
49. Valsky DV, Lipschuetz M, Cohen SM, et al. Persistence of levator ani sonographic defect detected by three-dimensional transperineal sonography in primiparous women. Ultrasound Obstet Gynecol 2015;46(6):724–9.
50. Van Delft KWM, Thakar R, Sultan AH, et al. The natural history of levator avulsion one year following childbirth: a prospective study. BJOG 2015;122(9):1266–73.
51. Van Delft K, Thakar R, Sultan AH, et al. Does the prevalence of levator ani muscle avulsion differ when assessed using tomographic ultrasound imaging at rest vs on maximum pelvic floor muscle contraction? Ultrasound Obstet Gynecol 2015; 46(1):99–103.

52. Dietz HP. Quantification of major morphological abnormalities of the levator ani. Ultrasound Obstet Gynecol 2007;29(3):329–34.
53. Konstantinovic ML, de Ridder D, Steensma AB, et al. Prevalence of major levator abnormalities in symptomatic patients with an underactive pelvic floor contraction. Int Urogynecol J 2010;21(7):861–7.
54. Dietz HP, Pattillo Garnham A, Guzmán Rojas R. Is it necessary to diagnose levator avulsion on pelvic floor muscle contraction? Ultrasound Obstet Gynecol 2017; 49(2):252–6.
55. Dietz HP, Shek KL. Tomographic ultrasound imaging of the pelvic floor: which levels matter most? Ultrasound Obstet Gynecol 2009;33(6):698–703.
56. Kashihara H, Shek KL, Dietz HP. Can we identify the limits of the puborectalis/pubovisceralis muscle on tomographic translabial ultrasound? Ultrasound Obstet Gynecol 2012;40(2):219–22.
57. Dietz HP, Bernardo MJ, Kirby A, et al. Minimal criteria for the diagnosis of avulsion of the puborectalis muscle by tomographic ultrasound. Int Urogynecol J 2011; 22(6):699–704.
58. Dietz HP, Shek C, De Leon J, et al. Ballooning of the levator hiatus. Ultrasound Obstet Gynecol 2008;31(6):676–80.
59. Dietz HP, Stankiewicz M, Atan IK, et al. Vaginal laxity: what does this symptom mean? Int Urogynecol J 2018;29(5):723–8.
60. Rodrigo N, Wong V, Shek KL, et al. The use of 3-dimensional ultrasound of the pelvic floor to predict recurrence risk after pelvic reconstructive surgery. Aust N Z J Obstet Gynaecol 2014;54(3):206–11.

# Nongynecologic Causes of Pelvic Pain: Ultrasound First

Mahan Mathur, MD[a,*], Leslie M. Scoutt, MD[b]

**KEYWORDS**

• Appendicitis • Diverticulitis • Urolithiasis • Pelvic congestion syndrome
• Inflammatory bowel disease • Bowel obstruction

**KEY POINTS**

- Ultrasonography (US) is often the first-line imaging study used to evaluate women who present with pelvic pain.
- Non-gynecologic causes of pelvic pain are important to recognize on US, because a delay in diagnosis can cause significant morbidity and mortality.
- US evaluation of nongynecologic causes of pelvic pain often requires a variety of transducers, changes in patient position, and use of graded compression technique (particularly if a pathologic condition of the bowel is suspected).

## INTRODUCTION

Pelvic pain is a common, nonspecific presenting complaint in women of all ages. A thorough history and physical examination, combined with evaluation of laboratory data and imaging studies, is mandatory to narrow the differential diagnosis. If a gynecologic cause is suspected, ultrasonography (US) is the first-line imaging study of choice owing to its high sensitivity and specificity for detection of gynecologic pathology in the pelvis, lack of ionizing radiation, relatively low cost, and widespread availability. However, in a subset of cases, nongynecologic entities, most commonly gastrointestinal (GI) or urinary tract in origin, may present with pelvic pain that is clinically indistinguishable from the more common gynecologic causes of pelvic pain. Whereas other imaging modalities such as computed tomography (CT) and MRI have been traditionally considered to be better suited for evaluation of these entities, it is imperative to recognize the appearance of nongynecologic causes of pelvic pain on US because pelvic US may be the first imaging study obtained, and a delay in diagnosis can result in significant morbidity and/or mortality. Furthermore, as concerns

Disclosure: The authors have nothing to disclose.
[a] Section of Body Imaging, Yale School of Medicine, 20 York Street, PO Box 208042, New Haven, CT 06520-8042, USA; [b] Section of Ultrasound, Yale School of Medicine, 20 York Street, PO Box 208042, New Haven, CT 06520-8042, USA
* Corresponding author.
*E-mail address:* mahan.mathur@yale.eu

Obstet Gynecol Clin N Am 46 (2019) 733–753
https://doi.org/10.1016/j.ogc.2019.07.007
0889-8545/19/

escalate regarding the risk of ionizing radiation and health care costs, it has become increasingly accepted to practice an "ultrasound first" approach to the imaging evaluation of women presenting with pelvic pain. Although one may not be able to accurately identify all GI and urinary tract causes of pelvic pain with US, a definitive diagnosis can be made in some cases, thereby avoiding the risks and cost of CT and MRI.

This article reviews the sonographic appearance of a variety of nongynecologic causes of pelvic pain and elucidates specific maneuvers that can be used to optimize their assessment with US.

## APPENDICITIS

Acute appendicitis (AA) is among the most common surgical emergencies in adults, with an estimated lifetime incidence in the United States ranging from 7% to 14%.[1,2] In the nonpregnant adult, CT remains the imaging gold standard.[3] Although the reported sensitivity, specificity, and accuracy of US for the diagnosis of AA has improved over the last decade, US remains highly operator dependent and is often limited by the body habitus of the patient, the position of the appendix, and overlying gas-filled loops of the bowel. As a result, reported sensitivities and specificities of US range from 44% to 100% and 47% to 99%, respectively.[4] However, owing to the lack of ionizing radiation, US remains of value as the initial imaging modality of choice in pediatric patients, young adults, and pregnant women.[5,6]

US evaluation of the appendix is generally performed with the patient in the supine position using the graded compression technique.[7] A high-frequency linear transducer (a low-frequency transducer may be necessary in larger patients or if the appendix has a more atypical location) is used to apply gentle pressure at or close to the region of the patient's point of maximal tenderness to displace adjacent air-filled loops of bowel without causing guarding.[8] Alternatively, the appendix can be located by tracking in the transverse plane inferiorly from the cecum or superiorly from the psoas and iliac vessels. In pregnant women, evaluation of the right upper quadrant and/or a posterior approach may be necessary because of displacement of the appendix by the gravid uterus. Additional maneuvers, such as posterior manual compression, upward graded compression, or left lateral oblique decubitus positioning have been described as useful adjuncts to visualize the appendix.[9]

On grayscale imaging, a normal appendix appears as a blind-ending, compressible, aperistaltic tubular structure arising from the cecum, with an outer-wall dimeter less than 6 mm (**Fig. 1**). The lumen may contain fluid, gas, or debris, and the wall will demonstrate the characteristic striated gut signature. Grayscale imaging features of AA include a noncompressible, dilated appendix, with an outer-wall to outer-wall diameter of greater than 6 mm, corresponding to the point of maximal tenderness (**Fig. 2**).[10] Some studies have reported higher specificities with a cutoff of greater than 7 mm.[11] Additional findings include the presence of an appendicolith (hyperechoic intraluminal structure with posterior shadowing), adjacent fluid, and/or hyperechogenicity of the periappendiceal tissue because of inflammation (**Fig. 3**).[10] Hypervascularity of the appendiceal wall and/or adjacent tissues may also be observed on color Doppler imaging (**Fig. 4**).[10]

The presence of AA on US should indicate initiation of treatment (operative resection vs nonoperant management with antibiotics). However, nonvisualization of the

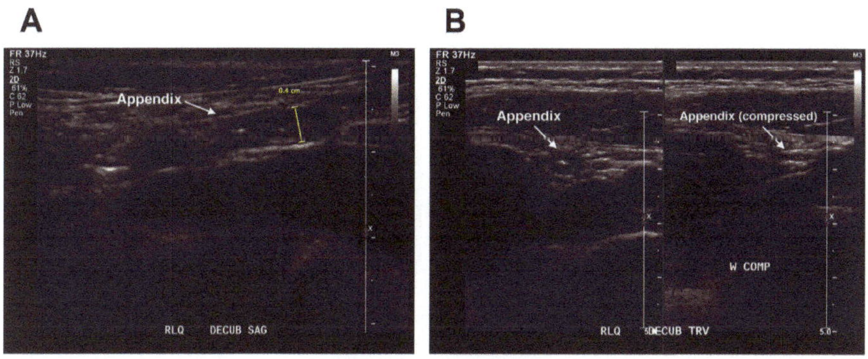


**Fig. 1.** Normal appendix. An 18-year-old woman with right lower quadrant (RLQ) pain. (*A*) Grayscale image of the RLQ demonstrates a nondilated blind-ending tubular structure (*yellow line*/calipers) with outer-wall diameter of 4 mm. (*B*) Transverse grayscale split-screen image performed without and with compression ("W COMP") demonstrates complete compressibility of the structure. No adjacent hyperemia was seen on color Doppler image (not shown) and no free fluid was identified.

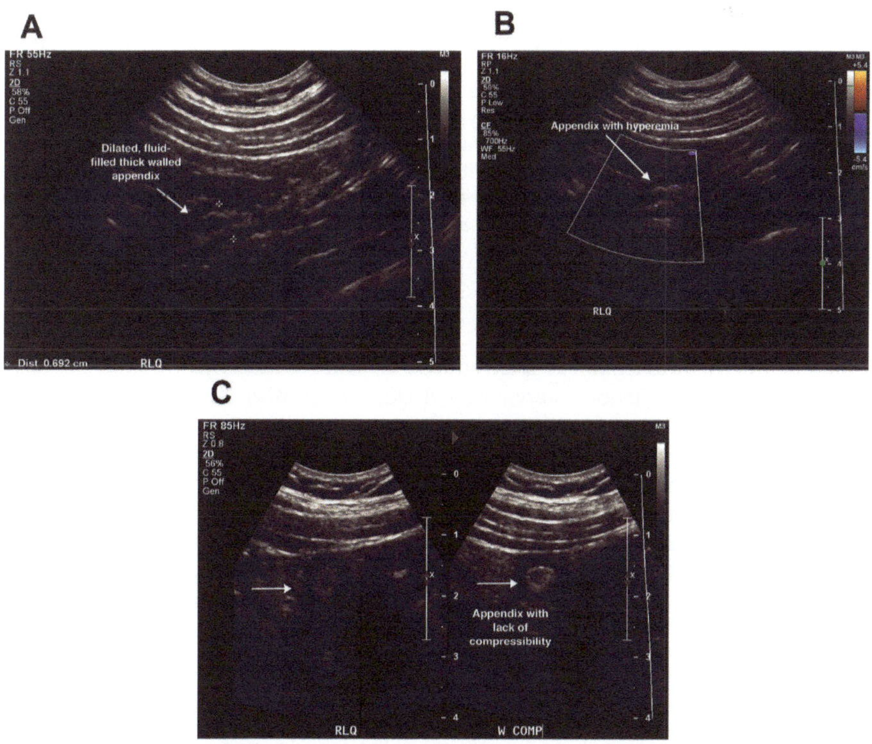


**Fig. 2.** Acute appendicitis. 22 year-old female with right lower quadrant pain. (*A*) Gray-scale image of the right lower quadrant (RLQ) demonstrates a dilated, thick walled fluid-filled appendix (*arrow and calipers*) with outer wall diameter of 7 mm. (*B*) Color Doppler image demonstrates minimal hyperemia (*arrow*). (*C*) Transverse gray-scale split screen image of the appendix (*arrow*) performed without and with compression ("W COMP") demonstrates no compressibility. Findings corresponded to the patient's point of maximal tenderness.

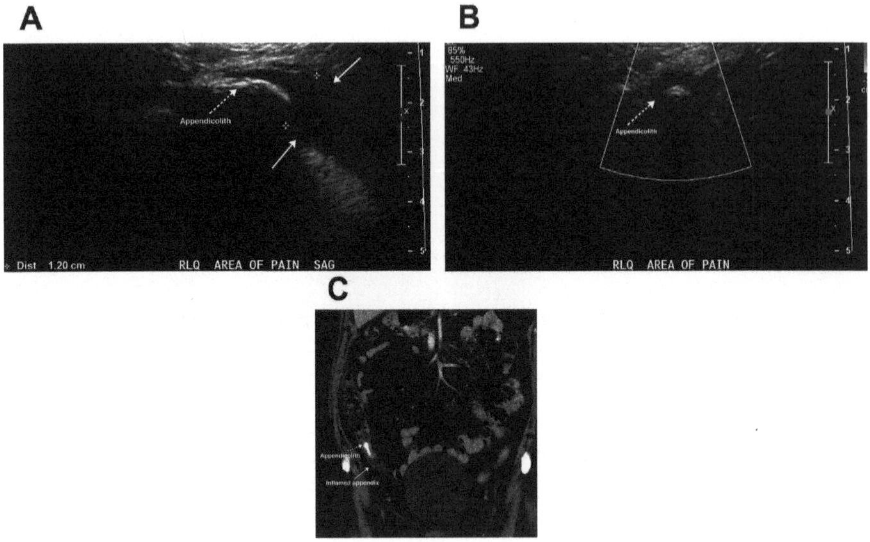


**Fig. 3.** Acute appendicitis with appendicolith. A 72-year-old woman with right lower quadrant (RLQ) pain. (*A*) Sagittal grayscale image of the RLQ demonstrates distended fluid-filled appendix (*solid arrows* and calipers), which measures 1.2 cm in diameter outer-wall to outer-wall. A curvilinear echogenic focus with posterior shadowing (*dashed arrow*) is noted within the lumen, compatible with an appendicolith. (*B*) Transverse color Doppler image demonstrates minimal hyperemia and increased echogenicity of the surrounding fat with the appendicolith (*dashed arrow*) again noted. (*C*) Coronal CT scan of the abdomen and pelvis performed with intravenous contrast confirms acute appendicitis. Note appendicolith (*dashed arrow*) at the junction of the appendix and cecum and distended distal appendix (*solid arrow*), as well as increased stranding in the periappendiceal fat.

appendix does not exclude AA and requires clinical reassessment before obtaining more imaging studies (short-interval repeat US, CT, or MRI). Some studies have reported that nonvisualization of the appendix may have high negative-predictive value to exclude AA in specific patient populations and clinical settings, particularly if secondary signs of inflammation, such as free fluid, phlegmon, and periappendiceal inflammatory changes, are absent.[12,13]

The presence of extraluminal gas (echogenic foci with “dirty” shadowing), an extruded appendicolith, frank abscesses, and/or extraluminal fluid/fluid or air/fluid levels is suggestive of perforation.[10] Abscesses manifest as hypoechoic fluid collections with thick hyperemic walls containing low-level echoes (consistent with debris or purulent material) and sometimes gas (echogenic foci with dirty shadowing). Perforation is more common in the pregnant patient because of both delay in diagnosis and immunologic changes reducing the host response to combat and wall off infection. In one study, complicated appendicitis (gangrenous appendicitis with or without perforation) was associated with loss of the normal echogenic submucosal layer in the wall of the appendix.[14] Rarely can all the above findings, with the exception of noncompressibility, be detected on transvaginal US allowing for the correct diagnosis of AA (**Fig. 5**).

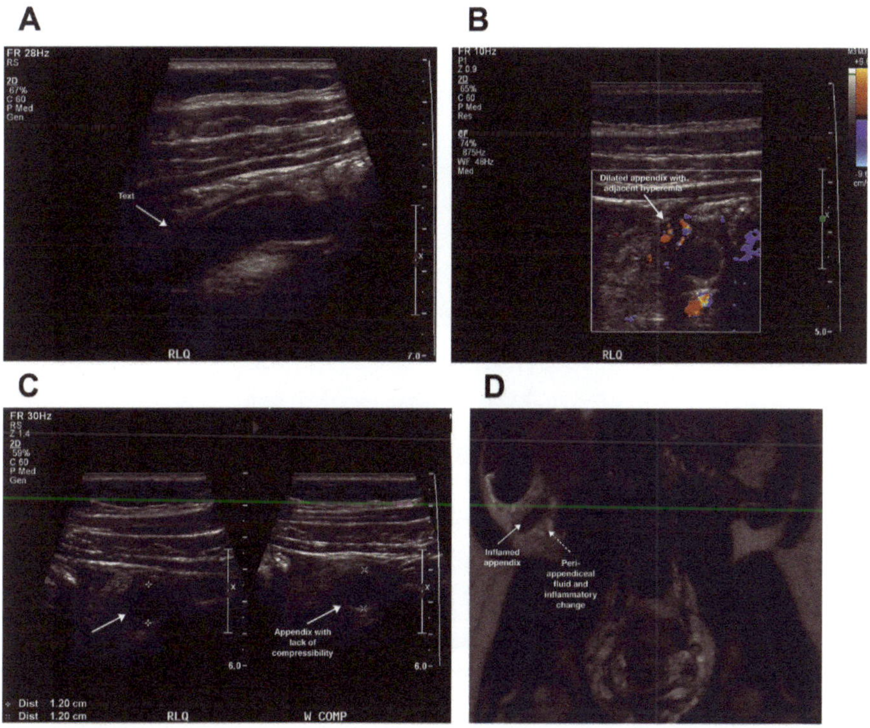


**Fig. 4.** Acute appendicitis in a pregnant patient. A 30-year-old pregnant woman with right lower quadrant (RLQ) pain. (*A*) Grayscale image of the RLQ demonstrates the presence of a dilated, fluid-filled appendix (*arrow*), with increased echogenicity of the surrounding pelvic fat and surrounding hyperemia on (*B*) transverse color Doppler image. (*C*) Transverse grayscale split-screen image performed without and with compression ("W COMP") demonstrates no compressibility of the appendix (*arrows*). (*D*) Coronal T2-weighted MR image performed for preoperative planning demonstrates a dilated and thick-walled blind-ending tubular structure (*solid arrow*) containing a thin central sliver of hyperintense T2 signal (fluid) with surrounding ill-defined T2 signal in the periappendiceal fat representing edema and inflammatory change (*dashed arrow*) compatible with acute appendicitis.

## SMALL BOWEL OBSTRUCTION

In patients with clinically suspected small bowel obstruction (SBO), the American College of Radiology appropriateness criteria recommends obtaining CT of the abdomen and pelvis with intravenous contrast as the first-line imaging test.[15] However, given that CT imaging is not always readily available and is associated with radiation exposure and relatively high cost, there has been interest in assessing the use of US in evaluating patients with suspected SBO.[16] In a recent systemic review of 11 studies, US demonstrated a sensitivity of 92.4% (95% CI, 89.0%–94.7%) and a specificity of 96.6% (95% CI, 88.4%–99.1%) for the diagnosis of SBO.[16] Whereas US may be helpful in establishing the nonspecific diagnosis of an SBO, it is inferior to CT imaging with regard to determining the level of the obstruction (transition point) and the cause of the obstruction, both of which are important for patient management.[17]

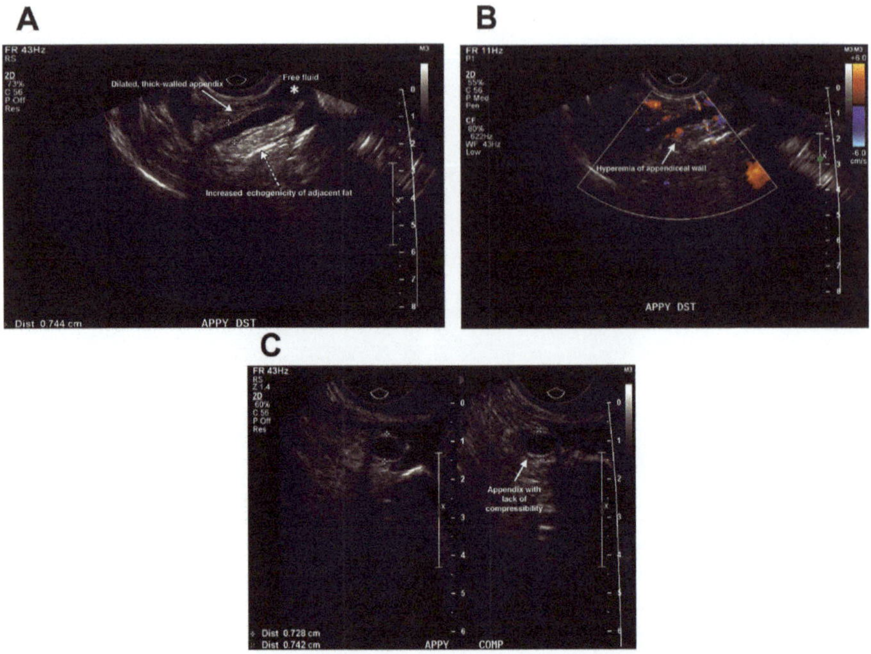


**Fig. 5.** A 23-year-old woman with right lower quadrant pain. (*A*) Grayscale transvaginal image of the right lower quadrant demonstrates a dilated, thick-walled, and fluid-filled appendix (*solid arrow*) with outer-wall diameter >7 mm. There is increased echogenicity of the surrounding fat (*dashed arrow*) as well as surrounding free fluid (*asterisk*). (*B*) Color Doppler transvaginal image demonstrates associated hyperemia in the appendiceal wall and surrounding tissue. (*C*) Grayscale transvaginal split-screen image performed without and with compression ("COMP") demonstrates no compressibility. During surgery, the patient was found to have acute appendicitis without perforation.

With the patient in the supine position, a 3.5 to 5 MHz curved transducer is typically used to obtain a general overview of the abdomen, with higher-frequency linear transducers reserved for more detailed evaluation of specific loops of the bowel.[18] On grayscale imaging, normal small bowel wall thickness is less than 3 mm and normal luminal diameter is less than 3 cm.[18] The normal bowel wall demonstrates alternating hyperechoic and hypoechoic layers that reflect the mucosa, submucosal, and muscularis (hypoechoic) layers (**Fig. 6**A). The valvulae conniventes (thin, closely spaced linear echoes projecting into the lumen from the bowel wall) and haustra (wider and more spread apart linear echoes that involve the serosa) differentiate small and large bowel, respectively (**Fig. 6**B, C).[19] Air in the bowel lumen is echogenic with "dirty" shadowing, whereas fluid is anechoic or hypoechoic with increased through transmission.

SBO manifests as distended loops of bowel (>3 cm) over a length of more than 10 cm, with variable wall thickness and abnormally increased peristalsis, which causes a "to-and-fro" or whirling motion of bowel contents (**Fig. 7**).[20] The presence of intraperitoneal free fluid, wall thickness greater than 4 mm, and/or diminished to absent peristalsis in a previously demonstrated obstructed loop of bowel has been

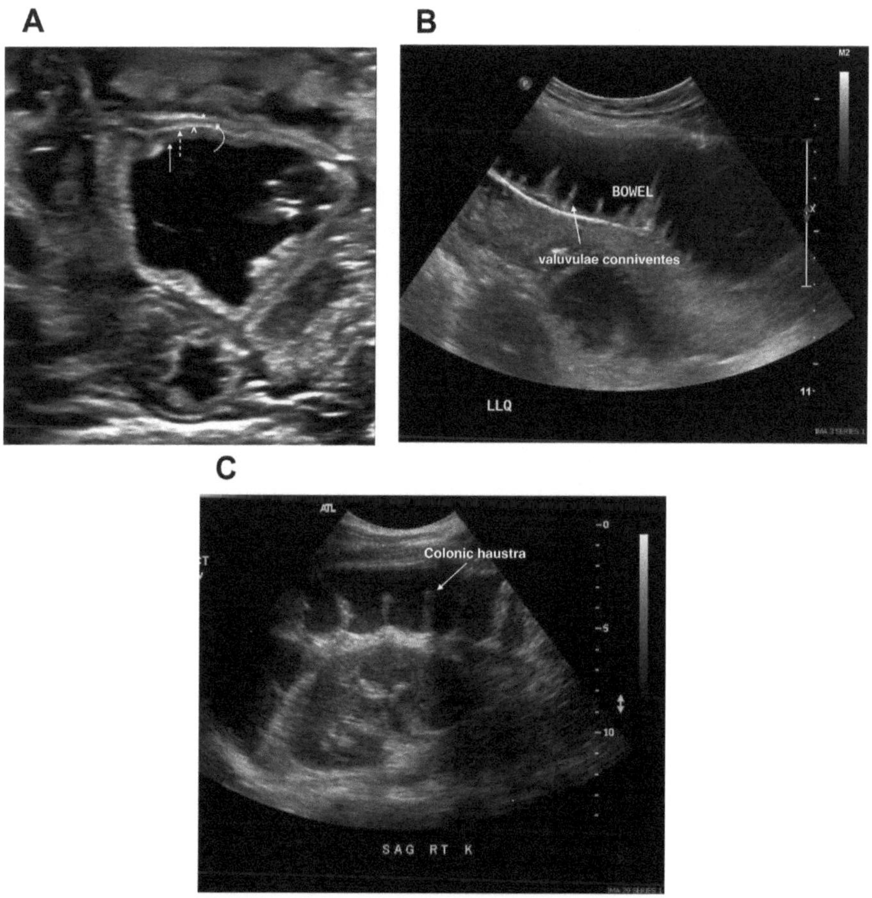


**Fig. 6.** Normal ultrasonographic appearance of bowel. (*A*) Grayscale transabdominal image demonstrates the characteristic bowel gut signature, which consists of alternating layers of hyper- and hypoechogenicity (*solid arrow*, mucosa; *dashed arrow*, muscularis mucosa; *arrowhead*, submucosa; *curved arrow*, muscularis propria; *asterisk*, serosa). (*B*) Normal valvulae conniventes manifest as thin, closely spaced linear echoes projecting into the lumen from the bowel wall (*solid arrow*). (*C*) Normal colonic haustra are wider and more spread apart than valvulae conniventes (*solid arrow*).

reported to be associated with the need for surgery.[16,21] Disruption of the mucosal lining and lack of bowel wall perfusion (which can be assessed using color Doppler imaging) with or without intramural air indicate ischemia, and the presence of free air (focal or diffuse extraluminal areas of increased echogenicity with posterior dirty shadowing) indicates a perforation (**Fig. 8**).[16]

## INFLAMMATORY BOWEL DISEASE

Inflammatory bowel disease (IBD) is a chronic, idiopathic, inflammatory condition of the GI tract which encompasses 2 disorders: Crohn disease (CD) and ulcerative colitis (UC).[22] Whereas CT is more commonly used to evaluate patients with IBD in the United States, MRI and US are preferred in Europe.[23] In one meta-analysis, US

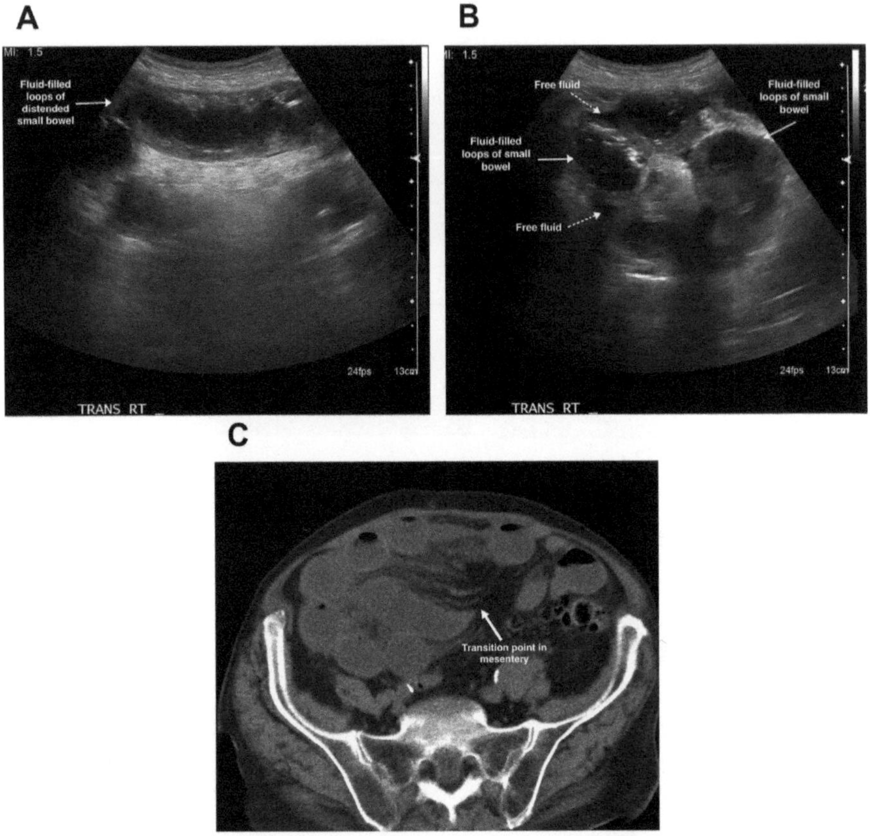


**Fig. 7.** Small bowel obstruction. A 55-year-old woman with diffuse abdominal and pelvic pain. (*A, B*) Grayscale images demonstrate numerous fluid-filled loops of distended bowel (*solid arrows*). The bowel wall is thick and irregular without visualization of the valvulae conniventes and poor mucosal definition; findings somewhat worrisome for ischemia. Bright echogenic intraluminal foci are consistent with intraluminal and possibly intramural air. A small amount of interloop fluid (*dashed arrows* in *B*) is also present. (*C*) Noncontrast CT scan performed subsequently confirms the presence of a small bowel obstruction with transition point in the mesentery (*solid arrow*). Exploratory laparotomy revealed a closed loop small bowel obstruction with necrotic bowel, necessitating resection.

sensitivity and specificity for the diagnosis of CD ranged from 75% to 94% and 67% to 100%, respectively.[24] Despite the operator-dependent variability of US, one study concluded that bowel sonography signs used to diagnose CD can be standardized, because most show fair to good reproducibility.[25] In addition, complications of CD, such as fistula, stenosis, and abscess can also be detected with high accuracy on US, with a sensitivity and specificity of up to 90% and 99% for abscesses in one study.[26]

Low-frequency (3.5–5 MHz) transducers are used to evaluate extraintestinal pathologic conditions, while high-frequency (5–17 MHz) transducers provide increased spatial and contrast resolution of the intestinal wall.[23] Unless performed urgently, patients should be scanned either in the preprandial state in the morning, or after at least 4 hours of fasting to decrease peristalsis and reduce intraluminal air.[23]

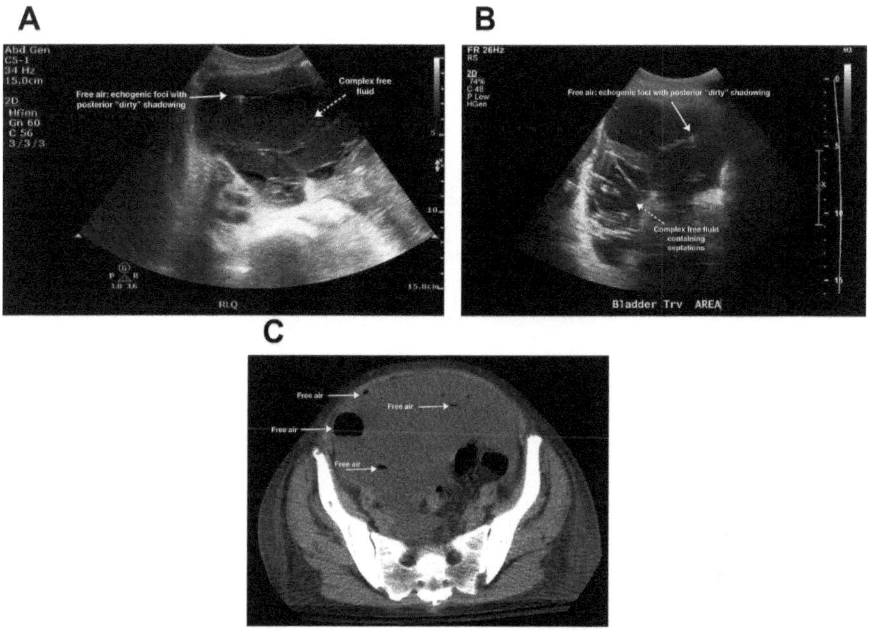


**Fig. 8.** Free air. A 47-year-old woman with pelvic pain status after diagnostic paracentesis. (*A, B*) Grayscale images of the right lower quadrant (RLQ) demonstrate complex fluid that contains numerous low-level echoes and septations (*dashed arrows*). In addition, numerous echogenic foci are noted with posterior "dirty" shadowing compatible with extraluminal gas (*solid arrows*). (*C*) Findings of ascites and free air (*solid arrows*) were confirmed on a subsequent noncontrast CT. Note that the complexity of the ascites is better appreciated on US than on CT.

On grayscale imaging, CD manifests as bowel wall thickening >3 to 4 mm (**Fig. 9**). In one meta-analysis, a cutoff of 3 mm yielded a sensitivity and specificity of 89% and 96%, respectively, for the detection of CD, while a cutoff of greater than 4 mm yielded a sensitivity and specificity of 87% and 98%, respectively.[27] There are conflicting data associating the degree of bowel wall thickening with clinical disease activity and severity.[28,29] The bowel wall stratification pattern may be preserved or disrupted, with "skip" lesions manifesting with both patterns along a single loop of bowel.[30] Chronic inflammation results in deposition of fat within the submucosal layers of the bowel wall resulting in increased echogenicity on grayscale imaging.[31] Adjacent extraintestinal findings include free fluid, reactive lymphadenopathy, and increased echogenicity and vascularity of the mesenteric fat.[23]

On color Doppler imaging, actively inflamed loops of bowel demonstrate increased vascularity,[23] with several studies demonstrating this as a useful parameter to distinguish between active disease and remission.[32,33] Contrast-enhanced US (CEUS) can depict transmural enhancement and can assess bowel wall vascularity more accurately than color Doppler imaging, particularly the smaller vessels that arise secondary to neoangiogenesis in the setting of inflammation.[31] Active inflammation also results in increased mesenteric vascularization ("comb" sign), a finding that can also be depicted using CEUS.[31] Following pharmacologic therapy, CEUS can objectively quantify the reduction in bowel wall vascularity, thereby differentiating responders

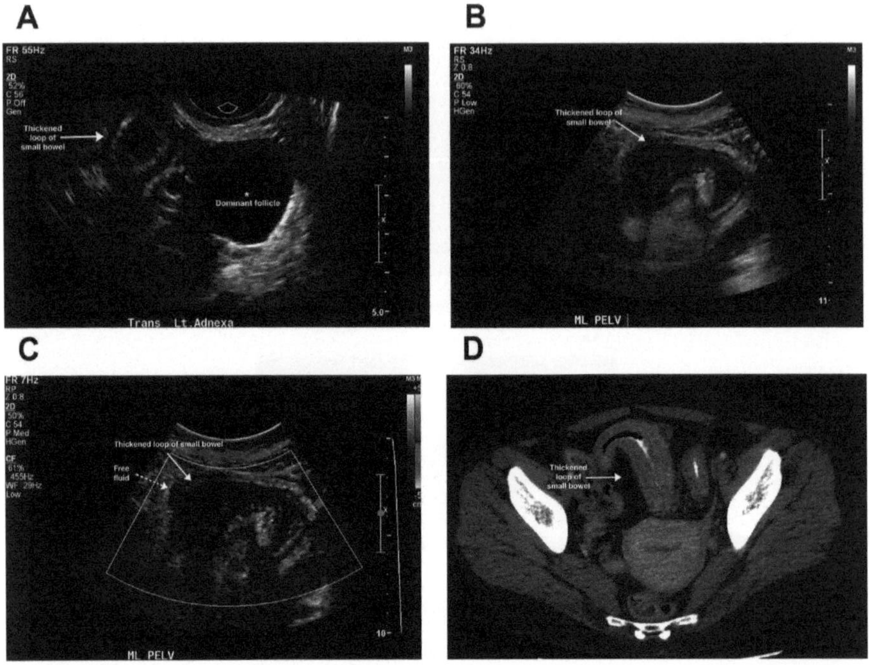


**Fig. 9.** Crohn disease. A 27-year-old woman with pelvic pain. (*A*) Grayscale transvaginal image of the left adnexa demonstrates a dominant follicle (*asterisk*), medial to which there is a thickened loop of bowel (*arrow*). Whereas the striated appearance of the bowel wall is still maintained, the mucosal and submucosal layers are particularly thick and echogenic. (*B*) Additional grayscale and (*C*) color Doppler images demonstrate the thickened loop of the bowel (*solid arrows*), as well as minimal hyperemia and increased echogenicity of the surrounding fat. There is also a small amount of adjacent free fluid seen on (*C*) (*dashed arrow*) as well as on the subsequent CT scan. (*D*) Contrast-enhanced CT confirms a thick-walled loop of ileum (*arrow*) consistent with active ileitis in this patient with a history of Crohn disease.

to medical therapy from nonresponders in patients with active CD.[34] Another study reported excellent accuracy for the diagnosis of postoperative CD recurrence with CEUS.[35]

The role of US in the diagnosis and monitoring of UC is less well established.[23] Grayscale imaging typically demonstrates moderate wall thickening (usually <9 mm), which involves the mucosa and submucosa.[30] There may be slight increased echogenicity of the submucosa because of fat deposition. However, the muscularis propria and pericolonic fat are spared.[30] Irregularity of the mucosa owing to trapping of gas bubbles in pseudopolyps may be observed.[36] Unlike CD, bowel wall stratification is generally preserved in patients with UC because of the lack of transmural involvement, although it may be disrupted in more severe disease.[23,30] The presence of increased bowel wall vascularity on color Doppler imaging has been associated with clinical and endoscopic activity of UC.[37,38] There are contradictory data regarding the role of color and power Doppler imaging to monitor response to treatment.[39,40] Toxic megacolon may be suspected with increased colonic dilatation (>6 cm), thin walls (<2 mm), and fluid-filled loops of bowel.[41]

## DIVERTICULITIS

Although the American College of Radiology appropriateness criteria recommends obtaining a CT scan in patients with suspected diverticulitis, it should be noted that US is used as the first-line imaging modality in some European and most developing countries.[42,43] Two meta-analyses comparing US and CT for the diagnosis of acute diverticulitis demonstrated sensitivities of 92% and 90% for US versus 94% and 95% for CT.[44,45] The same studies demonstrated specificities of 90% and 90% for US versus 99% and 96% for CT.[44,45] US can also detect complications such as abscesses and fistulas, although there are limited data regarding the efficacy of US in this setting.[10]

No specific patient preparation is needed, although a moderately fluid-filled bladder may be beneficial to image the lower sigmoid colon.[10] A low-frequency (at least 5 Mhz) curvilinear array transducer is generally used to image at lower depths.[8] Interrogation begins at the point of maximal tenderness and subsequently proceeds using the graded compression technique.[10]

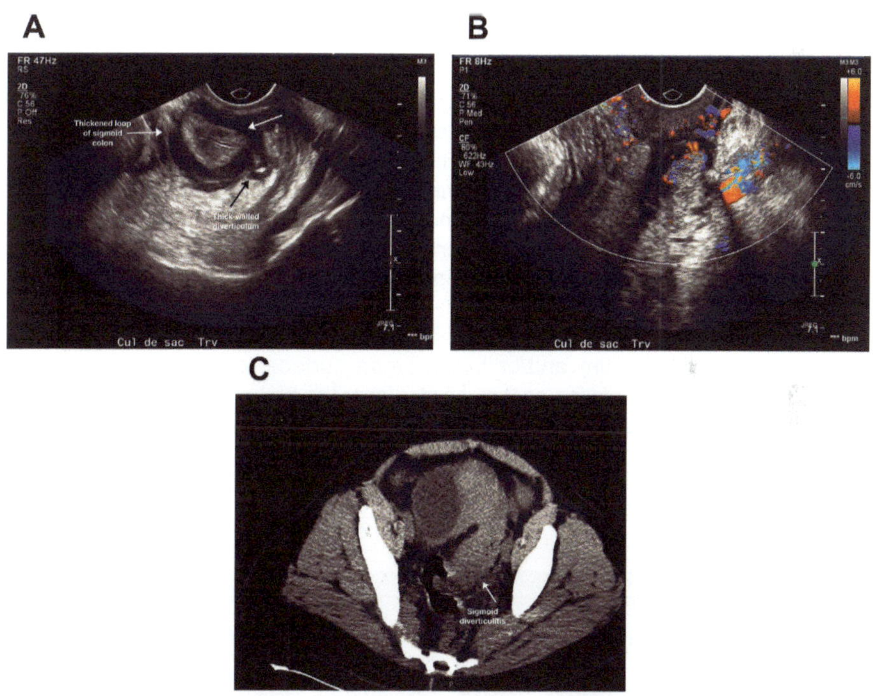


**Fig. 10.** Sigmoid Diverticulitis. A 47-year-old woman with left lower quadrant pain. (*A*) Grayscale transverse transvaginal image of the cul de sac demonstrates a thickened loop of bowel (*white arrows*) with a large, thick-walled diverticulum (*black arrow*). The outer hypoechoic muscularis layer of the bowel wall is hypertrophied and especially thick, as is often the case in patients with diverticulosis. Echogenic material within the lumen of the diverticulum reflects a small amount of gas. Increased echogenicity of the pericolonic soft tissues is also noted, consistent with inflammation of the surrounding pelvic fat. (*B*) Color Doppler transverse image demonstrates surrounding hyperemia of the soft tissues, compatible with inflammation. (*C*) Noncontrast CT scan of the pelvis demonstrates thickened, enlarged sigmoid diverticula (*arrow*) with adjacent inflammatory change, compatible with sigmoid diverticulitis. The adjacent wall of the sigmoid colon is also thickened.

On grayscale imaging, colonic diverticula appear as curvilinear protrusions off the colonic wall with variable amounts of internal echogenicity and posterior shadowing (depending on the presence of gas, feces, and/or fluid).[46] These findings may be associated with slight thickening of the muscularis propria layer because of hypertrophy of the circular smooth muscle.[10] Diverticulitis manifests as an enlarged, hypoechoic diverticulum with an ill-defined margin. The diverticular wall may be thick.[10] Associated circumferential or asymmetric thickening of the adjacent colon with hyperemia on color Doppler imaging is often present.[46] The pericolonic soft tissues demonstrate reactive fluid and hyperemia, whereas the adjacent fat is noncompressible and echogenic because of surrounding inflammation (**Fig. 10**).[10,46] Diverticulitis-related abscesses manifest as hypoechoic collections containing debris or gas bubbles, whereas fistulas appear as more band-like regions of decreased echogenicity.[10] Contrast-enhanced US has been reported to accurately differentiate abscess (avascular due to internal purulent material) from phlegmon (solid with internal vascularity), which may be occasionally difficult to distinguish based on grayscale and color Doppler imaging findings alone.[47]

## PERITONEAL CARCINOMATOSIS

Peritoneal carcinomatosis (PC) refers to the spread of tumor into the peritoneal cavity.[48] Secondary causes, because of metastases from gynecologic and gastrointestinal primary malignancies, are more common than primary peritoneal tumors with 71%, 17%, and 10% of patients with ovarian, gastric, and colorectal malignancies demonstrating carcinomatosis at the time of presentation.[48,49] Clinically, patients with PC may present with abdominal distension and bloating because of the presence of ascites, with one study reporting the presence of PC in 53.3% of patients with malignancy-related ascites.[50]

On grayscale imaging, tumor implants may manifest as nodular, hypoechoic lesions attached to the peritoneum and/or bowel/organ surface, or as sheet-like diffuse masses termed omental caking as they spread over the bowel (**Fig. 11**).[51] When ascites is present, it outlines the peritoneal nodules making them easier to detect. Color

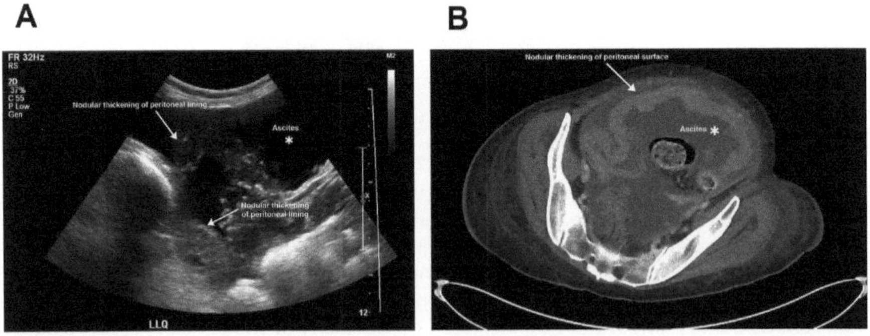


**Fig. 11.** Peritoneal carcinomatosis. A 57-year-old woman with left lower quadrant (LLQ) pain. (*A*) Grayscale imaging of the LLQ demonstrates ascites (*asterisk*) as well as nodular thickening of the peritoneal surface (*arrows*), which is highly concerning for carcinomatosis. (*B*) Subsequent contrast-enhanced CT scan confirms nodular thickening of the peritoneum (*arrow*) and extensive ascites (*asterisk*).

flow may be detected in the neoplastic tissue, allowing differentiation from hemorrhage and debris, with one study reporting detection of flow on power Doppler in 91% of tumor implants.[51] However, depending on the primary tumor, PC implants may be cystic. Detection of the thickened omentum as well as the extent of ascites may necessitate use of a transabdominal approach, in addition to transvaginal imaging (**Fig. 12**).[51]

## UROLITHIASIS

US has been reported to have variable accuracy in detecting urinary tract calculi, with one systematic review reporting a sensitivity and specificity of 45% and 94%, respectively, for the detection of ureteral calculi, and 45% and 88% for renal calculi.[52] However, US may be still be used as the first-line imaging modality to evaluate for urolithiasis because it is inexpensive, more readily available, and uses no ionizing radiation.[52] In addition, while US may miss small stones (<3 mm; which likely accounts for the overall poor sensitivity), it is an excellent means of detecting hydronephrosis, which dictates the management of patients with urolithiasis. US has also been shown to be accurate in following ureteral calculi within 35 mm of the uretero-vesicular junction (UVJ).[53] No specific patient preparation is required, although, in one study, sensitivity, specificity, and accuracy for the detection of ureteral calculi were reported to be

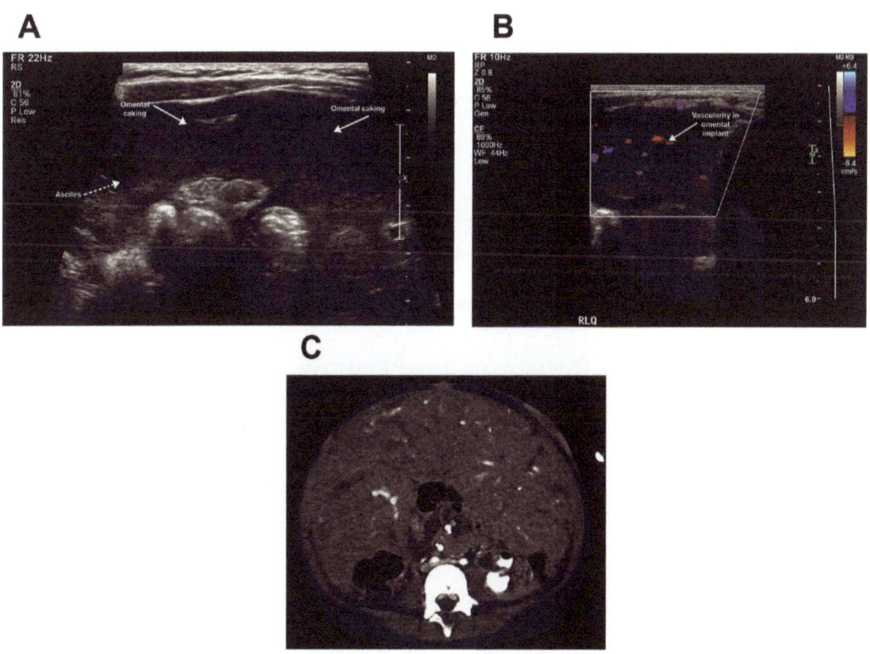


**Fig. 12.** Extensive peritoneal carcinomatosis. An 18-year-old woman with pelvic pain. (*A*) Grayscale image demonstrates diffuse omental caking (*solid arrows*). There is also a small amount of anechoic ascites (*dashed arrow*). (*B*) Color Doppler image demonstrates vascularity (*arrow*) in one of the implants. (*C*) Subsequent contrast-enhanced CT confirms diffuse, extensive peritoneal carcinomatosis with contrast enhancement of numerous vessels.

98.3%, 100%, and 98.4%, respectively, with the use of preprocedural patient fasting for 8 hours and intravenous hydration with normal saline immediately before scanning.[54]

On US, urolithiasis manifests as sharply marginated echogenic foci with posterior acoustic shadowing. Scanning with harmonics and spatial compounding will increase the grayscale sensitivity for the detection of renal calculi. However, spatial compounding will largely eliminate posterior acoustic shadowing, Hence, patients should be scanned with and without spatial compounding to maximize detection of calculi.

On color Doppler imaging, twinkle artifact may be noted posterior to the calculus, manifesting as a tapering multicolor signal similar to the color pattern of aliasing (**Fig. 13**).[55] This has been reported in 78% to 97% of urinary track calculi and may precede the detection of the stone itself on grayscale imaging in 70% of cases.[56,57] In addition, careful attention should be paid to the uretero-pelvic junction and UVJ because stones are most likely to lodge in these locations. In women, transvaginal imaging of the UVJ can be performed, with the higher-frequency

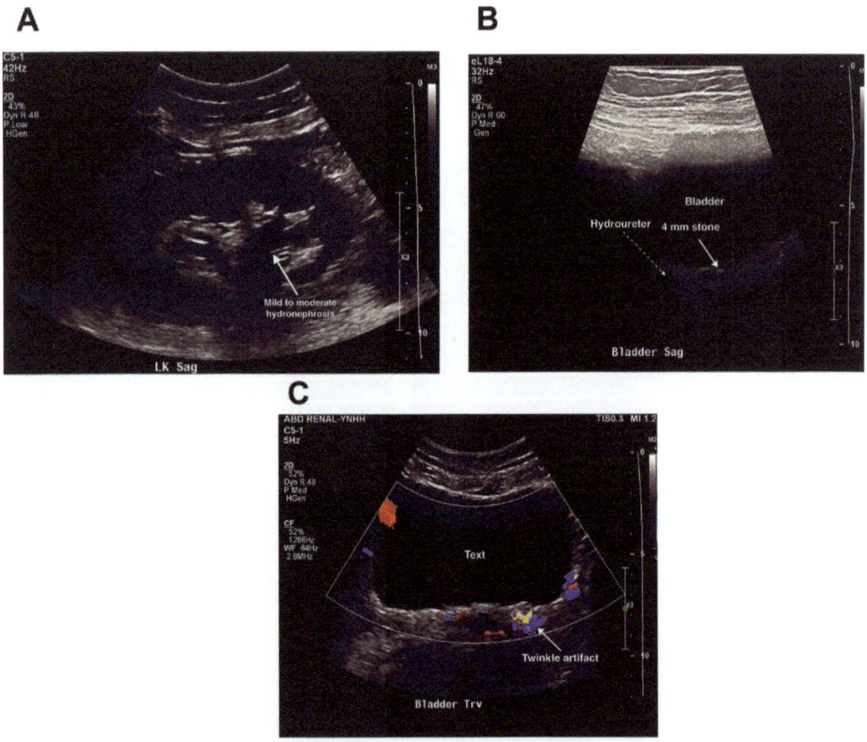


**Fig. 13.** Obstructing left ureteral calculus. 42 year-old female with left flank and groin pain. (*A*) Gray-scale longitudinal image of the left kidney (LK) demonstrates mild to moderate hydronephrosis (*arrow*). (*B*) Sagittal gray-scale evaluation of the left distal ureter reveals a 4 mm echogenic calculus (*arrow*) with posterior acoustic shadowing and upstream hydroureter (*dashed arrow*). On transverse color Doppler image (*C*) twinkle artifact (*arrow*) is noted posteriorly. A left ureteral jet was not observed in the bladder (*arrow*) suggesting complete obstruction.

transvaginal probe significantly improving the sensitivity of US for the detection of UVJ stones (**Fig. 14**).

With urinary tract obstruction, hydroureteronephrosis will be present, with or without adjacent perinephric fluid. An absent or an asymmetric low-level ureteral jet in the bladder may be noted at the UVJ on color Doppler imaging ipsilateral to an obstructing ureteral calculus (**Fig. 15**).[58] However, if the ureteral calculus is non-obstructing, the jet will be present. Of note, the sonographer should observe the bladder for up to 5 minutes with color Doppler before concluding that the jet is absent.

## PELVIC CONGESTION SYNDROME

Pelvic congestion syndrome (PCS) is a poorly understood disorder of the pelvic venous circulation resulting in chronic pelvic pain, defined as intermittent or constant pain of at least 3 to 6 months duration, not associated with pregnancy or sexual intercourse, and not limited to a specific period of the menstrual cycle.[59] Imaging findings are used to document the characteristic pelvic venous changes

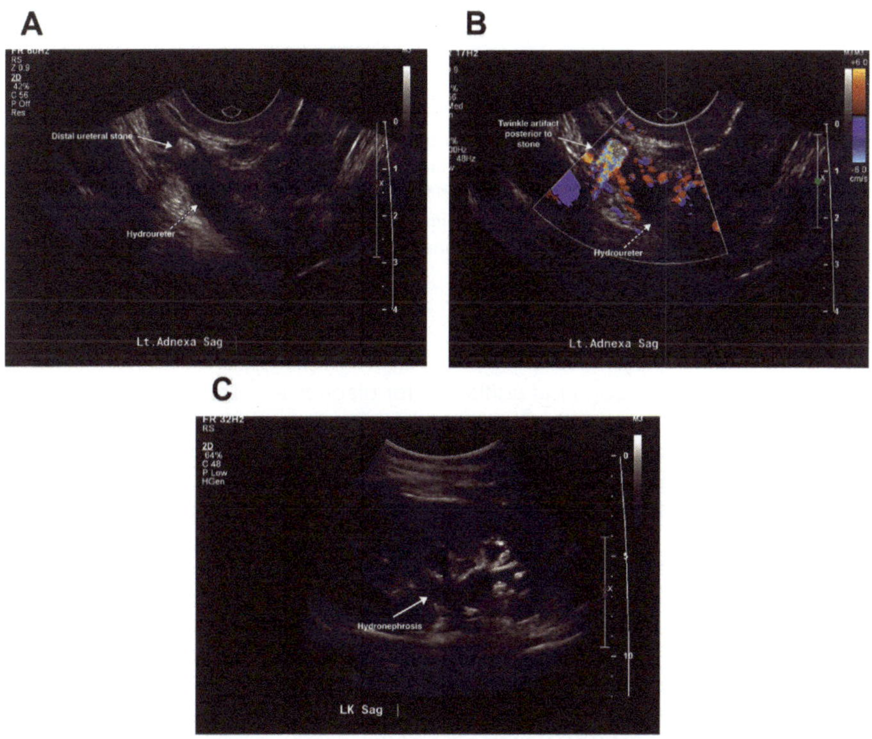


**Fig. 14.** A 41-year-old woman with left lower quadrant pain. (*A*) Grayscale transvaginal image of the left adnexa demonstrates a rounded, sharply marginated echogenic structure (*arrow*) with posterior twinkle artifact on transvaginal color Doppler image (*B*) (*arrow*) within a tubular, avascular anechoic structure (*dashed arrows* in *A* and *B*). Findings are compatible with a distal left ureteral stone with upstream hydroureter. (*C*) Transabdominal grayscale image of the left kidney (LK) reveals moderate hydronephrosis (*arrow*).

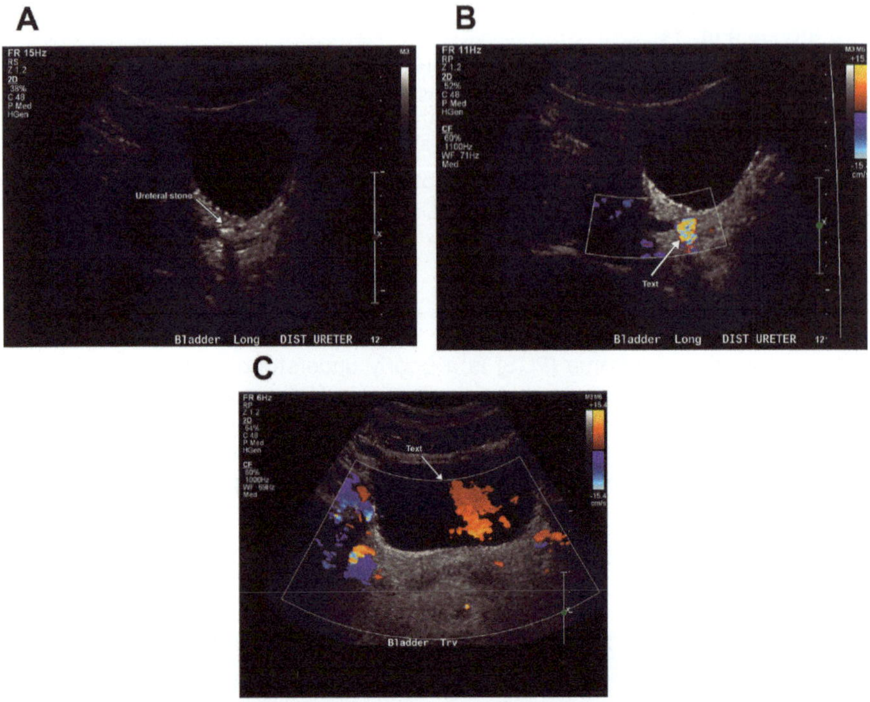


**Fig. 15.** Left ureteral calculus with partial obstruction. A 34-year-old woman with left groin pain and nausea. (*A*) Longitudinal grayscale image of the left distal ureter demonstrates a 4-mm echogenic calculus (*arrow*) with posterior acoustic shadowing and upstream mild hydroureter. (*B*) Longitudinal color Doppler image of the distal left ureter demonstrates twinkle artifact (*arrow*) posterior to the stone. (*C*) Transverse color Doppler image of the bladder demonstrates a left ureteral jet (*arrow*), which excludes complete ureteral obstruction.

that are necessary, although not sufficient, for diagnosis.[59] Transabdominal and/or transvaginal sonography with Doppler evaluation may be performed, with the latter preferred because it allows better visualization of the pelvic vasculature.[60] Imaging the patient in the semi-upright position or on performing a Valsalva maneuver improves venous filling and may enable better visualization of pelvic varicosities.[60]

Reported sonographic findings include dilatation greater than 4 mm of the left ovarian vein, which normally drains into the left renal vein with slow ($\leq$3 cm/s) or retrograde flow, dilated arcuate veins that communicate with the tortuous and engorged pelvic venous plexus across the myometrium, usually at the lower uterine segment and increased flow in the varices on spectral or color Doppler following a Valsalva maneuver (**Figs. 16** and **17**).[61] Polycystic changes of the ovaries have also been described, although the significance of this finding is uncertain.[61,62] PCS can be effectively treated with coil embolization with or without sclerotherapy. However, not all patients respond and response is not always durable. Therefore, it is likely that not all pelvic varices are symptomatic or directly related to an individual woman's chronic pelvic pain. (Note that this has been disputed often in the literature.)

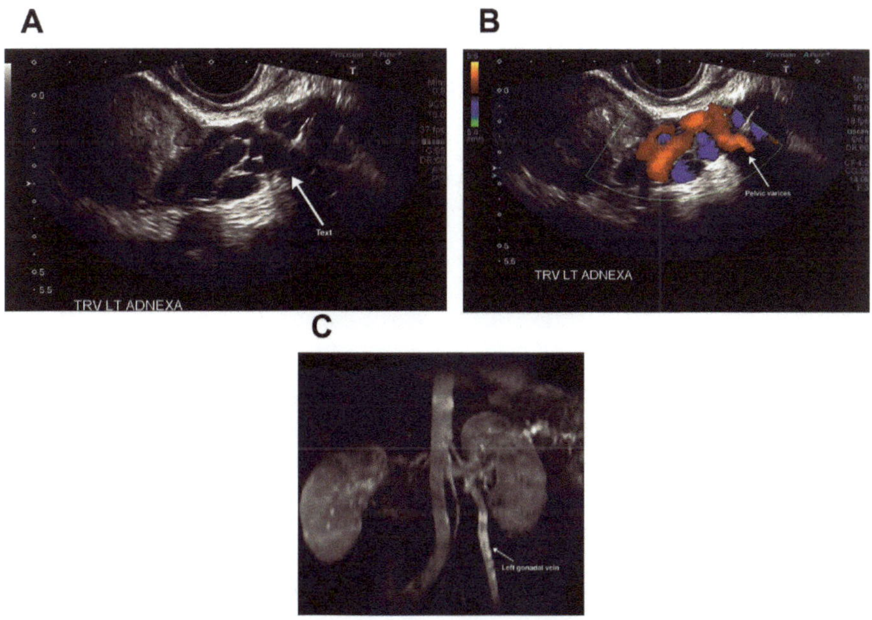


**Fig. 16.** Pelvic congestion syndrome. A 34-year-old woman with pelvic fullness. (*A*) Grayscale and (*B*) color Doppler transvaginal transverse images of the left adnexa demonstrate multiple enlarged tubular structures that fill in with color Doppler (*arrows*), consistent with pelvic varices. Spectral Doppler tracing (not shown) confirmed venous waveforms. (*C*) Coronal T1-weighted postcontrast MRI of the abdomen demonstrates reflux into the enlarged left gonadal vein (*arrow*) draining into the left renal vein.

## SUMMARY

US, using a combination of grayscale, color Doppler, and power Doppler imaging, is often the first-line imaging modality used to evaluate women who present with acute or chronic pelvic pain. Advantages include low cost, widespread availability, and lack of ionizing radiation. Whereas the role of US in the evaluation of gynecologic causes of pelvic pain is well appreciated, it is increasingly used, particularly in Europe and Asia, as the initial imaging modality of choice even when GI and urinary tract pathologic conditions are suspected, for these same reasons. It is imperative to recognize the US findings of nongynecologic causes of pelvic pain because a delay in diagnosis can result in significant morbidity and mortality. Use of transducers of various frequencies is crucial to image at the appropriate depth, with both transabdominal and transvaginal imaging approaches; imaging of patients in different positions is important to increase sensitivity and to detect certain entities. For evaluation of most pathologic conditions of the bowel, the graded compression technique should be used because it displaces adjacent air-filled loops of the bowel, thus eliminating artifact from overlying bowel gas and prevents guarding. This permits evaluation of deeper structures and helps identify the point of maximum tenderness, which can serve to localize the pathologic condition in the pelvic region and focus the examination. Future directions include the increasing use of CEUS, particularly in cases of IBD.

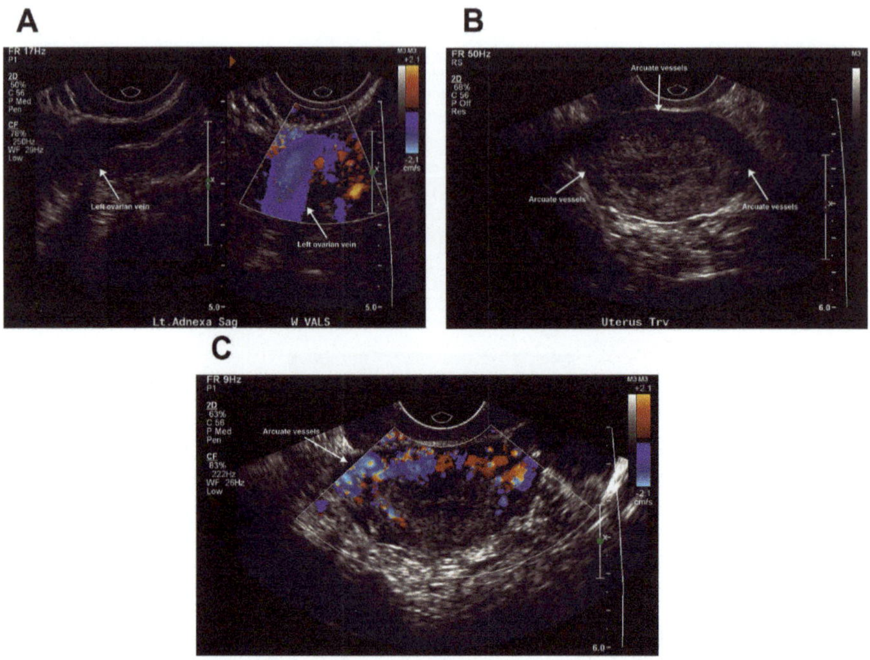


**Fig. 17.** Pelvic congestion syndrome. 32 year-old female with pelvic pain and heaviness. (*A*) Split screen gray-scale and color Doppler with Valsalva transvaginal image demonstrates a dilated left ovarian vein with color flow filling the lumen (*arrow*). Low level intraluminal echoes are noted on the gray-scale image, a finding indicative of slow flow. Transverse gray-scale (*B*) and color Doppler (*C*) transvaginal images of the uterus demonstrate prominent dilatated arcuate vessels at the periphery of the myometrium (*arrows in B*) that fill in with color (*C*). Dilated uterine arcuate vessels that directly connect to pelvic varices are believed to be highly specific for pelvic congestion syndrome.

## REFERENCES

1. Addiss DG, Shaffer N, Fowler BS, et al. The epidemiology of appendicitis and appendectomy in the United States. Am J Epidemiol 1990;132(5):910–25.
2. Weiss AJ, Elixhauser A, Andrews RM. Characteristics of operating room procedures in U.S. Hospitals, 2011: statistical brief #170. Healthcare Cost and Utilization Project (HCUP) statistical briefs. Rockville (MD): Agency for Healthcare Research and Quality (US); 2006.
3. Garcia EM, Camacho MA, Karolyi DR, et al. ACR appropriateness criteria® right lower quadrant pain-suspected appendicitis. J Am Coll Radiol 2018;15(11S): S373–87. Available at: https://acsearch.acr.org/docs/69357/Narrative/. Accessed February 4, 2019.
4. Pinto F, Pinto A, Russo A, et al. Accuracy of ultrasonography in the diagnosis of acute appendicitis in adult patients: review of the literature. Crit Ultrasound J 2013;5(1):S2.
5. Jacobs JE. CT and sonography for suspected acute appendicitis: a commentary. AJR Am J Roentgenol 2006;186(4):1094–6.
6. Sartelli M, Baiocchi GL, Di Saverio S, et al. Prospective observational study on acute appendicitis worldwide (POSAW). World J Emerg Surg 2018;13(1):19.

7. Puylaert J. Acute appendicitis: US evaluation using graded compression. Radiology 1986;158(2):355–60.
8. Nylund K, Maconi G, Hollerweger A, et al. EFSUMB recommendations and guidelines for gastrointestinal ultrasound-part 1: examination techniques and normal findings (long version). Ultraschall Med 2017;38(03):e1–15.
9. Lee JH, Jeong YK, Park KB, et al. Operator-dependent techniques for graded compression sonography to detect the appendix and diagnose acute appendicitis. AJR Am J Roentgenol 2005;184(1):91–7.
10. Dirks K, Calabrese E, Dietrich CF, et al. EFSUMB position paper: recommendations for Gastrointestinal Ultrasound (GIUS) in acute appendicitis and diverticulitis. Ultraschall Med 2019;40(2):163–75.
11. Chicaiza HP, Malia L, Mulvey CH, et al. Revisiting the appendiceal diameter via ultrasound for the diagnosis of acute appendicitis. Pediatr Emerg Care 2018; 34(11):757–60.
12. Cohen B, Bowling J, Midulla P, et al. The non-diagnostic ultrasound in appendicitis: is a non-visualized appendix the same as a negative study? J Pediatr Surg 2015;50(6):923–7.
13. Estey A, Poonai N, Lim R. Appendix not seen: the predictive value of secondary inflammatory sonographic signs. Pediatr Emerg Care 2013;29(4):435–9.
14. Xu Y, Jeffrey RB, Chang ST, et al. Sonographic differentiation of complicated from uncomplicated appendicitis: implications for antibiotics-first therapy. J Ultrasound Med 2017;36(2):269–77.
15. Katz DS, Baker ME, Rosen MP, et al. ACR appropriateness criteria® suspected small-bowel obstruction. American College of Radiology; 2013. Available at: https://acsearch.acr.org/docs/69476/Narrative/.
16. Gottlieb M, Peksa GD, Pandurangadu AV, et al. Utilization of ultrasound for the evaluation of small bowel obstruction: a systematic review and meta-analysis. Am J Emerg Med 2018;36(2):234–42.
17. Suri S, Gupta S, Sudhakar P, et al. Comparative evaluation of plain films, ultrasound and CT in the diagnosis of intestinal obstruction. Acta Radiol 1999; 40(4):422–8.
18. Hefny AF, Corr P, Abu-Zidan FM. The role of ultrasound in the management of intestinal obstruction. J Emerg Trauma Shock 2012;5(1):84.
19. Fleischer AC, Dowling AD, Weinstein ML, et al. Sonographic patterns of distended, fluid-filled bowel. Radiology 1979;133(3):681–5.
20. Silva AC, Pimenta M, Guimaraes LS. Small bowel obstruction: what to look for. Radiographics 2009;29(2):423–39.
21. Grassi R, Romano S, D'Amario F, et al. The relevance of free fluid between intestinal loops detected by sonography in the clinical assessment of small bowel obstruction in adults. Eur J Radiol 2004;50(1):5–14.
22. Kappelman MD, Rifas-Shiman SL, Kleinman K, et al. The prevalence and geographic distribution of Crohn's disease and ulcerative colitis in the United States. Clin Gastroenterol Hepatol 2007;5(12):1424–9.
23. Strobel D, Goertz RS, Bernatik T. Diagnostics in inflammatory bowel disease: ultrasound. World J Gastroenterol 2011;17(27):3192.
24. Fraquelli M, Colli A, Casazza G, et al. Role of US in detection of Crohn disease: meta-analysis. Radiology 2005;236(1):95–101.
25. Fraquelli M, Sarno A, Girelli C, et al. Reproducibility of bowel ultrasonography in the evaluation of Crohn's disease. Dig Liver Dis 2008;40(11):860–6.

26. Neye H, Ensberg D, Rauh P, et al. Impact of high-resolution transabdominal ultrasound in the diagnosis of complications of Crohn's disease. Scand J Gastroenterol 2010;45(6):690–5.
27. Dong J, Wang H, Zhao J, et al. Ultrasound as a diagnostic tool in detecting active Crohn's disease: a meta-analysis of prospective studies. Eur Radiol 2014;24(1):26–33.
28. Calabrese E, Petruzziello C, Onali S, et al. Severity of postoperative recurrence in Crohn's disease: correlation between endoscopic and sonographic findings. Inflamm Bowel Dis 2009;15(11):1635–42.
29. Ripollés T, Martínez MJ, Barrachina MM. Crohn's disease and color Doppler sonography: response to treatment and its relationship with long-term prognosis. J Clin Ultrasound 2008;36(5):267–72.
30. Maconi G, Nylund K, Ripolles T, et al. EFSUMB recommendations and clinical guidelines for intestinal ultrasound (GIUS) in inflammatory bowel diseases. Ultraschall Med 2018;39(3):304–17.
31. Lu C, Merrill C, Medellin A, et al. Bowel ultrasound state of the art: grayscale and Doppler ultrasound, contrast enhancement, and elastography in Crohn Disease. J Ultrasound Med 2019;38(2):271–88.
32. Drews B, Barth T, Hänle M, et al. Comparison of sonographically measured bowel wall vascularity, histology, and disease activity in Crohn's disease. Eur Radiol 2009;19(6):1379–86.
33. Neye H, Voderholzer W, Rickes S, et al. Evaluation of criteria for the activity of Crohn's disease by power Doppler sonography. Dig Dis 2004;22(1):67–72.
34. Quaia E, Sozzi M, Angileri R, et al. Time-intensity curves obtained after microbubble injection can be used to differentiate responders from nonresponders among patients with clinically active Crohn disease after 6 weeks of pharmacologic treatment. Radiology 2016;281(2):606–16.
35. Paredes JM, Ripollés T, Cortés X, et al. Contrast-enhanced ultrasonography: usefulness in the assessment of postoperative recurrence of Crohn's disease. J Crohns Colitis 2013;7(3):192–201.
36. Bru C, Sans M, Defelitto MM, et al. Hydrocolonic sonography for evaluating inflammatory bowel disease. AJR Am J Roentgenol 2001;177(1):99–105.
37. Bavil AS, Somi MH, Nemati M, et al. Ultrasonographic evaluation of bowel wall thickness and intramural blood flow in ulcerative colitis. ISRN Gastroenterol 2012;2012:370495.
38. Civitelli F, Di Nardo G, Oliva S, et al. Ultrasonography of the colon in pediatric ulcerative colitis: a prospective, blind, comparative study with colonoscopy. J Pediatr 2014;165(1):78–84.e2.
39. Rogoveanu I, Săftoiu A, Cazacu S, et al. Color Doppler transabdominal ultrasonography for the assessment of the patients with inflammatory bowel disease during treatment. Rom J Gastroenterol 2003;12(4):277–81.
40. Yamaguchi T, Yoshida S, Tanaka S, et al. Predicting the clinical response to cytapheresis in steroid-refractory or-dependent ulcerative colitis using contrast-enhanced ultrasonography. Scand J Gastroenterol 2009;44(7):831–7.
41. Maconi G, Sampietro GM, Ardizzone S, et al. Case report: ultrasonographic detection of toxic megacolon in inflammatory bowel diseases. Dig Dis Sci 2004;49(1):138–42.
42. Galgano SJ, McNamara MM, Peterson CM, et al. ACR appropriateness criteria® left lower quadrant pain-suspected diverticulitis. J Am Coll Radiol 2018. Available at: https://acsearch.acr.org/docs/69356/Narrative/. Accessed January 29, 2019.

43. Sartelli M, Catena F, Ansaloni L, et al. WSES guidelines for the management of acute left sided colonic diverticulitis in the emergency setting. World J Emerg Surg 2016;11(1):37.
44. Andeweg CS, Wegdam JA, Groenewoud J, et al. Toward an evidence-based step-up approach in diagnosing diverticulitis. Scand J Gastroenterol 2014; 49(7):775–84.
45. Laméris W, van Randen A, Bipat S, et al. Graded compression ultrasonography and computed tomography in acute colonic diverticulitis: meta-analysis of test accuracy. Eur Radiol 2008;18(11):2498.
46. Rodgers PM, Verma R. Transabdominal ultrasound for bowel evaluation. Radiol Clin 2013;51(1):133–48.
47. Ripollés T, Martínez-Pérez MJ, Paredes JM, et al. Contrast-enhanced ultrasound in the differentiation between phlegmon and abscess in Crohn's disease and other abdominal conditions. Eur J Radiol 2013;82(10):e525–31.
48. Coccolini F, Gheza F, Lotti M, et al. Peritoneal carcinomatosis. World J Gastroenterol 2013;19(41):6979.
49. Coakley FV, Choi PH, Gougoutas CA, et al. Peritoneal metastases: detection with spiral CT in patients with ovarian cancer. Radiology 2002;223(2):495–9.
50. Runyon BA, Hoefs JC, Morgan TR. Ascitic fluid analysis in malignancy-related ascites. Hepatology 1988;8(5):1104–9.
51. Savelli L, De Iaco P, Ceccaroni M, et al. Transvaginal sonographic features of peritoneal carcinomatosis. Ultrasound Obstet Gynecol 2005;26(5):552–7.
52. Ray AA, Ghiculete D, Pace KT, et al. Limitations to ultrasound in the detection and measurement of urinary tract calculi. Urology 2010;76(2):295–300.
53. Moesbergen TC, de Ryke RJ, Dunbar S, et al. Distal ureteral calculi: US follow-up. Radiology 2011;260(2):575–80.
54. Park SJ, Yi BH, Lee HK, et al. Evaluation of patients with suspected ureteral calculi using sonography as an initial diagnostic tool: how can we improve diagnostic accuracy? J Ultrasound Med 2008;27(10):1441–50.
55. Aytaç SK, Özcan H. Effect of color Doppler system on the twinkling sign associated with urinary tract calculi. J Clin Ultrasound 1999;27(8):433–9.
56. Mitterberger M, Aigner F, Pallwein L, et al. Sonographic detection of renal and ureteral stones: value of the twinkling sign. Int Braz J Urol 2009;35(5):532–41.
57. Ripollés T, Martínez-Pérez MJ, Vizuete J, et al. Sonographic diagnosis of symptomatic ureteral calculi: usefulness of the twinkling artifact. Abdom Imaging 2013;38(4):863–9.
58. Burge H, Middleton W, McClennan B, et al. Ureteral jets in healthy subjects and in patients with unilateral ureteral calculi: comparison with color Doppler US. Radiology 1991;180(2):437–42.
59. Borghi C, Dell'Atti L. Pelvic congestion syndrome: the current state of the literature. Arch Gynecol Obstet 2016;293(2):291–301.
60. Phillips D, Deipolyi AR, Hesketh RL, et al. Pelvic congestion syndrome: etiology of pain, diagnosis, and clinical management. J Vasc Interv Radiol 2014;25(5): 725–33.
61. Park SJ, Lim JW, Ko YT, et al. Diagnosis of pelvic congestion syndrome using transabdominal and transvaginal sonography. AJR Am J Roentgenol 2004; 182(3):683–8.
62. Adams J, Reginald P, Franks S, et al. Uterine size and endometrial thickness and the significance of cystic ovaries in women with pelvic pain due to congestion. Br J Obstet Gynaecol 1990;97(7):583–7.

# Three-Dimensional Volume Imaging in Gynecology

Beryl R. Benacerraf, MD

**KEYWORDS**

• 3D ultrasonography • Ultrasound uterus • Infertility ultrasound • Volume ultrasound • Gynecologic imaging

**KEY POINTS**

- 3D ultrasonography allows the rapid acquisition of a volume containing innumerable images that can be generated in any orientation and reconstructed off sight by practitioners remote from the patient.
- Volumes contain large amounts of sonographic information that can be displayed in many ways. These include 3 orthogonal planes at right angles to each other, parallel cuts similar to computed tomography and MRI displays, inverse mode to see the cystic areas within the volume, and surface rendering of any interface.
- 3D ultrasonography of the pelvis enables the display of the coronal view of the uterus. This critical plane allows one to diagnose Mullerian duct anomalies, location of IUDs, and localization of fibroids, polyps, and adhesions.
- 3D is helpful to evaluate the adnexa and distinguish hydrosalpinges from septated ovarian cysts or other adnexal disorders.
- 3D ultrasonography can include Doppler to demonstrate mapping of blood flow, as well as measurements of any portion of the volume.

Three-dimensional (3D) volume imaging of the female pelvis among the key advances in women's imaging within the last 2 decades.[1] Volume imaging has been the basis for the display of computed tomography (CT) and MR images for a long time. Ultrasonography, on the other hand, has always been very operator dependent and time consuming, because 2D ultrasonography requires the manual acquisition of one image at a time, taken at the discretion of the person holding the transducer. Hence, the quality and information in standard ultrasound images rely on the expertise of the operator that produced them, similar to sending someone on vacation with a camera and reviewing the photos taken on the trip. Even a careful review of these 2D photos will often not reveal anything that was not observed and deliberately imaged by the operator. Furthermore, 3D sonography allows clinicians to review entire volumes after the patient has left and essentially rescan the pelvis, independently from

One Brookline Place, Brookline, MA 02445, USA
*E-mail address:* berylbenacerraf@post.harvard.edu

Obstet Gynecol Clin N Am 46 (2019) 755–781
https://doi.org/10.1016/j.ogc.2019.07.008

the way the operator initially viewed the anatomy.[1] Just a few volume acquisitions can provide complete images of the entire pelvis, which can be reviewed and rescanned electronically in any plane by a different or expert operator who is less dependent on the expertise of the sonographer who actually scanned the patient.[2]

## TECHNIQUE

Automated 3D transducers gather 2D ultrasound information from one side of the probe to the other at a constant rate of speed. The operator holds the probe still, and the transducer travels across the width of the housing to acquire the volume in a systematic and reproducible fashion. The speed of this mechanical acquisition varies inversely with the resolution of the image, a setting easily changed by the operator before initiating the automatic acquisition. The distance traversed during the acquisition will determine the width of the reconstructed planes, and this too needs to be selected as the sweep angle. Different types of processing as well as harmonics can also modify the appearance of the volume and, hence, the quality of the image.

Once the 3D volume has been acquired, it represents a large amount of sonographic data that can then be displayed in various ways. The most common way to present and evaluate a volume initially is the multiplanar image set of 3 orthogonal planes at right angles to each other, representing planes x, y, and z (**Fig. 1**).There is a small dot that indicates the intersection of these 3 planes, and the practitioner can navigate

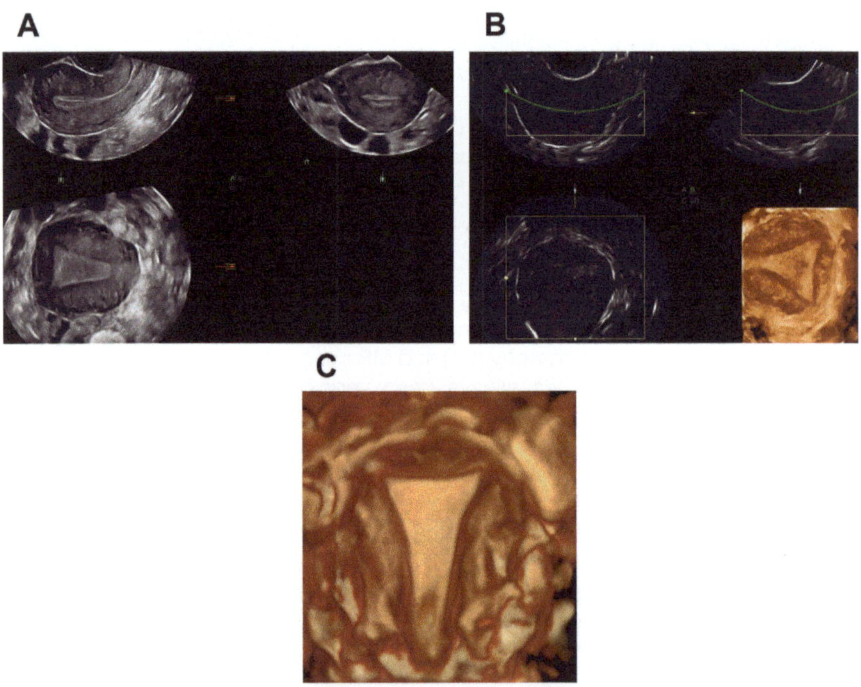


**Fig. 1.** (*A*) 3D volume of a normal uterus displayed using the 3 orthogonal planes. The lower left image shows the reconstructed coronal view of the uterus. (*B*) 3D volume of a normal uterus displayed using the 3 orthogonal planes, also including the rendered view in the lower right side of the image. (*C*) The rendered coronal view of the uterus using a thick slice technique to produce a rich and more detailed rendering of the endometrium and subendometrial regions.

through the volume using the 4 basic tools of rotation: x, y, z and cutting from one end of the data set to the other in parallel slices similarly to a CT or MRI scan. This type of display of these 3 orthogonal planes are usually the optimal way the volume data sets are initially presented to the operator for manipulation.[3] Any plane of orientation within the volume can be completely reconstructed from the volume data, including planes that cannot be acquired directly while scanning a patient either transabdominally or transvaginally. The most useful reconstructed plane within a 3D volume is the coronal view of the uterus and adnexa, similar to the appearance of these organs on a Netter anatomic diagram, where all of the anatomic information of the uterine surface and well as endometrial cavity shape is displayed[3,4] (see **Fig. 1**). The reconstructed coronal view of the pelvic organs may be the most informative view for diagnosing uterine and tubal disorder. Volumes of 3D information can also be used to display the internal surfaces of the uterine cavity by using the surface-rendering technique while distending the cavity with saline[5] (**Fig. 2**). The inverse mode is a tool used to display all the cystic portions within a volume, regardless of image plane, making this technique a very useful 3D rendition of portions of the volumetric information. By selecting the inverse mode, all of the cystic areas within the volume become opaque and the solid areas disappear, resulting in a cast of the fluid-containing sections[6,7] (**Fig. 3**). Volumetric measurements can be also made within the data set to allow quantitative measurements of portions of the anatomy.[8] The volume can be acquired with the Doppler function on, such that blood flow data can be integrated into the volume information. One can then interpret the Doppler information quantitatively using blood flow velocity and waveform or qualitatively with mapping.[9,10]

Tomographic ultrasound imaging (TUI) is another method by which the information within a volume can be displayed[1] (**Fig. 4**). Multiple tomographic cuts, equidistant from each other, can result in a display of many parallel 2D images traversing the entire volume, much like a CT or MRI display. These tomographic displays are accomplished by selecting a single plane from within the volume, and slicing through the entire volume from one end to the other in the same orientation. These techniques bring ultrasonography closer to other forms of cross-sectional imaging, such as CT and MRI.

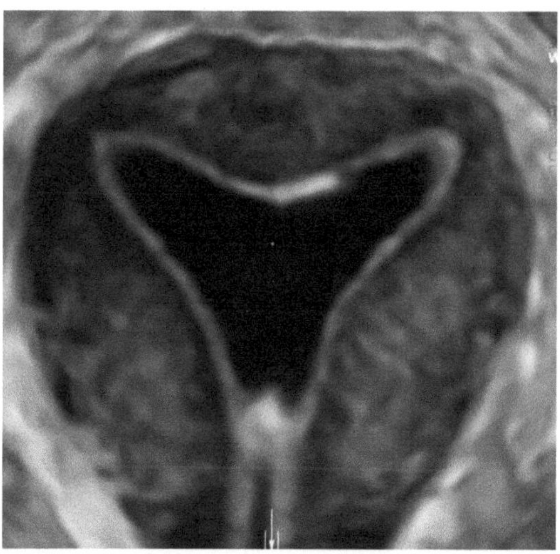

**Fig. 2.** The rendered coronal view of a normal uterus showing some saline in the cavity outlining a normal endometrium during a sonohysterogram.

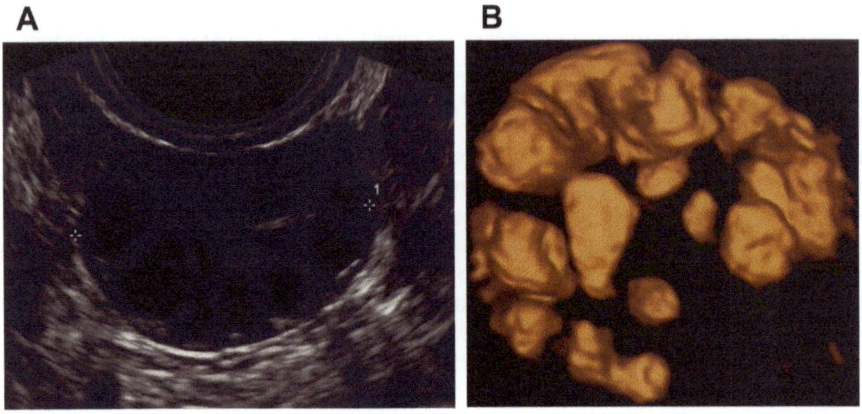


**Fig. 3.** (*A*) 2D ultrasound image of an ovary with a multitude of small follicles. (*B*) A volume image of the same ovary using the inverse mode that demonstrates each follicle as an individual element.

The entire pelvis can be imaged by acquiring several volumes (at least one of the uterus and one of each ovary), then displaying them using TUI or navigating through the volume doing a "virtual rescan" of the patient electronically so that the whole examination can be read offline or at a remote site. When the authors studied the feasibility of performing pelvic ultrasonography using this technique, they found that in comparison with a standard 2D examination, a full set of images could be

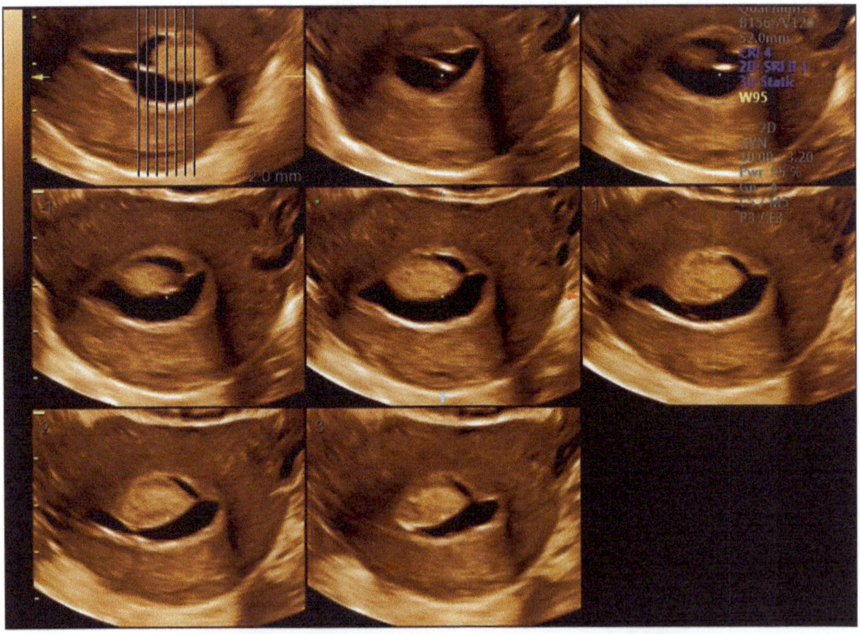

**Fig. 4.** 3D volume of a sonohysterogram showing a polyp surrounded by saline. The volume is displayed as parallel or tomographic cuts from one side of the uterus to the other, all information contained within one volume.

generated accurately and efficiently using displayed volume imaging.[2] The mean time needed to perform a 2D transvaginal scan was at least double the time needed to acquire and store 3D volumes that contained all the necessary anatomic information. The images read offline were of sufficient quality to render a report similar to the original reading of the standard 2D ultrasonogram done at the time of the patient's visit. Acquiring volumes to generate images offline could provide a means of standardizing the way sonographic images are archived in the future, rather than generating 2D images one at a time without the ability to go back and rescan.

Four-dimensional (4D) sonography represents real-time 3D imaging, motion being the fourth dimension.[1] Most current ultrasound machines still have mechanical 3D transducers whereby a multitude of 2D slices are rapidly acquired, resulting in a choppy 4D display. The speed of the frame rate varies inversely with the resolution of the image. Matrix array transducers that can acquire volumes electronically without having to sweep mechanically from one end of the transducer housing to the other are likely to improve the resolution of 4D ultrasonography. The mechanical aspect of volume imaging must be replaced by volume acquisitions that can be accomplished far more rapidly, at full resolution.[1]

## SURFACE RENDERING WITHIN A VOLUME

When there is fluid within a volume, a surface-rendering display can be used at the interface between the fluid and a solid surface to obtain a view of the solid surface under the fluid. Sonohysterography imaged with the 3D rendering technique can demonstrate the surface of the uterine cavity much like a virtual hysteroscopy, showing polyps or intracavitary fibroids in detail[11,12] (**Fig. 5**). 3D surface imaging can demonstrate the internal texture of an ovarian cyst, thus showing the mural nodularity in cystic masses such as ovarian neoplasms (**Fig. 6**).

When using the surface-rendering technique, the electronic scalpel can carve away portions of the images, revealing the anatomy of interest. Cutting away these layers of echoes from in front of the target area is best accomplished by rotating

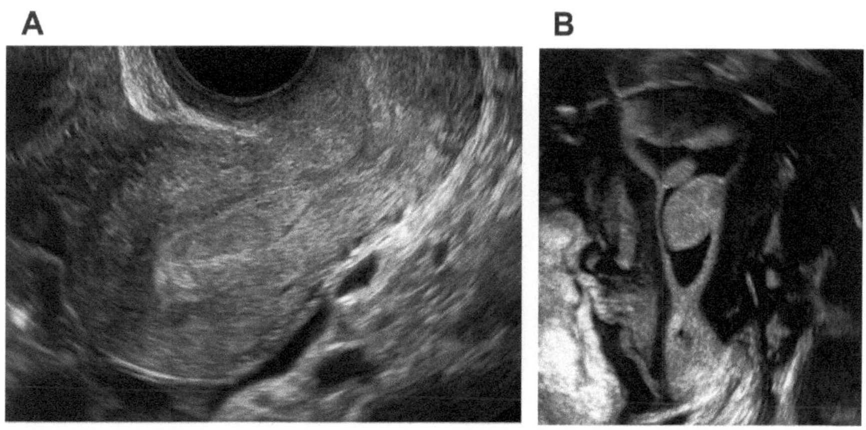


**Fig. 5.** (*A*) 2D image of a uterus taken in long axis showing an abnormally heterogeneous endometrium in a patient with abnormal bleeding. (*B*) After saline was placed into the uterine cavity, a 3D volume was acquired; this is the reconstructed coronal view of the cavity showing 2 endometrial polyps.

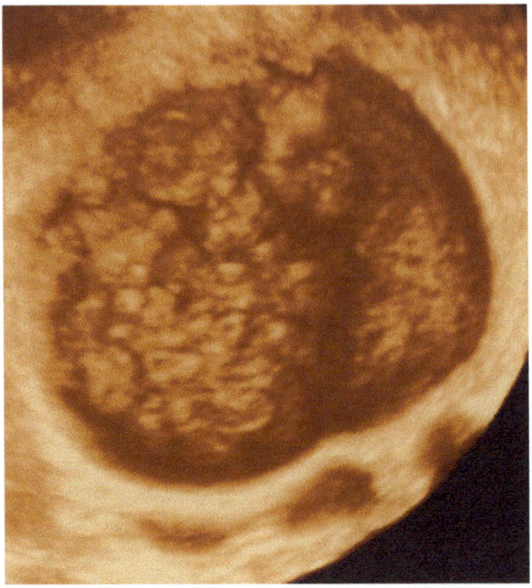

Fig. 6. Surface-rendering image from a volume containing a cystic mass. Cutting the volume in half electronically results in this view of the inside of the cyst showing the abundant nodularity on the inner surface of this borderline ovarian tumor.

the volume in different directions to reach the best cutting plane to demonstrate the anatomy. One can slice an entire volume in half with the electronic scalpel, then pry the 2 parts apart to reveal the inner surface of the cyst contained inside the volume (see **Fig. 6**).

Finally, the practitioner can render just a thin portion of the volume by using a thick slice technique that shows a thicker slice of anatomy than standard 2D imaging. This technique emphasizes the edge enhancement of structures and provides an image rich in contrast (**Fig. 7**).

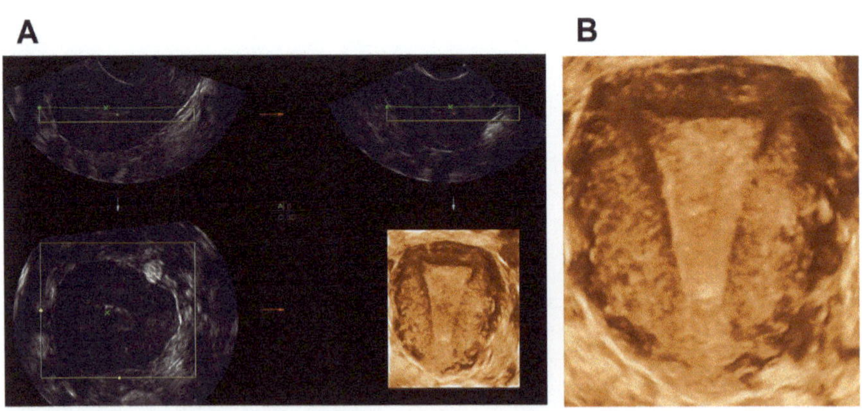


Fig. 7. (*A*) Standard display of a volume containing the entire uterus showing the 3 orthogonal views of the uterus, including the reconstructed thick slice-rendered view of the coronal view of the uterus (*lower right*). (*B*) Enlarged view of the reconstructed rendered view of the coronal orientation of the uterus shown in (*A*).

## CORONAL VIEW OF THE PELVIS

### *The Uterus*

3D ultrasonography provides the ability to display planes that cannot be acquired by direct transducer application to the patient. Hence, these planes are reconstructed from within the volume and include the coronal view, which is the most useful view of the uterus diagnostically.[4,13]

Anatomy books, such as Netter's, use the coronal view of the pelvis to display the anatomy of the uterus, ovaries, and tubes. Traditional 2D ultrasound technology cannot provide this orientation to view the female pelvis, since imaging from inside the vagina or the surface of the abdomen does not provide a direct path to this view. Now, however, this coronal view can be reconstructed using 3D ultrasonography, and demonstrate the shape of the uterine cavity as well as the outline of the outer surface of the uterus, an image that neither 2D ultrasonography alone nor hysterosalpingography can provide (see **Fig. 1**). Abuhamad and colleagues[3] demonstrated the z-technique of manipulating a volume, a simple method by which practitioners can learn to manipulate the volume and obtain the coronal view of the uterus in less than 30 seconds.

Several studies have demonstrated the overall effectiveness of the coronal view of the uterus in clinical practice and suggest that the coronal image of the uterus and endometrial cavity should be a part of routine pelvic sonography.[4,13] Andreotti and colleagues[13] found that the 3D reconstructed view of the endometrium and adjacent myometrium provided additional information in 53% of patients who had abnormal findings by 2D sonography. The authors also demonstrated that the 3D coronal view of the uterus added value to the standard 2D ultrasonogram in 24% of all gynecologic cases, especially among patients with abnormal initial 2D sonography and those with endometrium thicker than 5 mm.[4] The normally echogenic endometrium provides a visual contrast to the darker myometrium for displaying intracavitary uterine fibroids and polyps (**Fig. 8**). The thicker the endometrium, the better the image quality showing the uterine cavity on 3D coronal view and the presence of intracavitary lesions. 3D coronal views of the uterus are particularly helpful in patients who have abnormal 2D imaging of the uterus or in patients who present with infertility.[4] The 3D coronal view is able to better characterize the Mullerian duct anomaly, and in some cases detect a defect not previously suspected by the traditional 2D views.

### *Uterine Anomalies*

One of the most important contributions of the coronal display of the uterus is the ability to detect Mullerian duct abnormalities that may affect fertility. Uterine anomalies are associated with a higher proportion of infertility and first-trimester pregnancy loss compared with women with a normal uterus.[14] Hence, the correct diagnosis of these abnormalities is the key to proper management. An MR image is no longer needed to map out uterine shape abnormalities now that volume sonography is available. Currently, 3D reconstruction of the coronal view is a quick, easy, and accurate way to display these clinically important uterine shape abnormalities.[15–18] (**Fig. 9**)

Many septate uteri have mistakenly been diagnosed as bicornuate when viewing standard 2D sonographic images. The incidence of the septate is far higher than that of bicornuate uterus; however, uteri with 2 islands of endometrium separated by myometrium in standard transverse views were often erroneously called a bicornuate uterus. 3D ultrasonography can easily and accurately differentiate between these 2 very different entities using the coronal view of the uterus[19] (**Figs. 10** and **11**). The correct diagnosis of a septate uterus is key because of the higher associated

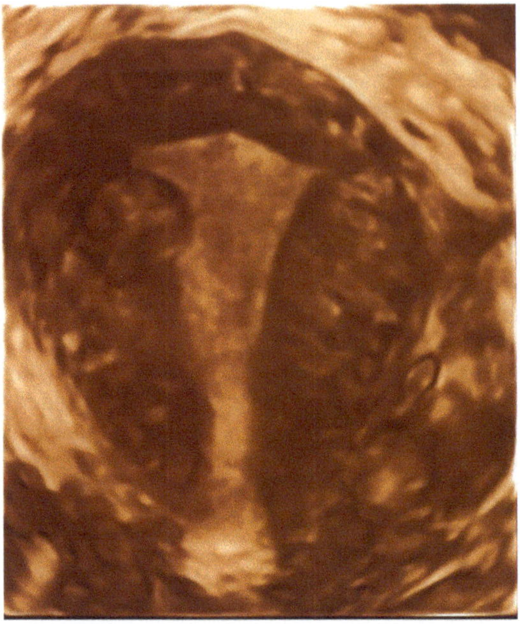

**Fig. 8.** Reconstructed rendered coronal view of a uterus that contains a partly submucous fibroid along the right side of the uterine cavity.

incidence of infertility and spontaneous first-trimester miscarriage when compared with the bicornuate uterus. The septate uterus present important surgical treatment options with good success, whereas the bicornuate uterus usually does not require surgery[19] (**Fig. 12**). The arcuate uterus is controversial, being considered a normal

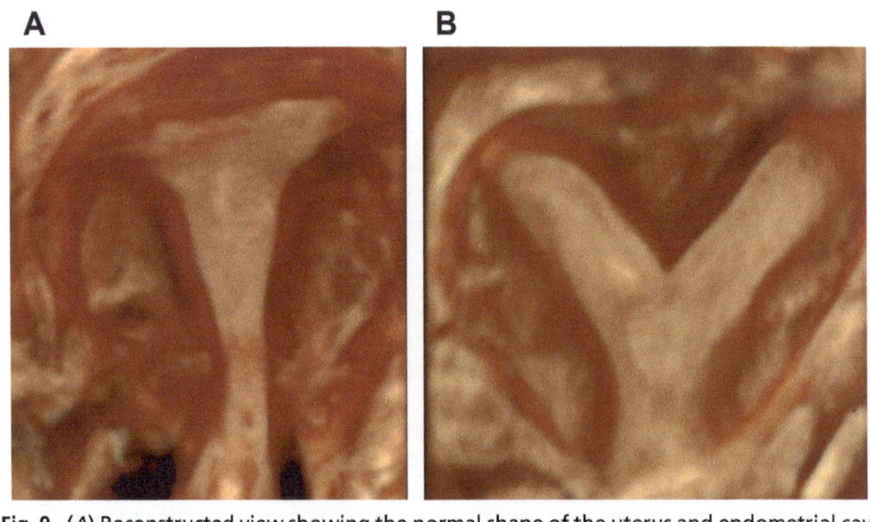


**Fig. 9.** (*A*) Reconstructed view showing the normal shape of the uterus and endometrial cavity. (*B*) Reconstructed view of a subseptate uterus showing that the septum extends approximately halfway down into the cavity. There is a single cervix.

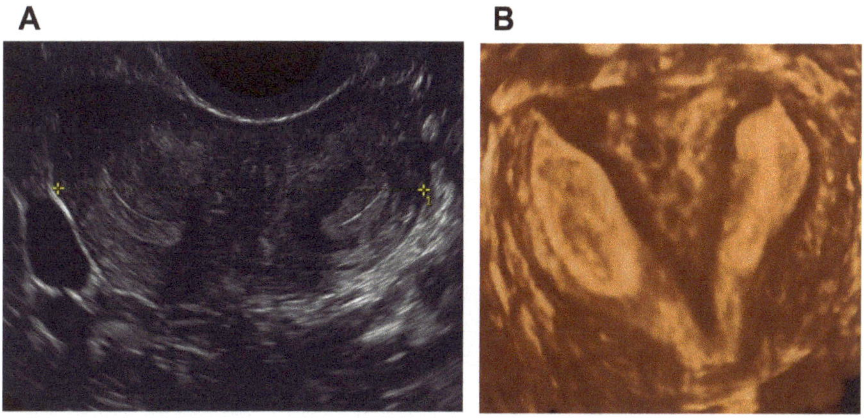


**Fig. 10.** (*A*) 2D image of a septate uterus taken in transverse section showing 2 islands of endometrium indicating 2 different horns. This view cannot demonstrate whether the uterus is septate or bicornuate without a reconstructed coronal display. (*B*) The coronal display shows that the uterus is septate and not bicornuate because the serosal surface is flat.

variant by some, whereas others claim that it is associated with a higher incidence of second-trimester losses and preterm labor compared with women with normal uteri (**Fig. 13**). Other types of uterine shape abnormalities may include a combination of bicornuate and septate uteri, including duplications of the cervix, and rudimentary horns that may or may not connect with the main uterine cavity (**Fig. 14**). Complex uterine abnormalities can be mapped out with a 3D coronal reconstruction of the uterus, thus providing an accurate diagnosis without the need for MRI[16,18] (**Fig. 15**).

### *Uterine Polyps and Fibroids*

The coronal view has great value for detecting the presence of endometrial polyps and intracavitary fibroids.[4] Polyps are rounded masses with a sharp interface between the polyp and the rest of the endometrium. Polyps are sometimes easier to find with the reconstructed coronal view than with the traditional 2D imaging of the endometrial

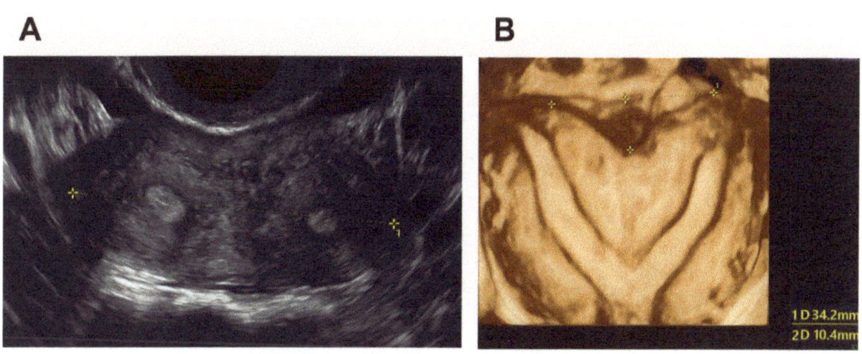


**Fig. 11.** (*A*) 2D image of a bicornuate uterus taken in transverse section showing 2 islands of endometrium indicating 2 different horns. This view cannot demonstrate whether the uterus is septate or bicornuate without a reconstructed coronal display. (*B*) The coronal display shows that the uterus is bicornuate with a 10-mm indentation on the serosal surface of the uterus (*calipers*).

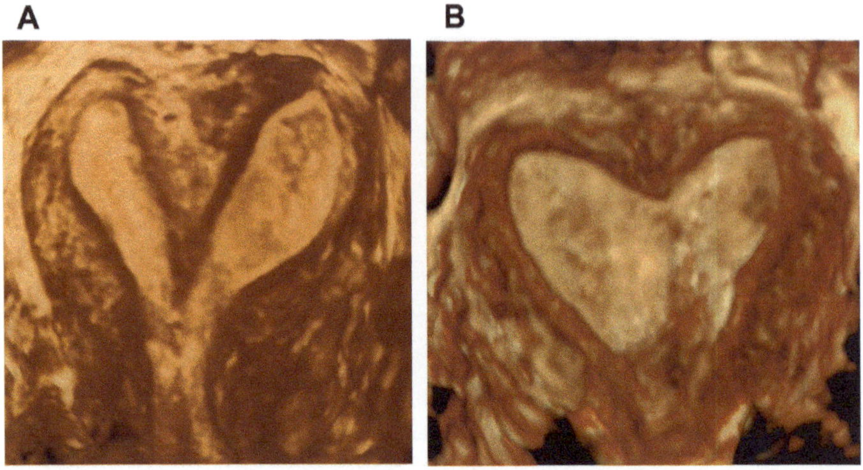

**Fig. 12.** Before and after surgery to repair a septum. (*A*) Coronal view of the uterus preoperatively demonstrates a complete septum. (*B*) Postoperative result of the same uterus shows that there is still a small indentation at the uterine fundus, but much improved.

cavity, because the display of the uterine cavity shows the entirety of the cavity including both cornua and cervix in the same image (see **Fig. 15**; **Fig. 16**). The coronal display permits a better grasp of the position of the polyp within the cavity. Doppler can demonstrate blood flow with the polyp, and this feeder vessel can be displayed in 3D reconstructed views, providing additional benefit in diagnosing polyps

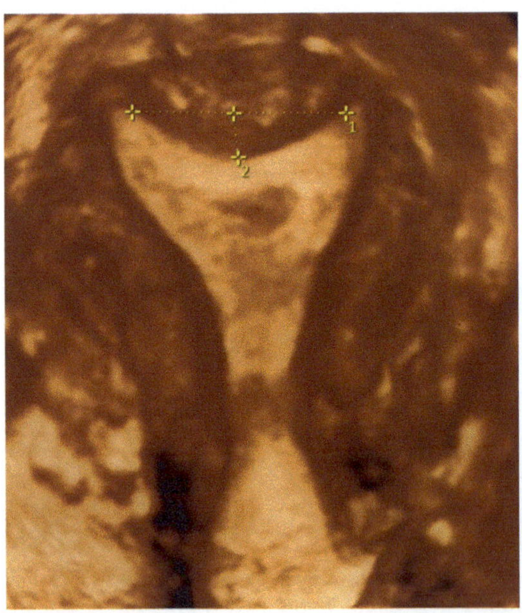

**Fig. 13.** The coronal display shows that the uterus is arcuate, which indicates a slight indentation of less than 10 mm at the top of the cavity. The significance of this finding is controversial because many consider this a normal variant. Surgery is not typically recommended.

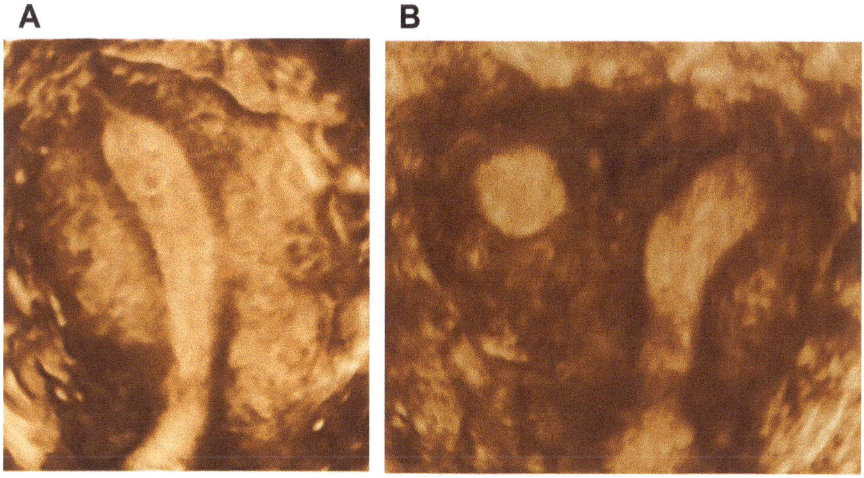

Fig. 14. Unicornuate uterus. (*A*) Coronal view of a right unicornuate uterus with no significant rudimentary horn. (*B*) Coronal view of a left unicornuate uterus with a rudimentary horn that contains endometrial tissue but no connection to the cervix. A pregnancy in that noncommunicating horn would likely result in catastrophic rupture.

(**Figs. 17** and **18**). Adenomyosis is easier to see with the 3D reconstructed coronal view because of the irregular junctional zone and cystic/linear areas along the junctional zone representing endometrial glands in the subendometrial region[20] (**Fig. 19**).

The location of fibroids within the uterus is a very important application for 3D ultrasonography and the coronal view.[4,13] The coronal view of the uterus is key in showing the correct location of fibroids in the uterus, including the proportion of submucosal component and the distance between the outside of the fibroid and the serosal surface, hence facilitating successful removal of fibroids with submucosal components (**Figs. 20** and **21**). Navigating through the volume can provide important measurements and demonstrate tangentially the correct plane to best display uterine lesions.

### *Asherman Syndrome*

Asherman syndrome is a condition characterized by extensive endometrial adhesions that can ultimately be severe enough to destroy the endometrial layer.[5] Repeated or

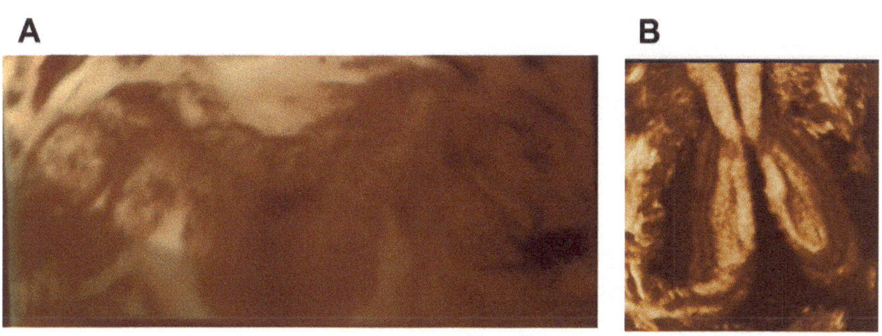

Fig. 15. (*A*) Uterus didelphys shown in a reconstructed coronal display demonstrating 2 completely separate uteri joined only at the cervix. (*B*) The cervix can also be double or septate, which is best displayed using a magnified detailed 3D reconstructed view of the lower uterine segment.

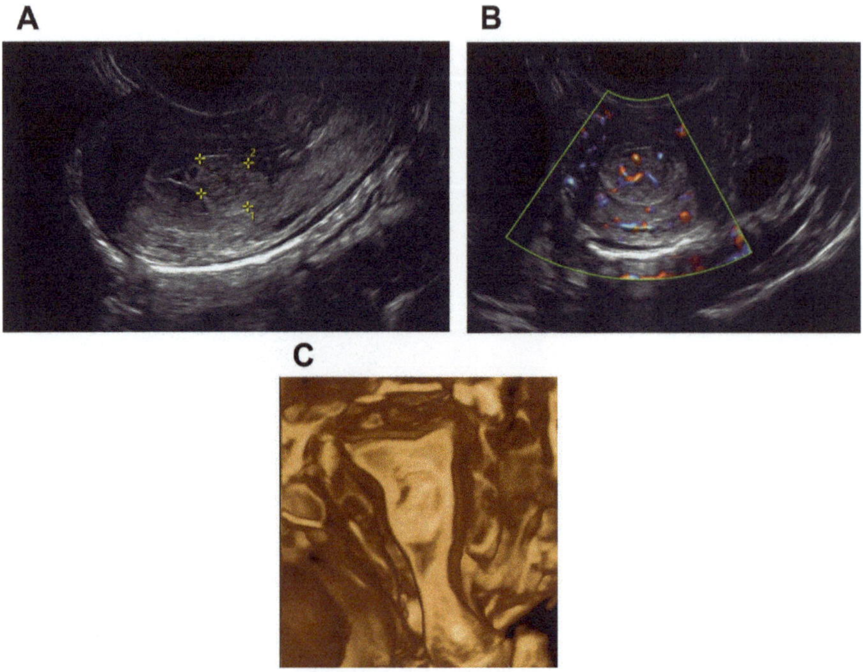

Fig. 16. Uterine polyp. (*A*) 2D image of a uterus taken in long axis showing an intracavitary polyp (*calipers*). (*B*) 2D transverse view of the same polyp using color Doppler showing the presence of blood in the polyp. (*C*) 3D coronal view of the same polyp showing its location mid uterus.

vigorous dilatation and curettage can cause these severe adhesions or synechiae, hence making the endometrium irregular, denuded, and poorly receptive to implant of a conceptus. Endometritis can also cause Asherman syndrome, with similar poor fertility results. When evaluating these patients sonographically, the endometrium is

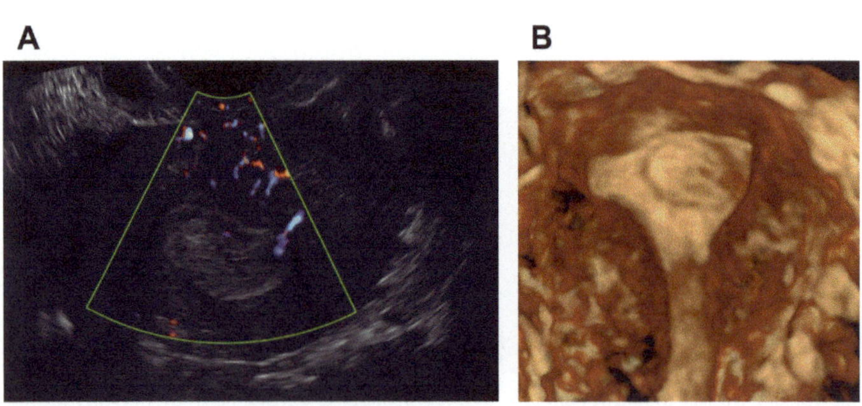

Fig. 17. (*A*) 2D transverse view of an endometrial polyp containing a feeding vessel. (*B*) 3D coronal view of the same polyp showing its exact location within the uterus cavity near the left cornu.

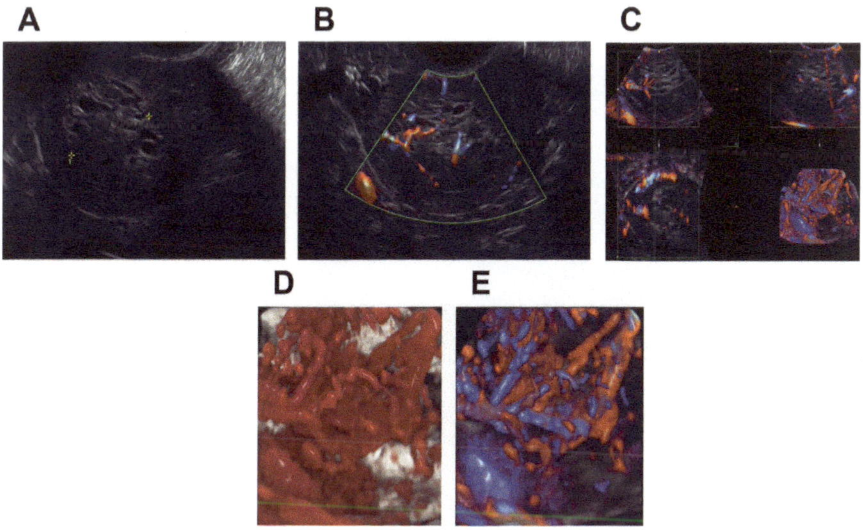


**Fig. 18.** Polyp with vascular flow. (*A*) 2D transverse view of a cystic endometrial polyp (*calipers*). (*B*) 2D view of the polyps with color Doppler showing the presence of blood flow. (*C*) 3D volume of uterine polyp with Doppler flow displayed using the 3 orthogonal planes. (*D, E*) Only the fully reconstructed 3D view demonstrates the entire blood supply of the polyp, including the branching of the vessels.

often thin and difficult to image. Sonohysterography may not be able to fully distend the uterine cavity because of the walls being adhered. The reconstructed coronal view of the uterus often demonstrated the numerous synechiae without the need to insert saline (**Fig. 22**). Sometimes an entire horn of the uterus can be obliterated, or the cavity may appear T-shaped and shaggy because of endometrial adhesions (**Figs. 23** and **24**).

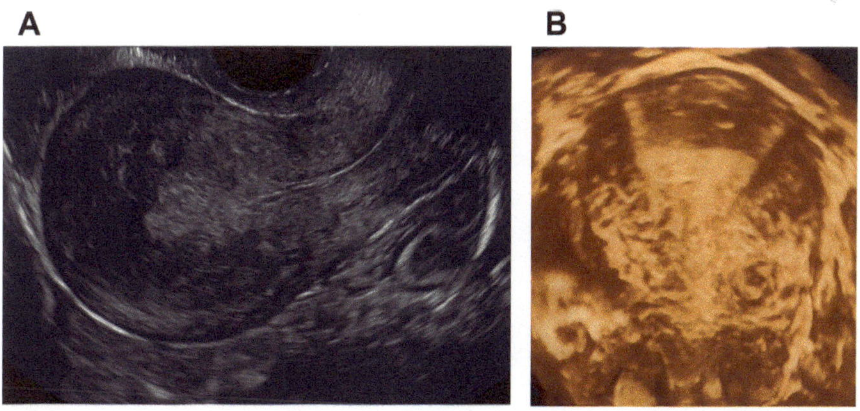


**Fig. 19.** Adenomyosis. (*A*) 2D image of the uterus taken in long axis showing complete obliteration of the junctional zone with blotchy/heterogeneous myometrial texture caused by adenomyosis. (*B*) 3D rendered coronal view of the same uterus showing the characteristic blurring of the junctional zone with wavy lines caused by dilated endometrial glands in the subendometrial region.

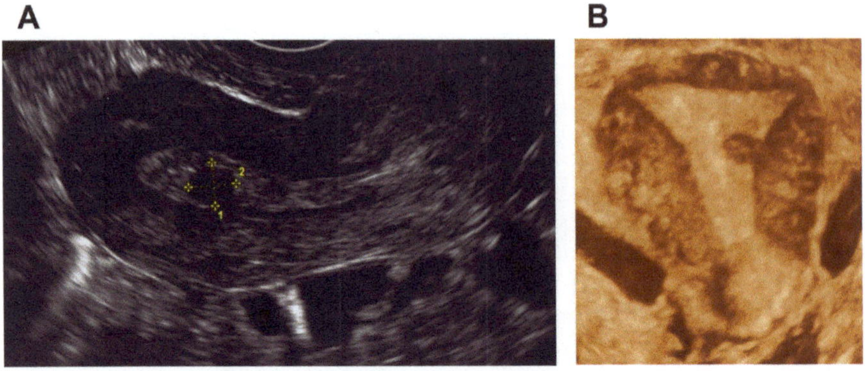


Fig. 20. Submucous fibroid. (*A*) 2D image of the uterus taken in long axis showing a tiny intracavitary fibroid. (*B*) The same fibroid seen on 3D coronal view showing that it is rising from the midlateral left wall of the uterine cavity.

## *Adenomyosis*

Adenomyosis is a condition characterized by the invasion of the myometrium, especially the subendometrial region, by endometrial glands that normally reside in the endometrium. As a result of this infiltration, the endometrial-myometrial junction becomes indistinct and the myometrium takes on a heterogeneous sonographic appearance. The uterus becomes tender, enlarged, and globular, containing cystic spaces and echogenic foci. 3D ultrasonography is well suited to show the abnormal endometrial-myometrial junction and the resulting subendometrial cysts and echogenic foci[20] (see **Fig. 19; Fig. 25**).

## *The Uterus and Intrauterine Device Placement*

The coronal view of the uterus provides valuable information regarding the presence of foreign bodies within the uterus.[21–25] The position of intrauterine devices (IUDs) has been especially challenging to observe accurately with traditional 2D ultrasonography,

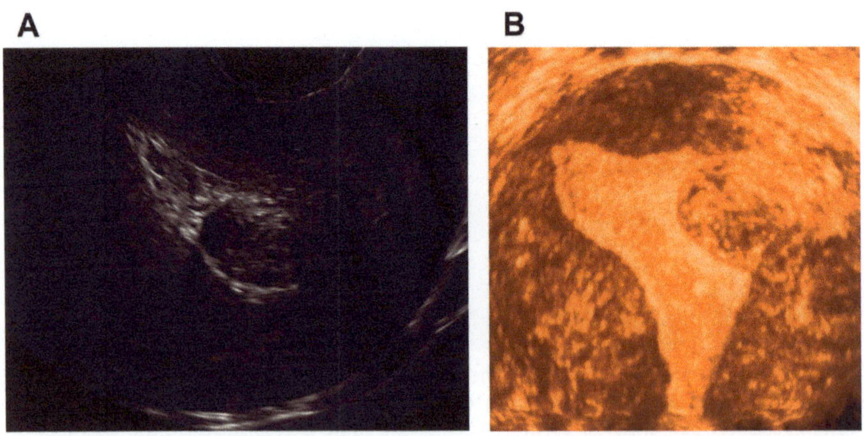


Fig. 21. Submucosal fibroid. (*A*) 2D image of the uterus showing an intracavitary fibroid. (*B*) The same fibroid seen on 3D coronal view showing that it is obliterating the left cornu.

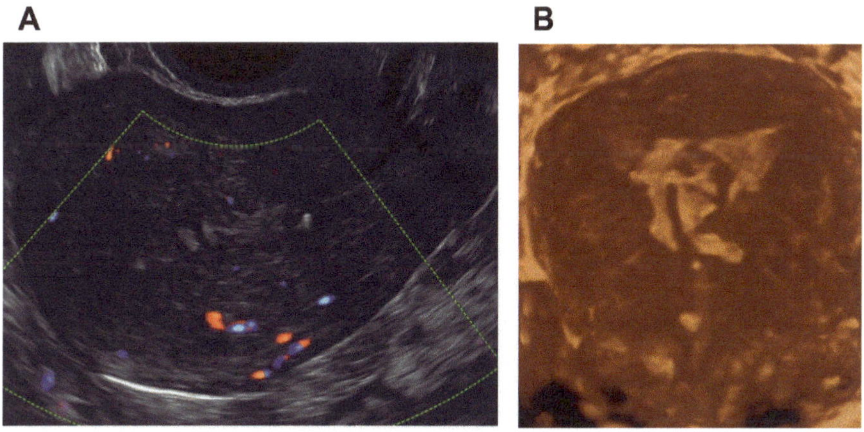


Fig. 22. Asherman syndrome. (*A*) 2D image of a uterus taken in long axis showing an abnormally irregular and interrupted endometrial echo. (*B*) 3D coronal view of the same uterus showing distinct synechiae criss-crossing the endometrial cavity.

and 3D coronal displays have made IUD localization much easier, especially the arms of the IUDs.[21–25](**Fig. 26**) Many IUDs are partly embedded within the myometrium, often unrecognized with traditional 2D ultrasonography. The arms of the IUDs are especially difficult to visualize accurately with 2D alone. When the IUD stem seems to be correctly placed when viewed by 2D ultrasonography alone, 3D reconstructed images may demonstrate that the arms are actually embedded, at least in part, within the myometrium (**Fig. 27**).

Although IUDs typically do not fit properly in a septate uterus, it is not uncommon to see an IUD in a uterus with Mullerian duct anomaly (**Fig. 28**).

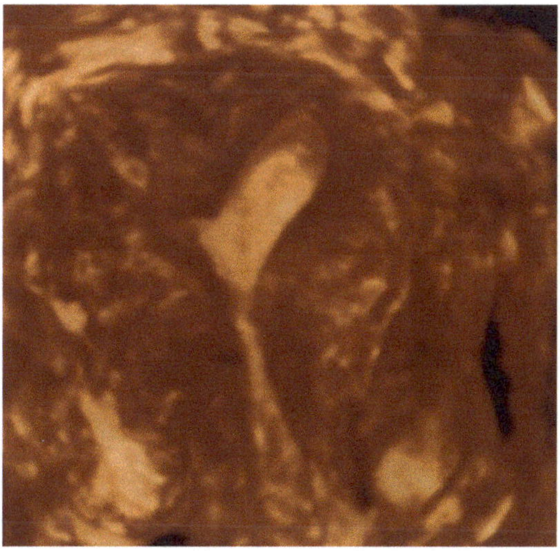

Fig. 23. Asherman syndrome. 3D coronal view of a heavily scarred uterine cavity. This patient had a hysterosalpingogram suggesting that her uterus was unicornuate; however, the right horn is heavily scarred because of prior failed pregnancies and could not be distended.

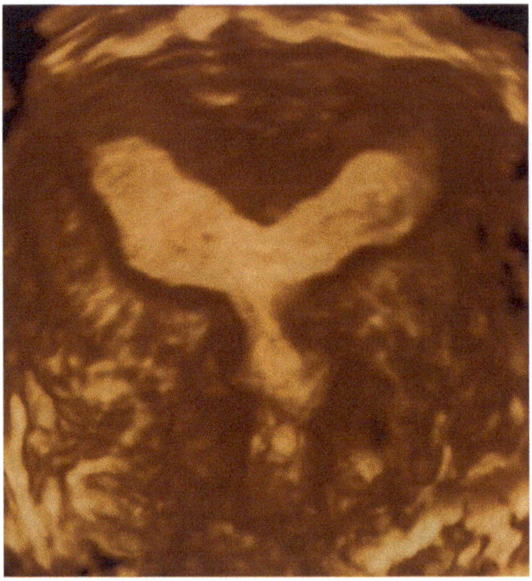

Fig. 24. Asherman syndrome. 3D coronal view of a heavily scarred uterine cavity resulting in a T-shaped uterus.

IUDs that are not in their correct location in the uterus are a common cause of pain and bleeding. The authors showed that 17% of IUDs were embedded in the myometrium or cervix when looking at ultrasonograms of 167 consecutive patients who had IUDs. Patients with embedded IUDs presented with a higher incidence of bleeding (35.7%) or pain (39.3%) compared with those with normally located IUDs (15.1% bleeding and 19.4% pain).[21] There were 75% of patients with imbedded IUDs who presented with bleeding or pain in comparison with 34.5% of patients whose IUDs were in the normal location ($P = .0001$). Twenty of 21 patients reported improvement of their symptoms of pain and/or bleeding after removal of their embedded IUD.

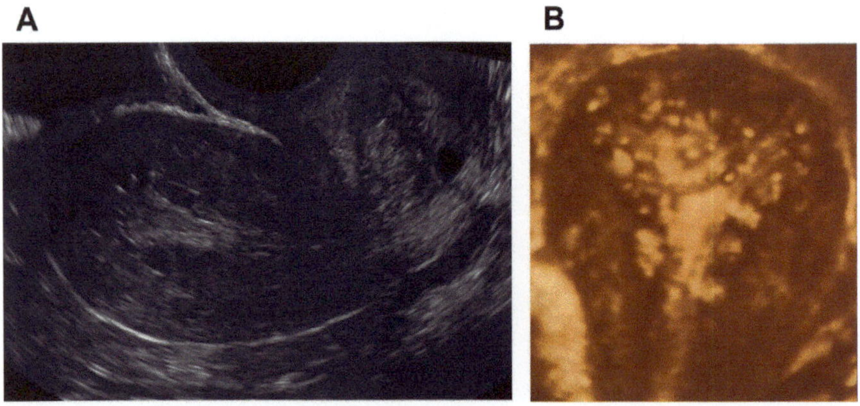


Fig. 25. Adenomyosis. (*A*) 2D image of the uterus taken in long axis showing obliteration of the junctional zone by subendometrial cysts. (*B*) 3D rendered coronal view of the same uterus shows the characteristic bubbling along the junctional zone representing the dilated endometrial glands in the subendometrial region in a patient with extensive adenomyosis.

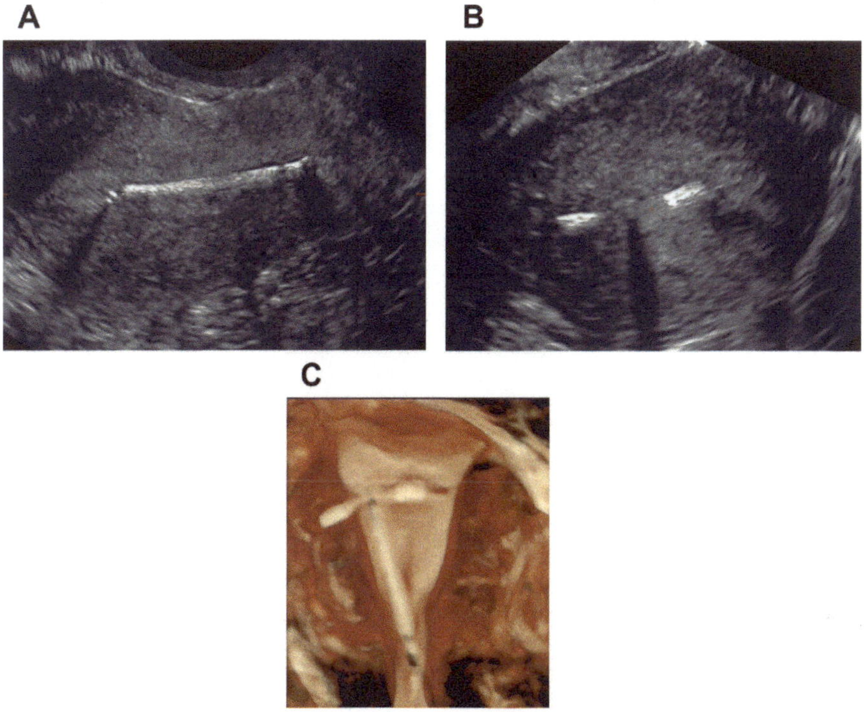


**Fig. 26.** (*A, B*) 2D Longitudinal and transverse views of the uterus containing an IUD. Based on these 2D images, the IUD appears to be in place. (*C*) 3D rendered coronal view of the same uterus shows that the right arm of the IUD is completely embedded in the myometrium in this patient who had pelvic pain.

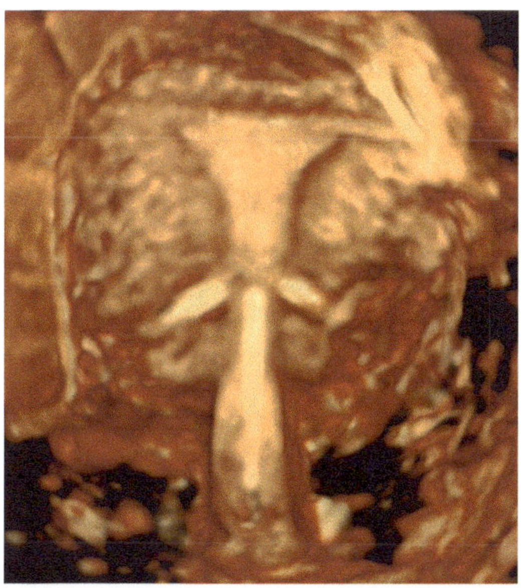

**Fig. 27.** 3D rendered coronal view of the uterus of a patient with pain. The IUD is not only low in the cervix, but both arms are embedded in the myometrium of the lower uterine segment.

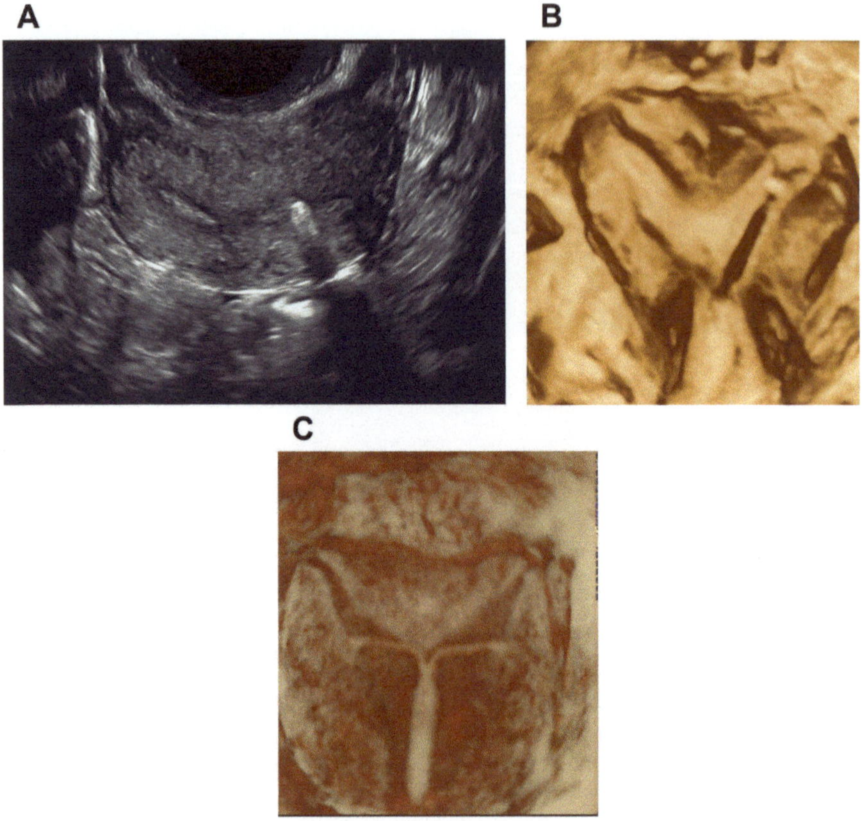


**Fig. 28.** (*A*) Transverse view of the uterus showing the shadow from an IUD in one side of the cavity. 2D imaging was not sufficient to understand the orientation and actual location of the IUD within the uterus. (*B*) 3D coronal view of the uterine cavity shows a septate cavity; the IUD is embedded in the left horn, almost perforating the myometrium. (*C*) Another septate uterus with an IUD where the IUD remains below the septum.

Artifacts can be confusing when looking at an IUD using reconstructed planes.[26] The shadow of the IUD can easily be mistaken for the actual IUD on a 3D reconstructed view unless the original 2D images are available for comparison. In a standard 2D view, the source of the shadow of the IUD is easily interpreted as the IUD itself. In a reconstructed plane from a 3D volume, a linear or T-shaped shadow cannot be interpreted because the IUD casting the shadow is in a different plane not displayed. It is important to obtain the entire volume so as to navigate through the volume and locate the IUD, sometimes by using its shadow; however, it is easy to misinterpret the location of the IUD if the shadow is mistaken for the device (**Fig. 29**).

## INVERSION ULTRASONOGRAPHY

Reconstructed views using 3D ultrasonography also provide helpful images in the adnexa. 3D inversion is a method by which the cystic areas within the volume can be displayed as a cast, and the solid areas disappear so that only the cystic spaces are visible. Hydrosalpinges criss-cross through multiple different planes of a section, making it challenging to image with standard 2D ultrasonography[6,7]

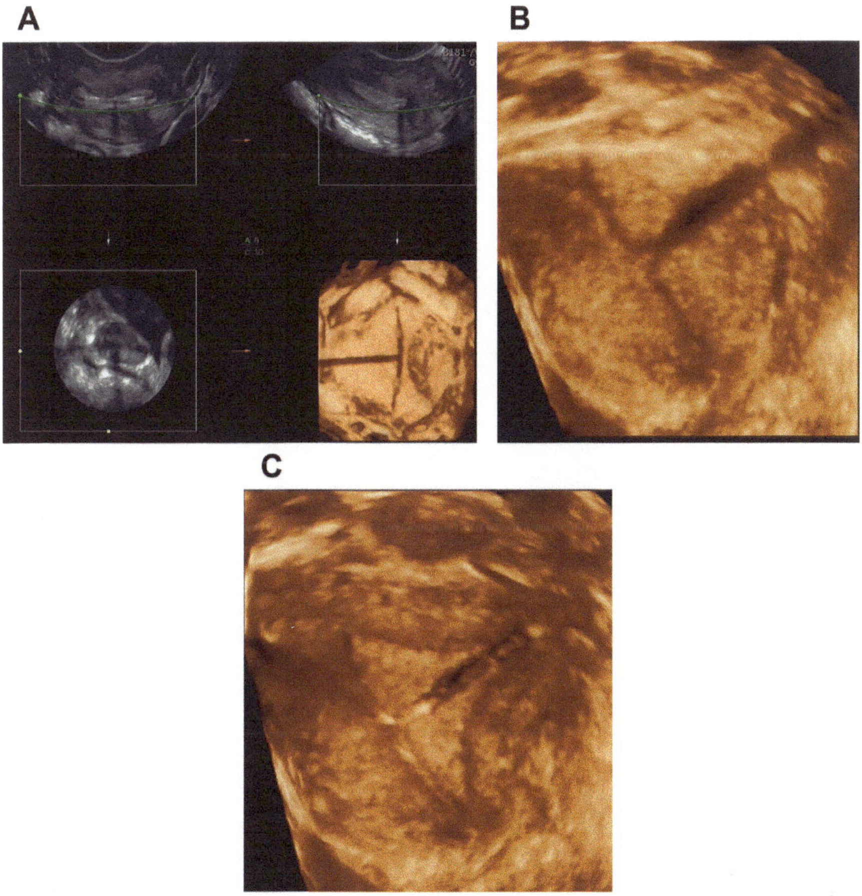


**Fig. 29.** (*A*) Standard display of a volume containing the entire uterus with an IUD in the cavity. The 3 orthogonal views of the uterus show that the region of interest chosen for the 3D reconstruction begins just below the IUD in the acquisition view (*upper left*). This explains why it is the shadow of the IUD being rendered rather than the IUD itself in the lower right window of the display. (*B*, *C*) These 2 rendered images of the coronal view of a uterus with an IUD show that the shadow is often easier to find than the IUD itself, especially if the IUD is in an unusual location. (*C*) The shadow can assist in finding the location of the IUD itself.

(**Fig. 30**). Usually a hydrosalpinx can be confused with a multiseptated cystic mass because the multiple planes of the section are not easily appreciated when using conventional 2D imaging. If a cystic mass is contained within a volume, the inverse mode is crucial to displaying the entire fluid-filled dilated tube as a cast as it traverses through several planes of the section. The inverse mode then produces an echogenic mold of the entire tube and displays the whole tube within the volume, regardless of plane (**Fig. 31**).

The volume can be rotated to display all of the sides of these cystic portions. Another helpful use for the inverse mode is evaluation of follicles within an ovary. The follicles become opaque on the image, and thus easier to count and measure simultaneously. Ovaries with polycystic ovarian syndrome are easily displayed by

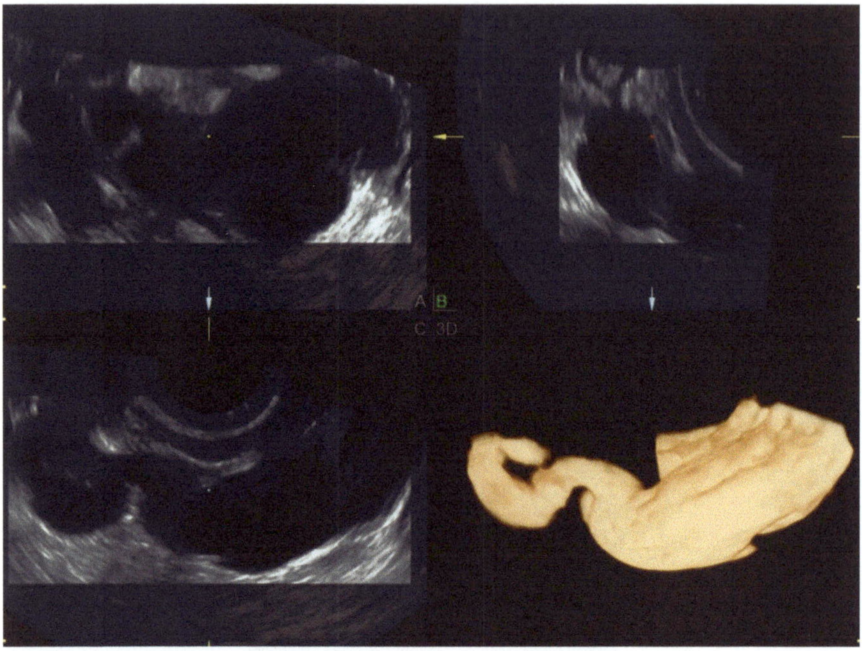


**Fig. 30.** 3D volume containing a hydrosalpinx. The 3 orthogonal views each show a single plane; however, the volume with inverse mode (*lower left*) shows the entire dilated tube contained within the volume.

the push of a button, showing the characteristic appearance of the follicles in the periphery of the ovary[27,28] (see **Fig. 3**). One can also use 3D inverse-mode display of the endometrial cavity with fluid during a sonohysterogram to view the endometrial cavity in its entirety. This technique provides positive contrast within the uterus, producing an image similar to a hysterosalpingogram (**Fig. 32**).

## SONOHYSTEROGRAPHY WITH THREE-DIMENSIONAL IMAGING

The efficiency and accuracy of sonohysterography is greatly enhanced when using a 3D volume to evaluate the uterine cavity, owing to its ability to acquire images that contain the entire uterine cavity using one volume. Multiple 3D volume acquisitions are typically done during sonohysterography so that the procedure is done faster (**Fig. 33**). Several 3D volumes of the uterus are acquired as the saline is injected, and saved for later evaluation of the endometrial cavity. This technique is far more efficient than trying to obtain multiple single 2D images as the fluid is injected.[11,12,29,30] Comparing the accuracy of 3D multiplanar sonohysterography, 2D sonohysterography, and hysterosalpingography, Lev-Toaff and colleagues[29] showed that the coronal plane reconstructed from a 3D volume was the most valuable image for displaying the relationship between the uterine cavity and lesions such as polyps and fibroids (**Fig. 34**).

When performing sonohysterography, 3D volume provides important benefits in comparison with using 2D ultrasonography for imaging the inside of the endometrial cavity. Ludwin and colleagues[30] showed that 3D sonohysterography was as diagnostically accurate as hysteroscopy. Another study, by Silvestre and colleagues,[12] also

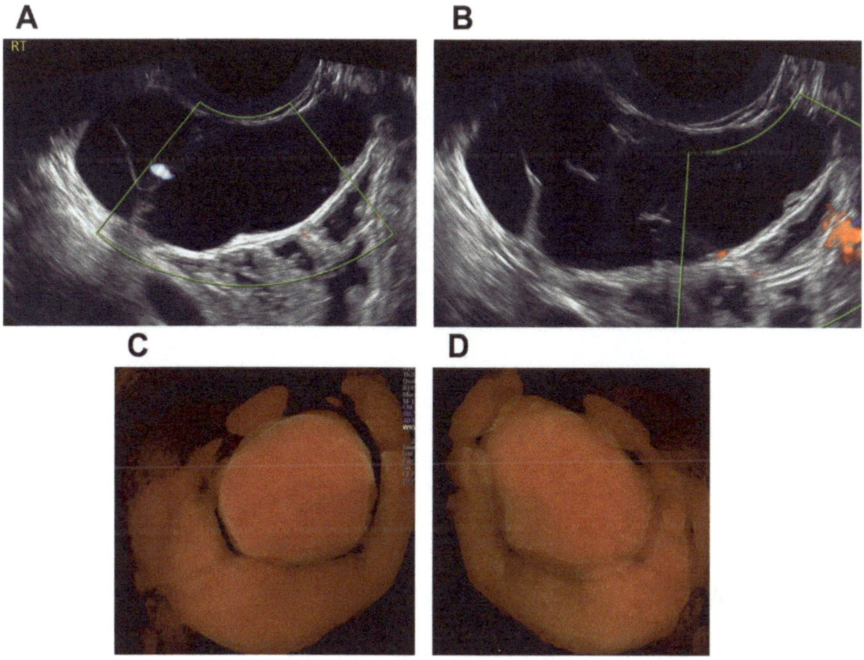


**Fig. 31.** (*A, B*) Two standard 2D views of a multiseptated cystic mass whose etiology was indeterminate based on the 2D images. (*C, D*). Two views of the entire volume using the inverse mode showing that the suspected multiseptated cystic mass actually represents a hydrosalpinx wrapped around an ovarian cyst.

showed that 3D sonohysterography allowed better and more reliable localization of polyps and fibroids within the uterine cavity than using 2D only. Hysterosalpingo-contrast-sonography, or HyCoSy, is quickly replacing hysterosalpingography for visualizing the uterine cavity and patency of fallopian tubes in patients with infertility.[5,30,31] Although air can be used as contrast to demonstrate tubal patency, commercial contrast agents remain in the tubes long enough to allow 3D acquisitions to show

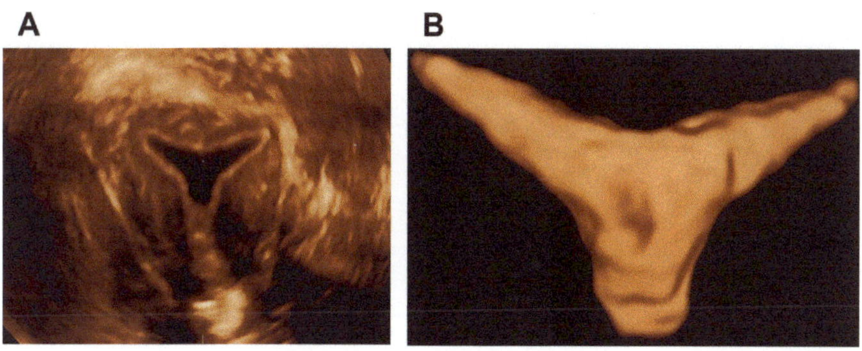


**Fig. 32.** (*A*) 3D coronal view of the uterus during a sonohysterogram showing fluid filling the endometrial cavity. (*B*) Same uterus shown from the same volume but using inverse mode, making a cast of the endometrial cavity.

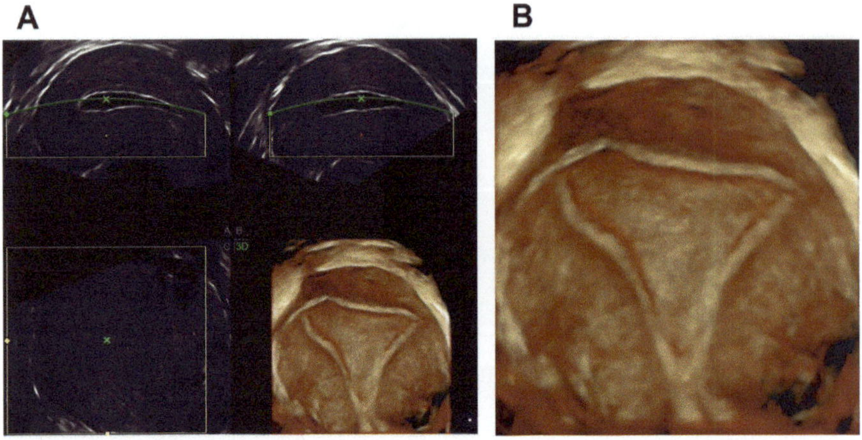

**Fig. 33.** (*A*) 3D volume with 3 orthogonal views and rendered coronal image of the uterus during a sonohysterogram showing fluid filling the endometrial cavity. (*B*) A magnified view of the fluid-filled uterine cavity.

the entire length of the tube in coronal view. Hysterosalpingography represents an excellent screening technique to determine the cause of postmenopausal bleeding before proceeding to the gold standard of hysteroscopy.[32]

## ASSESSMENT OF PREGNANCY LOCATION

2D ultrasonography is sufficient to locate most intrauterine pregnancies accurately. Some gestational sacs can be located eccentrically, near the cornua or the edges of the uterus, making it difficult to differentiate an interstitial pregnancy, angular pregnancy, and pregnancies with congenitally abnormal uteri using standard 2D images.[33] 3D ultrasonography provides the coronal and tangential views of the uterus, which can be crucial in accurately identifying the location of an interstitial pregnancy, demonstrating a tongue of myometrium between the pregnancy and

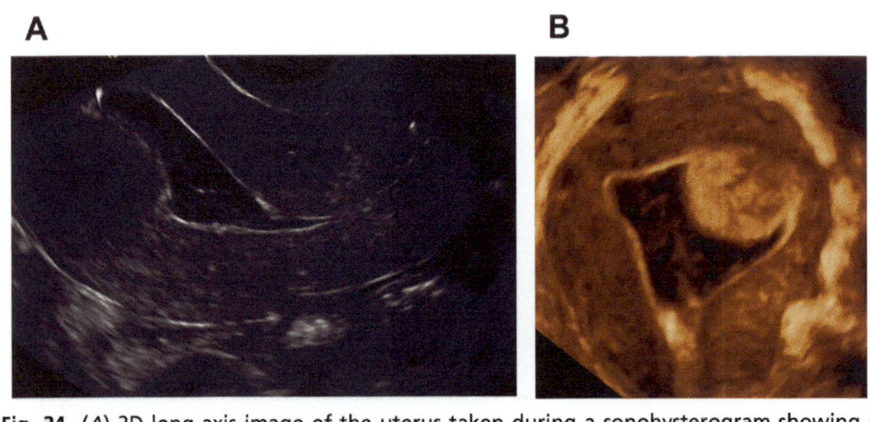

**Fig. 34.** (*A*) 2D long-axis image of the uterus taken during a sonohysterogram showing a posterior partly submucous fibroid. (*B*) 3D coronal view of the same uterus showing that the fibroid involves the left lateral and cornual aspect of the cavity.

the endometrial cavity (**Fig. 35**). An angular pregnancy is an implantation at the lateral angles of the uterine cavity near the cornu. Such pregnancies can be successful, although they are associated with a higher risk of bleeding and pregnancy loss. Although it may be very difficult to distinguish them from interstitial pregnancies, 3D ultrasonography with follow-up scans is key to locating such pregnancies more precisely.

## DOPPLER IN THREE DIMENSIONS

Doppler evaluation of blood flow using 3D displays provides a subjective evaluation of the morphology, location, and density of the vessels in ovarian or uterine masses.[34–38] 3D color Doppler provides mapping of the vascular architecture, revealing the location of vessels within the lesion and the clustering of irregular tumor vessels centrally within a malignant tumor (see **Fig. 18**). Quantification of the vascularity within a mass is obtained using the 3D volume with color flow on, and the region of interest can be outlined to calculate the vascular parameters within the area of interest. The Vascularization Index measures the percentage of color voxels within the area selected, thus essentially providing a vessel count. The Flow Index is a measure of the flow coursing through the mass when the volume was acquired. The Vascular Flow Index combines these 2 measurements to provide an assessment of the blood flow and vessel count within the area selected.

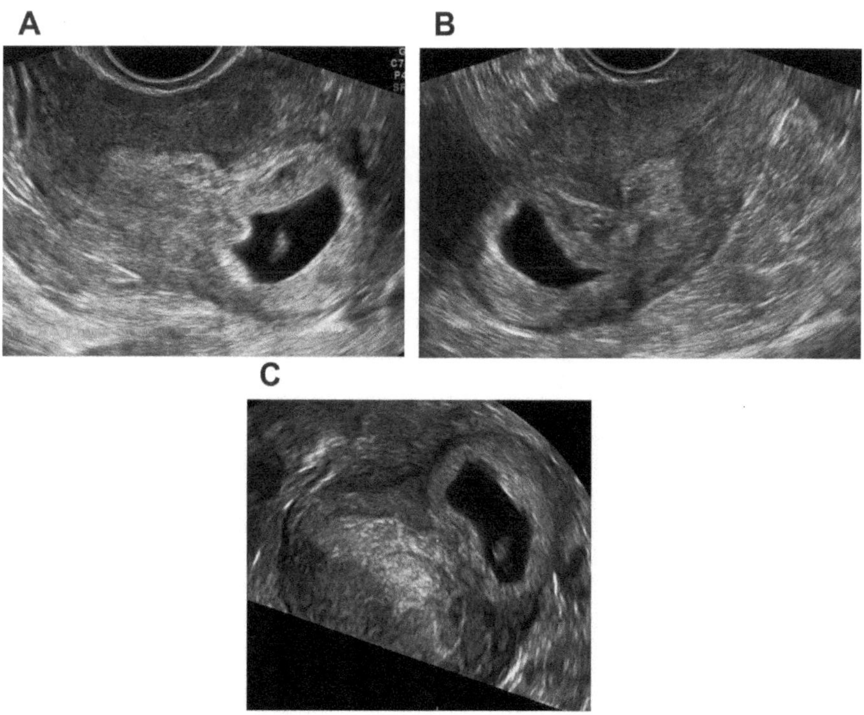


**Fig. 35.** Interstitial pregnancy. (*A, B*) 2D views of this early pregnancy show that it is located peripherally, but it is impossible to tell whether it is appropriately placed within the uterus. (*C*) 3D coronal view of the same uterus shows that the pregnancy is actually a left interstitial pregnancy. 3D allows manipulation of the volume to obtain the tangential view of the uterus to best demonstrate the location of the gestational sac.

3D color Doppler is also used to evaluate the vascularity within the uterus and the endometrium.[35–38] Investigators have demonstrated that 3D power Doppler is a tool to study the changes in the ovarian and endometrial and subendometrial vascularity during the normal menstrual cycle.[34,39] The endometrial and subendometrial vascularity increase throughout the follicular phase, and diminishing after follicular rupture, before escalating again after ovulation. There are also important color and power Doppler artifacts to consider, such as aliasing and motion, which may require several attempts at accurate volumes.

## VOLUME MEASUREMENT

3D ultrasonography can provide accurate measurements of regions within the volume.[37–41] The accuracy of volume measurements carried out on a 3D ultrasound data set in vitro are highly reliable to within 4% of the true volumes.[39] Studies indicate that 3D ultrasonography can provide accurate volume measurements compared with those done traditionally using 2D imaging.[41] 3D ultrasound data sets can also provide accurate measurements such as multiple follicles in an ovary, essential in patients undergoing assisted reproduction.[28] Such automated/semiautomated capabilities allow for faster workflow in infertility practices.[39]

## FUTURE DEVELOPMENTS

CT and MRI have used 3D volume imaging for decades, with reconstruction of volumes using many different types of displays. 3D volume imaging is, therefore, one of the most important advances in modern sonography, as 3D ultrasonography will challenge and replace other forms of cross-sectional pelvic imaging.[42] The ultrasound community must embrace this technology to further the use of ultrasonography in all aspects of imaging of the female pelvis. Currently, 3D ultrasonography with at least reconstruction of the coronal view of the uterus (and adnexa if indicated) should be part of many if not most of the pelvic ultrasonography scans performed today. Standard 2D sonography is no longer sufficient to demonstrate many of our patients' pelvic disorders. Gynecology practice is evolving away from hysterosalpingography and toward the use of 3D sonography and hysterosalpingography to evaluate uterine shape.[5,43] New techniques are also evolving for staging gynecologic cancers with 3D ultrasonography, including cervical tumors, and the degree of invasion of myometrium and cervix and surrounding tissues.[44,45]

Volume sonography as a technology is still young. Many of the current transducers are still mechanical, resulting in jerky 4D "real-time" ultrasonography, and the current trade-off between resolution and speed remains discouraging. Matrix technology, based on electronic transducers, is changing 3D ultrasound technology dramatically to provide the increased speed and improved image resolution needed in all planes, but still needs to improve. True real-time 4D ultrasonography should ultimately provide guidance for pelvic procedures such as follicular aspirations, abscess drainage, and guided dilatation and curettage, and also supply the basis of comprehensive pelvic imaging for most indications.

## REFERENCES

1. Benacerraf BR, Benson CB, Abuhamad AZ, et al. Three- and 4-dimensional ultrasound. In: obstetrics and gynecology: proceedings of the American Institute of Ultrasound in Medicine consensus conference. J Ultrasound Med 2005;24: 1587–97.

2. Benacerraf BR, Shipp TS, Bromley B. Improving the efficiency of gynecologic ultrasound using 3D volumes: a pilot study. J Ultrasound Med 2006;25:169–71.
3. Abuhamad AZ, Singleton S, Zhao Y, et al. The Z technique: an easy approach to the display of the mid-coronal plane of the uterus in volume sonography. J Ultrasound Med 2006;25:607–12.
4. Benacerraf BR, Shipp TD, Bromley B. Which patients benefit from a 3D reconstructed coronal view of the uterus added to standard routine 2D pelvic sonography? AJR Am J Roentgenol 2008;190:626–9.
5. Groszmann Y, Benacerraf BR. Complete evaluation of anatomy and infertility pelvic ultrasound examination. Fertil Steril 2016;105:1381–93.
6. Timor-Tritsch IE, Monteagudo A, Tsymbal T, et al. Three-dimensional inversion rendering: a new sonographic technique and its use in gynecology. J Ultrasound Med 2005;24:681–8.
7. Benacerraf BR. Three-dimensional ultrasound—the inverse mode display: a pictorial essay on applications in OB GYN imaging. AJR Am J Roentgenol 2006;187:965–71.
8. Riccabona M, Nelson TR, Pretorius DH. Three-dimensional ultrasound: accuracy of distance and volume measurements. Ultrasound Obstet Gynecol 1996;7:429–31.
9. Fleischer AC, Milam MR, Crispens MA, et al. Sonography depiction of intratumoral vascularity with 2- and 3-dimensional color Doppler techniques. J Ultrasound Med 2005;24:533–7.
10. Alcázar JL, Mercé LT, Manero MG. Three-dimensional power Doppler vascular sampling: a new method for predicting ovarian cancer in vascularized complex adnexal masses. J Ultrasound Med 2005;24:689–96.
11. de Kroon CD, Louwe LA, Trimbos JB, et al. The clinical value of 3-dimensional saline infusion sonography in addition to 2-dimensional saline infusion sonography in women with abnormal uterine bleeding: work in progress. J Ultrasound Med 2004;23:1433–40.
12. Sylvestre C, Child TJ, Tulandi T, et al. A prospective study to evaluate the efficacy of two- and three-dimensional sonohysterography in women with intrauterine lesions. Fertil Steril 2003;79:1222–5.
13. Andreotti RF, Fleischer AC, Mason LE. 3D sonography of the endometrium and adjacent myometrium: preliminary observations. J Ultrasound Med 2006;25:1313.
14. Raga F, Bonilla-Musoles F, Blanes J, et al. Congenital Mullerian anomalies: diagnostic accuracy of three-dimensional ultrasound. Fertil Steril 1996;65:523–8.
15. Jurkovic D, Geipel A, Gruboeck K, et al. Three-dimensional ultrasound for the assessment of uterine anatomy and detection of congenital anomalies: a comparison with hysterosalpingography and two-dimensional sonography. Ultrasound Obstet Gynecol 1995;5:233–7.
16. Bermejo C, Martinez Ten P, Cantarero R, et al. Three-dimensional ultrasound in the diagnosis of Mullerian duct anomalies and concordance with magnetic resonance imaging. Ultrasound Obstet Gynecol 2010;35:593–601.
17. Salim R, Woelfer B, Backos M, et al. Reproducibility of three-dimensional ultrasound diagnosis of congenital uterine anomalies. Ultrasound Obstet Gynecol 2003;21:578–82.
18. Faivre E, Fernandez H, Deffieux X, et al. Accuracy of three-dimensional ultrasonography in differential diagnosis of septate and bicornuate uterus compared with office hysteroscopy and pelvic magnetic resonance imaging. J Minim Invasive Gynecol 2012;19:101–6.

19. Woelfer B, Salim R, Banerjee S, et al. Reproductive outcomes in women with congenital uterine anomalies detected by three-dimensional ultrasound screening. Obstet Gynecol 2001;98:1099–103.
20. Exacoustos C, Brienza L, di Giovanni A, et al. Adenomyosis: three-dimensional sonographic findings of the junctional zone and correlation with histology. Ultrasound Obstet Gynecol 2011;37:471–9.
21. Benacerraf BR, Shipp TD, Bromley B. Three-dimensional ultrasound detection of abnormally located intrauterine contraceptive devices which are a source of pelvic pain and abnormal bleeding. Ultrasound Obstet Gynecol 2009;34:110–5.
22. Moschos E, Twickler DM. Does the type of intrauterine device affect conspicuity on 2D and 3D ultrasound? AJR Am J Roentgenol 2011;196:1439–43.
23. Valsky DV, Cohen SM, Hochner-Celnikier D, et al. The shadow of the intrauterine device. J Ultrasound Med 2006;25:613–6.
24. Peri N, Graham D, Levine D. Imaging of intrauterine contraceptive devices. J Ultrasound Med 2007;26:1389–401.
25. Benacerraf BR, Shipp TD, Lyons JG, et al. What is the width of the normal uterine cavity in premenopausal women and does it vary with parity? Obstet Gynecol 2010;116:305–10.
26. Nelson TR, Pretorius DH, Hull A, et al. Sources and impact of artifacts on clinical three-dimensional ultrasound imaging. Ultrasound Obstet Gynecol 2000;16:374–83.
27. Raine-Fenning N, Jayaprakasan K, Deb S, et al. Automated follicle tracking improves measurement reliability in patients undergoing ovarian stimulation. Reprod Biomed Online 2009;18:658–63.
28. Deutch TD, Joergner I, Matson DO, et al. Automated assessment of ovarian follicles using a novel three-dimensional ultrasound software. Fertil Steril 2009;92:1562–8.
29. Lev-Toaff AS, Pinheiro LW, Bega G, et al. Three-dimensional multiplanar sonohysterography: comparison with conventional two-dimensional sonohysterography and X-ray hysterosalpingography. J Ultrasound Med 2001;20:295–306.
30. Ludwin A, Ludwin I, Kudla M, et al. Diagnostic accuracy of three-dimensional sonohysterography compared with office hysteroscopy and its interrater/intrarater agreement in uterine cavity assessment after hysteroscopic metroplasty. Fertil Steril 2014;101:1392–9.
31. Kupesic S, Plavsic BM. 2D and 3D hysterosalpingo-contrast-sonography in the assessment of uterine cavity and tubal patency. Eur J Obstet Gynecol Reprod Biol 2007;133:64–9.
32. Lagana AS, Ciancimino L, Mancuso A, et al. 3D sonohysterography vs hysteroscopy: a cross-sectional study for the evaluation of endouterine diseases. Arch Gynecol Obstet 2014;290:1173–8.
33. Tanaka Y, Mimura K, Kanagawa T, et al. Three-dimensional sonography in the differential diagnosis of interstitial, angular, and intrauterine pregnancies in a septate uterus. J Ultrasound Med 2014;33:2031–5.
34. Jokubkiene L, Sladkevicius P, Rovas L, et al. Assessment of changes in volume and vascularity of the ovaries during the normal menstrual cycle using three-dimensional power Doppler ultrasound. Hum Reprod 2006;21:2661–8.
35. Raine-Fenning NJ, Campbell BK, Clewes JS, et al. The interobserver reliability of three-dimensional power Doppler data acquisition within the female pelvis. Ultrasound Obstet Gynecol 2004;23:501–8.

36. Alcazar JL, Galvan R. Three-dimensional power Doppler ultrasound scanning for the prediction of endometrial cancer in women with postmenopausal bleeding and thickened endometrium. Am J Obstet Gynecol 2009;200:44.e1-6.
37. Merce LT, Alcazar JL, Lopez C, et al. Clinical usefulness of 3-dimensional sonography and power Doppler angiography for diagnosis of endometrial carcinoma. J Ultrasound Med 2007;26:1279–87.
38. Odeh M, Vainerovsky I, Grinin V, et al. Three-dimensional endometrial volume and 3-dimensional power Doppler analysis in predicting endometrial carcinoma and hyperplasia. Gynecol Oncol 2007;106:348–53.
39. Raine-Fenning NJ, Campbell BK, Clewes JS, et al. The reliability of virtual organ computer-aided analysis (VOCAL) for the semiquantification of ovarian, endometrial and subendometrial perfusion. Ultrasound Obstet Gynecol 2003;22:633–9.
40. Alcazar JL, Merce LT, Manero MG, et al. Endometrial volume and vascularity measurements by transvaginal 3-dimensional ultrasonography and power Doppler angiography in stimulated and tumoral endometria: an interobserver reproducibility study. J Ultrasound Med 2005;24:1091–8.
41. Yaman C, Jesacher K, Polz W. Accuracy of three-dimensional transvaginal ultrasound in uterus volume measurements; comparison with two-dimensional ultrasound. Ultrasound Med Biol 2003;29:1681–4.
42. Sakhel K, Benson C, Platt L, et al. Begin with the basics: role of 3D ultrasound as a first-line imaging technique in the cost-effective evaluation of gynecologic pelvic disease. J Ultraosund Med 2013;32:381–8.
43. Bocca S, Oehninger S, Stadtmauer L, et al. A study of the cost, accuracy, and benefits of 3D sonography compared with hysterosalpingography in women with uterine abnormalities. J Ultrasound Med 2012;31:81–5.
44. Jantarasaengaram S, Praditphol N, Tansathit T, et al. Three-dimensional ultrasound with volume contrast imaging for preoperative assessment of myometrial invasion and cervical involvement in women with endometrial cancer. Ultrasound Obstet Gynecol 2014;43:569–74.
45. Byun JM, Kim YN, Jeong DH, et al. Three-dimensional transvaginal ultrasonography for locally advanced cervical cancer. Int J Gynecol Cancer 2013;23:1459–64.

# Ultrasound in Early Pregnancy

## Viability, Unknown Locations, and Ectopic Pregnancies

Emily W. Scibetta, MD[a,*], Christina S. Han, MD[b,c]

**KEYWORDS**

- Ectopic pregnancy • Gestational sac • Miscarriage • Early pregnancy loss
- Pseudosac

**KEY POINTS**

- Despite significant advances in early obstetric ultrasound, complications of ectopic pregnancy still account for 6% of all maternal deaths in the United States and remain the leading cause of maternal death secondary to hemorrhage.
- Ultrasound is critical in the evaluation and management of early pregnancy loss, pregnancy of unknown location, and ectopic pregnancies. In some cases, both transabdominal and transvaginal routes should be used for complete evaluation.
- In an asymptomatic woman with early pregnancy, there is no demonstrated benefit in routine screening for ectopic pregnancy. Evaluation for cesarean scar pregnancies should be considered in women with a previous cesarean delivery.
- The sensitivity of transvaginal ultrasonography for the diagnosis of ectopic pregnancy ranges from 73% to 93% and depends on the gestational age and the expertise of the ultrasonographer.
- Diagnostic criteria for early pregnancy loss have expanded in recent years to ensure false positive results do not lead to inappropriate evacuation of desired pregnancies. The patient, her desire to continue pregnancy, and her willingness to postpone interventions must be included in the diagnostic process and decision making to individualize these guidelines to patient circumstances.

Disclosures: The authors have nothing to disclose.
[a] Department of Obstetrics and Gynecology, Harbor-UCLA, 1000 W Carson St, Torrance, CA 90509, USA; [b] Division of Maternal-Fetal Medicine, University of California at Los Angeles, 10833 Le Conte Avenue, Room 27-139 CHS, Los Angeles, CA 90095-1740, USA; [c] Center for Fetal Medicine and Women's Ultrasound, 6310 San Vicente Boulevard, Suite 520, Los Angeles, CA 90048, USA
* Corresponding author. 300 Hillmont Avenue, Ventura, California 93003.
*E-mail address:* Emily.scibetta@gmail.com

Obstet Gynecol Clin N Am 46 (2019) 783–795
https://doi.org/10.1016/j.ogc.2019.07.013 

## INTRODUCTION

A *pregnancy of unknown location (PUL)* is defined by a positive beta-subunit of the human chorionic gonadotropin (β-hCG) test with no clear evidence of either an intrauterine or an ectopic pregnancy on transvaginal ultrasound. The differential diagnosis in PUL includes early, normal intrauterine pregnancy, early pregnancy loss, and ectopic pregnancy. Up to 25% of identified pregnancies will end in early pregnancy loss, and 1% to 2% will be ectopic pregnancy.[1]

These 3 diagnoses have been increasingly inserted into the political discourse on reproductive rights over the past decade, but it is important to remember that in the clinical setting, accurate diagnosis and prompt management of acute situations, such as ectopic pregnancies, are integral in decreasing morbidity and mortality of the woman. Despite significant advances in early obstetric ultrasound, complications of ectopic pregnancy still account for 6% of all maternal deaths in the United States and remain the leading cause of maternal death secondary to hemorrhage.[1,2] Early identification and appropriate surveillance in these women to rule out ectopic pregnancy are critical to decreasing maternal mortality and are the primary focus of this article.

## NORMAL EARLY PREGNANCY

Early diagnosis of a normal intrauterine pregnancy is best established with transvaginal ultrasonography with an empty maternal bladder. Approximately 1 week after fertilization, the blastocyst should implant eccentrically in 1 side of the uterine decidua, although this structure is not yet visible on ultrasound. A small, anechoic, well-circumscribed fluid collection known as a *gestational sac* can be identified by 4 to 5 weeks' gestation with transvaginal ultrasound (**Fig. 1**A). The normal gestational sac measures only 2 to 3 mm in the fifth week of pregnancy. The sac is typically surrounded by 2 concentric echogenic rims known as the *double decidual sign* (**Fig. 1**B).

An early intrauterine pregnancy can be confirmed on 2-dimensional ultrasound with the identification of a bright, echogenic ring with anechoic center, known as the "yolk sac" (**Fig. 1**C). The yolk sac is typically present by the fifth week of gestation. The embryo is often visible by 6 weeks of gestation. It can be seen on transvaginal ultrasonography as a linear echogenic structure adjacent to the yolk sac (**Fig. 1**D). A measurement of the embryo or "fetal pole" from crown to rump confirms the gestational age of the pregnancy. Fetal cardiac activity should be noted by 6 to 7 weeks' gestational age. **Table 1** shows the progression of normal early pregnancy findings and associated gestational ages.

## EARLY PREGNANCY LOSS: DIAGNOSTIC CRITERIA

Early pregnancy loss is defined as a nonviable pregnancy at less than 13 weeks' gestation identified by appropriate size criteria, such as a fetal pole without cardiac activity, or loss of normal ultrasound finding progression on transvaginal imaging.[3,4] Early pregnancy loss occurs after 25% of positive pregnancy tests and at least 10% of clinically recognized pregnancies.[5] More than 80% of spontaneous pregnancy loss occurs before 12 weeks' gestation.[6] Of these early losses, 50% are anembryonic gestations.[6] Of the remaining embryonic early pregnancy loss, another 40% to 50% have been attributed to aneuploidy.[7]

In desired pregnancies, it is critical to ensure appropriate criteria have been met before offering intervention to avoid undesired loss of a viable pregnancy, or missed diagnosis of other pregnancy complications, such as ectopic, molar pregnancy, birth

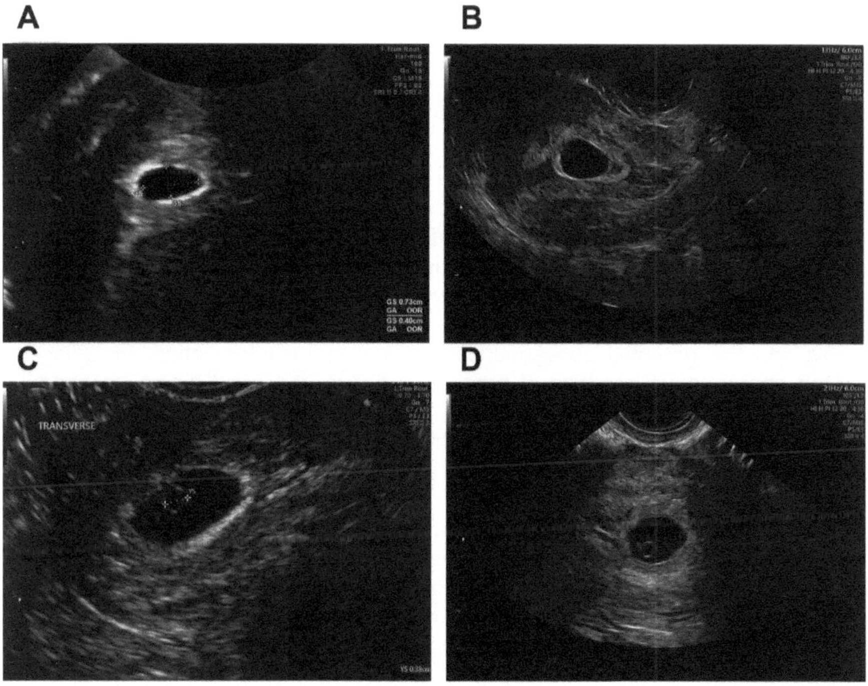


**Fig. 1.** Early normal pregnancies. (*A*) Early gestational sac located in an eccentric position in the decidua, (*B*) double decidual sign, (*C*) gestational sac with echogenic well-circumscribed yolk sac, and (*D*) fetal pole seen adjacent to a yolk sac.

defects, or cesarean scar pregnancy. When pregnancy loss is suspected, but not confirmed, it is appropriate to offer follow-up imaging in 7 to 10 days, or sooner if clinical picture evolves (ie, worsening bleeding or pain). If pregnancy loss is reliably confirmed, the patient can be definitively counseled on the diagnosis of pregnancy loss and offered management options, such as expectant management, prostaglandin and mifepristone administration, or surgical evacuation. Detailed discussion of management options is beyond the scope of this article.

### *Ultrasound Findings*

Ultrasound is the preferred modality for diagnosis of early pregnancy loss. Diagnostic criteria for early pregnancy loss have expanded in recent years to ensure

**Table 1**
**Progression of early normal pregnancy findings**

| | Gestational Age at Diagnosis by Transvaginal Ultrasound, wk |
|---|---|
| Gestational sac | 5 |
| Yolk sac | 5–6 |
| Fetal pole | 6 |
| Cardiac activity | 6–7 |

false positive results do not lead to inappropriate evacuation of desired pregnancies. The criteria discussed in this article were defined by Doubilet and colleagues,[8,9] on behalf of the Society of Radiologists in Ultrasound Multispecialty Panel on Early First Trimester Diagnosis of Miscarriage and Exclusion of a Viable Intrauterine Pregnancy and endorsed by the American College of Obstetricians and Gynecologists (ACOG). In order to achieve a specificity approaching 100%, diagnostic criteria for early pregnancy loss, as defined by these organizations, include increasingly conservative criteria, which can be applied indiscriminately to all ultrasound facilities. It is important to note that ACOG encourages practitioners to individualize their counseling and diagnosis of early pregnancy loss to meet an individual patient's needs, including the woman's desire to continue the pregnancy; her willingness to postpone intervention to achieve 100% certainty of failure of pregnancy; and the potential consequences of waiting for intervention, including unwanted spontaneous passage of pregnancy tissue, the need for an unscheduled visit or procedure, and patient anxiety. A shared decision-making model, engaging the patient and provider in a discussion of risks, benefits, and patient priorities, should be used in the diagnostic process and decision making to individualize these guidelines to patient circumstances.[3]

Early pregnancy loss can be subdivided into anembryonic and embryonic gestations. *Anembryonic gestation* is defined as an enlarged gestational sac with no visualization of fetal pole. The diagnostic criteria for anembryonic gestation require a mean sac diameter (MSD) greater than or equal to 25 mm on transvaginal ultrasound[3,10] (**Fig. 2**A). *Embryonic demise* is defined as a sufficiently sized fetal pole with no cardiac activity visualized (**Fig. 2**B). Although cardiac activity is widely accepted to be visible once the linear fetal pole can be seen, the size necessary to definitively rule out cardiac activity has expanded over the years. For many years, 5 mm was considered an appropriate cutoff for identification of cardiac activity. However, a 2011 metaanalysis showed that the small sample size in initial studies was not sufficient to establish specificity greater than 90%.[11] In addition, an interobserver variability of up to 15% on crown-rump-length measurements identified by Pexsters and colleagues[12] suggests the less stringent criteria were warranted.[10] Following these studies, new criteria for crown-rump length greater than or equal to 7 mm were established. Additional sonographic criteria for diagnosis of early pregnancy loss are listed in **Box 1**.

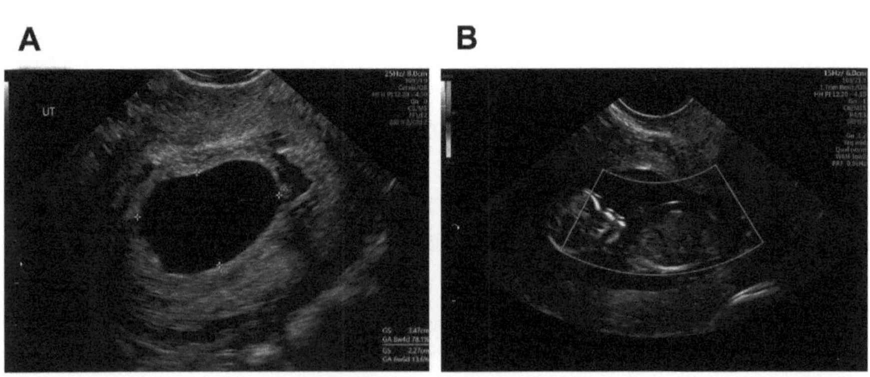


**Fig. 2.** Early pregnancy loss. (*A*) An empty gestational sac measuring >25 mm MSD with no yolk sac or fetal pole and (*B*) an embryo with no fetal cardiac activity seen on Doppler imaging. UT, uterus.

**Box 1**
**Ultrasound criteria for diagnosis of early pregnancy loss**

Enlarged gestational sac with no embryo: MSD ≥25 mm

Embryo with no cardiac activity: crown-rump length ≥7 mm

Absence of embryo with heartbeat 14 days or more after ultrasound confirming gestational sac WITHOUT yolk sac

Absence of embryo with heartbeat 11 days or more after ultrasound confirming gestational sac WITH yolk sac

Empty uterine cavity in patient with vaginal bleeding and previously confirmed intrauterine pregnancy by at least gestational sac and yolk sac

*Adapted from* Early Pregnancy Loss. Practice Bulletin No. 150. American College of Obstetricians and Gynecologists. Obstet Gynecol 2015;125:1258-67; and Rodgers SK, Chang C, DeBardeleben JT, et al. Normal and Abnormal US Findings in Early First-Trimester Pregnancy: Review of the Society of Radiologists in Ultrasound 2012 Consensus Panel Recommendations. Radiographics 2015;35(7):2135-48.

## PREGNANCY OF UNKNOWN LOCATION AND ECTOPIC PREGNANCY

Ectopic pregnancy is defined as a pregnancy implanted in a location other than the endometrial cavity. The most common location is tubal, which can be further classified as fimbrial, ampullary, or isthmic (**Fig. 3**A, B). Five percent to 10% of nonuterine pregnancies implant outside the tube, including the ovary, interstitium, cervix, peritoneal cavity, rudimentary uterine horns (also known as cornual), or cesarean section scar. In incredibly rare cases, posthysterectomy pregnancies have been described.[10] Appropriate management of suspected ectopic pregnancy must balance an incorrect early diagnosis that leads to disruption of a normal, desired intrauterine pregnancy against the risk of delayed confirmation of ectopic pregnancy with increased morbidity and mortality in the patient with a rupture of the ectopic pregnancy.

### *Epidemiology of Ectopic Pregnancy*

Approximately 2% of pregnancies in the United States are ectopic.[1] The actual burden of disease is difficult to confirm because the Centers for Disease Control and Prevention tracking does not account for outpatient management of cases, but it appears the

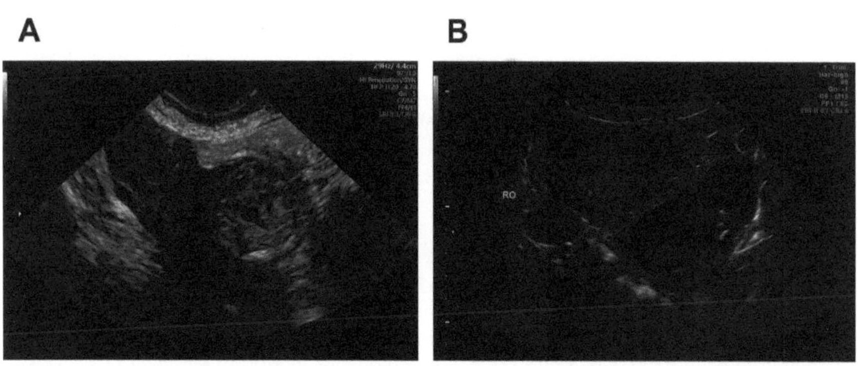


**Fig. 3.** Tubal pregnancies. (*A*) Early tubal ectopic pregnancy and (*B*) advanced tubal ectopic pregnancy in late first trimester. RO, right ovary.

overall burden of disease has been stable over recent decades.[2,13] Tubal ectopic pregnancy remains a significant risk for maternal death and morbidity. It is still the main cause of pregnancy-related death owing to hemorrhage. Overall, tubal pregnancy accounts for a surprising 6% of maternal deaths in the United States.[2,14]

The risk of recurrence of ectopic pregnancy is approximately 10% in women with 1 prior ectopic pregnancy and as high as 25% with 2 or more prior ectopic pregnancies.[15] Heterotopic pregnancy, defined as an intrauterine gestation with concurrent ectopic pregnancy, carries a natural incidence of 1 in 30,000, but assisted reproductive technology (ART) has increased the incidence to 1 in 7000 after ovulation induction.[16] This risk is considered even higher after in vitro fertilization, with incidence documented as high as 1 case per 100 for women who underwent in vitro fertilization.[17] Additional risk factors for ectopic pregnancy are listed in **Table 2**.

### *Pathophysiology*

Risk factors for tubal pregnancy include any exposure that could damage the fallopian tubes, such as prior ectopic pregnancy, prior tubal surgery, history of pelvic inflammatory disease, and salpingitis node isthmica. Other risk factors include smoking, endometriosis, abdominal surgery, smoking, history of sexually transmitted infection, endometriosis, in utero exposure to diethylstilbestrol, and the use of ART. Although pregnancy risk is low with intrauterine devices (IUD) in place, if a pregnancy occurs with an IUD in situ, the risk of ectopic pregnancy is much higher. Approximately 50% of patients with ectopic pregnancy carry no known risk factors. Thus, a high index of suspicion is warranted in any woman of reproductive age who presents with abdominal pain, vaginal bleeding, or evidence of hemodynamic instability.

### *Pregnancy of Unknown Location: Clinical Evaluation*

Up to one-half of all pregnant women have signs and symptoms, such as pain or bleeding, that are suggestive of early pregnancy loss in the first trimester.[18] Every patient with early pregnancy bleeding and/or abdominal pain should be evaluated with the goal of early identification of ectopic pregnancy. There is no demonstrated benefit in screening asymptomatic, clinically stable women for ectopic pregnancy.[19] Consideration can be made for screening for cesarean scar pregnancies in women with 1 or more prior cesarean deliveries (see Ilan E. Timor-Tritsch and colleagues' article, "Cesarean Scar Pregnancy: Diagnosis and Pathogenesis," and Ilan E. Timor-Tritsch

**Table 2**
**Risk factors for ectopic pregnancy**

| Major Risk Factors | Minor Risk Factors |
|---|---|
| History of tubal surgery, including reconstructive surgery and tubal sterilization | Endometriosis |
| In utero exposure to diethylstilbestrol | Previous abdominal surgery |
| ART | Tobacco smoking |
| IUDs | |
| History of pelvic inflammatory disease | |
| Previous ectopic pregnancy | |
| Salpingitis nodosa isthmica | |
| History of tubal sterilization | |

*Adapted from* Baltarowich OH, Scoutt LM. Ectopic Pregnancy. In: Norton ME, Scoutt LM, Feldstein VA, editors. Callen's Ultrasonography in Obstetrics and Gynecology, 6th edition. Philadelphia: Elsevier; 2017; with permission.

and colleagues' article, "Cesarean Scar Pregnancy: Patient Counselling and Management," in this issue).

Initial management depends on the clinical stability of the patient and thorough history and physical examination. For patients who present with a positive pregnancy test, signs of shock, and evidence of intraabdominal bleeding, immediate surgical management is warranted. In these cases, patients may present with rebound tenderness on abdominal examination, hypotension, tachycardia, and evidence of free fluid on ultrasound. Ultrasound identification of free fluid is best established by FAST (focused assessment with sonography in trauma) scan to identify fluid in the pericolic gutters and posterior cul-de-sac. Occasionally, an ectopic pregnancy with chronic insidious bleeding will appear as organized, expansive clot on ultrasound. With appropriate surgical training, urgent surgical management is often accomplished with laparoscopy. Some resource-limited settings may call for exploratory laparotomy.

For stable patients, quantitative serum β-hCG levels combined with transvaginal ultrasound assessment is the standard of care. Approximately 40% of ultrasounds at first presentation in symptomatic first-trimester patients will be inconclusive because of a failed pregnancy before development of a gestational sac or because the pregnancy is too early to be readily identified.[20] Because of this, triaging patients into appropriate categories for expedited follow-up is critical.

### *Clinical Evaluation: Role of Ultrasound*

Ultrasound is critical in the diagnosis of PUL. Appropriate understanding of normal signs in early intrauterine pregnancy and early pregnancy loss is important to rule out ectopic pregnancy. With reliable pregnancy dating, transvaginal ultrasonography should identify normal intrauterine pregnancies by 5.5 weeks of gestation close to 100% of the time.[21]

A standardized protocol should be implemented in each ultrasound laboratory. Given the known common locations for nonintrauterine pregnancies, the protocol for evaluation of patient with PUL should include clear imaging of the uterus (including bilateral cornua), cervix, bilateral ovaries and tubes, cul-de-sac, and nearby pelvic structures. Both transabdominal and transvaginal imaging may be necessary to evaluate the pelvis and lower abdomen adequately.

Clear evidence of ectopic pregnancy on ultrasound relies on characteristic extrauterine findings combined with no clear evidence of an intrauterine gestation except in a heterotopic pregnancy. These findings include a nonhomogenous mass separate from the ovary with or without a hyperechoic "ring sign" or a fetal pole with or without cardiac activity in an extrauterine location. Literature suggest that more than 60% of ectopic pregnancies present as a nonhomogenous mass separate from the ovary; approximately 20% present as a hyperechoic ring, and 13% will present with an obvious gestational sac, with or without a fetal pole.[22] Ectopic placental blood flow, commonly referred to as a ring of fire, can be seen with color Doppler within the periphery of an adnexal mass. This hypervascularity can be difficult to distinguish from typical findings in a corpus luteum, and thus, distinct diagnosis can be difficult.[6] The sensitivity of transvaginal ultrasonography for the diagnosis of ectopic pregnancy ranges from 73% to 93% and depends on the gestational age and the expertise of the ultrasonographer.[18]

If there is identification of a hypoechoic fluid collection without the double decidual sign or without clear identification of a yolk sac, commonly referred to as a pseudosac, an ectopic pregnancy cannot be ruled out. This pseudosac is often distinguished from a gestational sac by its midcavity position (as opposed to eccentric placement), lack of double decidual sign or yolk sac, and teardrop shape (**Fig. 4**A).

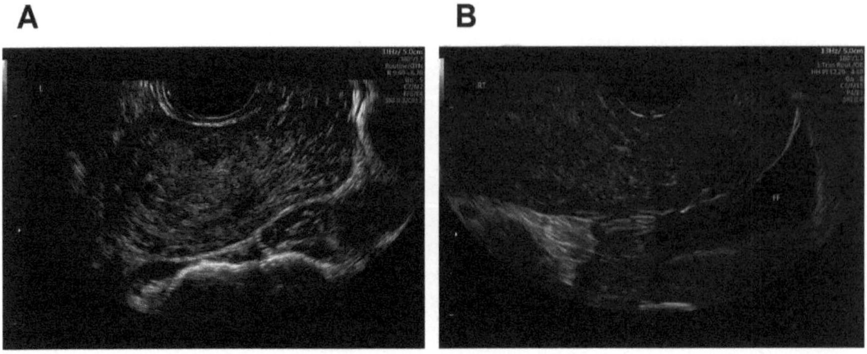

**Fig. 4.** Potential nonpregnancy findings in ectopic pregnancies. (*A*) A pseudosac in decidua and (*B*) a free fluid in the cul-de-sac. FF, free fluid; L, left; RT, right.

Although a scant amount of intraperitoneal fluid can be normal, significant intraabdominal fluid raises the suspicion for hemoperitoneum and thus adds diagnostic utility (**Fig. 4**B). Hemoperitoneum can be hypoechoic or of mixed echogenicity, evolving to become more hyperechoic as the clot organizes. Bleeding typically collects in gravity-dependent regions, most commonly in the cul-de-sac on pelvic imaging, where as little as 50 mL can be appreciated. Additional imaging of the pericolic gutters and pouch of Morrison near the liver can confirm the presence of significant intraabdominal bleeding that has overwhelmed the pelvis. Imaging via both the transabdominal and the transvaginal routes can also elicit peritoneal signs in cases of intraabdominal bleeding, with guarding and rebound tenderness on transabdominal imaging and cervical motion tenderness on transvaginal imaging.

Nontubal locations of ectopic pregnancy, including interstitial, cornual, ovarian, cervical, abdominal, and cesarean scar, account for approximately 5% of all ectopic pregnancies. Ultrasound findings in these cases are widely variable (**Fig. 5**A–D).

Interstitial pregnancies develop in the proximal fallopian tube immediately adjacent to the uterine myometrium (see **Fig. 5**A). The expansibility of this space allows the pregnancies to progress to later gestations than typical distal tubal pregnancies before rupturing. However, if rupture does occur, patients experience significantly greater blood loss and morbidity, with mortalities quoted as high as 2.5%.[6] Evaluation for a suspected interstitial pregnancy begins by identifying the interstitial segment of the tube, located in the transverse plane at the level of the uterine fundus. This segment is seen as a thin echogenic line extending from the lateral aspect of the endometrial cavity through the myometrium toward the uterine serosa.[15] An abnormal interstitial ectopic pregnancy is located within this line (see **Fig. 5**B), compared with a normal intrauterine pregnancy, which would be located medial to the line.

Cornual pregnancies specifically refer to a pregnancy implanted in a rudimentary horn of a patient with a Mullerian anomaly. Interstitial and cornual pregnancies can mirror the appearance of an eccentrically implanted gestational sac, making diagnosis by ultrasound challenging. Three ultrasound criteria for diagnosis of interstitial or cornual pregnancies include (1) empty uterine cavity, (2) a gestational sac separate from an empty endometrial cavity and greater than 1 cm distant from most lateral edge of uterine cavity, and (3) a thin less than 5 mm myometrial mantle surround the gestational sac.[23] Three-dimensional (3D) ultrasound can be invaluable in distinguishing a cornual or interstitial from an eccentric intrauterine pregnancy and is discussed later.

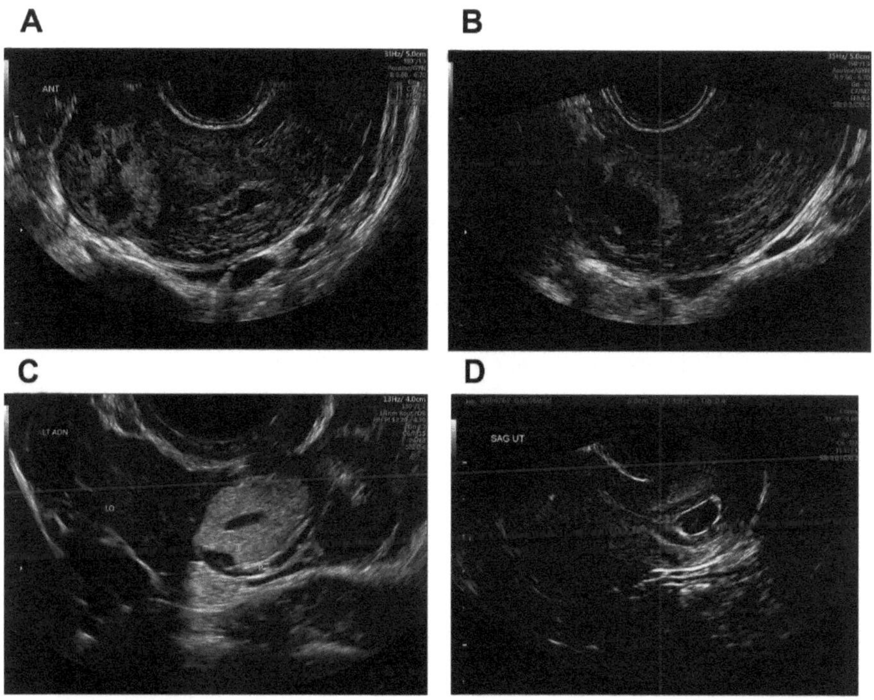


**Fig. 5.** Nontubal ectopic pregnancies. (*A*) An interstitial ectopic pregnancy, (*B*) interstitial line sign connecting the interstitial ectopic pregnancy, (*C*) ovarian ectopic pregnancy, and (*D*) cervical ectopic pregnancy. ANT, anterior; LO, left ovary; LT ADN, left adnexa; SAG UT, sagittal uterus.

Abdominal pregnancies are rare and defined as an intraperitoneal implantation separate from a pelvic organ location. The presentation of abdominal pregnancy is widely varied, nonspecific, and dependent on the gestational age at diagnosis. Some ultrasound findings include oligohydramnios (common, but nonspecific) and lack of myometrium surrounding fetus. A transabdominal scan with a full maternal bladder is very helpful in establishing the diagnosis. MRI may also be helpful as an adjunct in identifying implantation site in an abdominal pregnancy.

Ovarian pregnancies are difficult to distinguish from tubal ectopics by ultrasound, but may be diagnosed by the identification of ovarian cortex surrounding or contiguous with a mass that is suspicious for ectopic pregnancy (see **Fig. 5**C). Intraperitoneal fluid suggestive of hemoperitoneum may increase the index of suspicion, but can also represent a ruptured hemorrhagic cyst. Diagnosis is typically made surgically and even then can be difficult to distinguish on direct visualization from a bleeding corpus luteum cyst.

Cervical ectopic pregnancies are often diagnosed by transvaginal imaging, speculum examination, and palpation. The more cephalad the implantation, the greater the risk of bleeding in cervical ectopic pregnancies given their increased capacity to expand. Ultrasound findings may include an hourglass uterine shape with ballooning of the cervical canal, gestational tissue at the level of the cervix with no evidence of intrauterine gestational tissue, and a bridge of endocervical canal visualized between the empty endometrial canal and the cervical pregnancy[6] (see **Fig. 5**D). It is important to distinguish a cervical ectopic from an aborting conceptus or a cesarean scar pregnancy, because management of these 3 diagnoses are very different. A suction curettage in an unexpected cervical ectopic pregnancy or cesarean scar pregnancy can result in unexpected hemorrhage. Color Doppler will show copious peritrophoblastic flow in a cervical or cesarean scar pregnancy, whereas a pregnancy in transit through the cervical canal will have decreased flow.

### *Clinical Evaluation: Role of Three-Dimensional Ultrasound*

3D imaging may play an integral role in differentiating between normal and eccentrically located pregnancies, particularly in cases of abnormal uterine cavity (such as Mullerian abnormality or leiomayomatous uterus) and suspected interstitial, corneal, or cesarean scar pregnancies. In these cases, the ability to render multiple planes and postprocess an image allows for more exact localization of the suspected pregnancy relative to the endometrial cavity, as shown in **Fig. 6.**[17,19,24,25] 3D ultrasound is preferred over MRI because of lower cost and accessibility.

### *Clinical Evaluation: Role of Quantitative β-Human Chorionic Gonadotropin*

Without definitive evidence of ectopic pregnancy on ultrasound, it is inappropriate to manage PUL with only 1 β-hCG measurement. The common practice is to rule out normal intrauterine pregnancy based on a discriminatory zone in β-hCG measurement above which pregnancy should be identified transvaginally. This ultrasound evaluation is often coupled with an anticipated increase in β-hCG of at least 53% in 48 hours. The appropriate discriminatory zone has been expanded in recent years to avoid disruption of a normal intrauterine pregnancy in stable patients. ACOG generally accepts 3500 mIU/mL as the appropriately conservative level.[13]

### *Pregnancy of Unknown Location: Summary of Surveillance Strategies*

Conservative management with close follow-up is appropriate in women with PUL if they are clinically stable and have sufficient support in their life to follow up in clinic in 2 days and have safe, swift access to emergency facilities. A reasonable management strategy includes the following:

1. Obtain serum quantitative β-hCG levels on 2 occasions, 48 hours apart, sent to the same commercial laboratory. In a normal intrauterine pregnancy, serum β-hCG levels are expected to increase at least 53% to 66% over 48 hours.[26–28] An

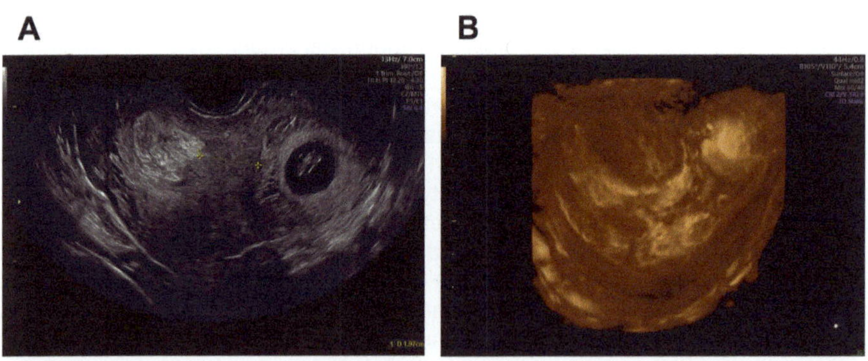


**Fig. 6.** Demonstration of utility of 3D ultrasound imaging. (*A*) Two-dimensional imaging at the level of the fundus in the transverse view with the sac seen to be located in the cornua without contiguity with the endometrial cavity. (*B*) 3D rendering of the same uterus in the coronal view revealing intact myometrium surrounding the normally located gestational sac located lateral to the uterine septum.

increase of less than 53% over 48 hours without definitive evidence of intrauterine pregnancy on pelvic ultrasound is suspicious for early pregnancy failure or ectopic pregnancy.

2. If β-hCG increases greater than 53% over 48 hours with a level greater than 3500 mIU/mL and there is still no evidence of intrauterine pregnancy, ectopic pregnancy is highly likely.
3. If no evidence of intrauterine pregnancy or ectopic pregnancy is identified after 48 hours and β-hCG is falling in a clinically stable patient, it is reasonable to continue expectant management because early intrauterine pregnancy loss cannot be excluded and methotrexate can be avoided. In a recent study evaluating expectant management in suspected ectopic pregnancy with β-hCG less than 2000 mIU/mL, there was no statistically significant difference in treatment success when methotrexate was compared with expectant management.[29]

The detailed management of ectopic pregnancies is not covered in this article, because it is outside the scope of an ultrasound volume. For the nonobstetrician imaging provider, it is, however, important to remember that ACOG recommends that Rhesus-D–negative patients with any form of early pregnancy loss receive anti-Rh(D) immunoglobulin.[13]

### *Role of Novel Biomarkers in Pregnancy of Unknown Location*

A significant focus of recent clinical inquiry has been on modeling novel serum biomarkers for early pregnancy outcomes. The goal has been to determine if biomarkers may be able to aid in determining the location or viability of an early gestation. The hope has been that these studies could aid in determination of best treatment plans.[24]

As reviewed above, in the absence of clear ultrasound evidence of an extrauterine gestation with elevated hCG, a firm diagnosis of ectopic pregnancy currently relies on serial β-hCG levels and usually multiple pelvic ultrasounds. Much to the continued frustration of gynecologists everywhere, ultrasound at first presentation of symptomatic women in early pregnancy is inconclusive in up to 40% of women. Although operator experience plays a major role, this is likely because the gestation is too early to be clearly identified or an early pregnancy loss has occurred with collapse of the gestational sac. Given the limited role of ultrasound at initial diagnosis in stable patients, the pursuit of novel biomarkers has intensified to prevent the morbidity of bleeding, infertility, or death of delayed diagnosis of ectopic pregnancy.

Novel markers of interest include ratio of β-hCG of day 0 and day 2, Activin A, pregnancy-associated plasma protein-A, pregnancy-specific beta-glycoprotein 1, metalloprotease-12, nucleic acid markers, markers of corpus luteal function, angiogenesis markers, endometrial function markers, and multiple marker tests. Despite the promise of many of these tests, prospective cohort studies of PUL will be required to validate these tests independently to the point of incorporation into clinical care.[20]

## SUMMARY

Ultrasound is the primary tool in the evaluation and management of PUL. The practitioner must keep in mind the differential diagnoses of early pregnancy loss, PUL, and ectopic pregnancies. Both transabdominal and transvaginal ultrasounds should be available, in addition to physical examination, for complete evaluation. Diagnostic criteria for early pregnancy loss have expanded in recent years to ensure false positive results do not lead to inappropriate evacuation of desired pregnancies. A shared decision-making model, engaging the patient and provider in a discussion of risks, benefits, and patient priorities should be used in the diagnostic process and decision making to individualize these guidelines to patient circumstances.

## REFERENCES


1. Centers for Disease Control and Prevention (CDC). Ectopic pregnancy–United States, 1990-1992. MMWR Morb Mortal Wkly Rep 1995;44:46–8.
2. Creanga AA, Syverson C, Seed K, et al. Pregnancy-related mortality in the United States, 2011-2013. Obstet Gynecol 2017;130(2):366–73.
3. Early pregnancy loss. ACOG Practice Bulletin No. 200. American College of Obstetricians and Gynecologists. Obstet Gynecol 2018;132:e197–207.
4. National Institute for Health and Clinical Excellence. Ectopic pregnancy and miscarriage: diagnosis and initial management in early pregnancy of ectopic pregnancy and miscarriage. NICE Clinical Guideline 154. Manchester (United Kingdom): NICE; 2012.
5. Wang X, Chen C, Wang L, et al. Conception, early pregnancy loss, and time to clinical pregnancy: a population-based prospective study. Fertil Steril 2003;79:577–84.
6. Cunningham FG, Leveno KJ, Bloom SL, et al. Williams Obstetrics, 25th edition. New York: McGraw-Hill Education; 2014.
7. Stephenson MD, Awartani KA, Robinson WP. Cytogenetic analysis of miscarriages from couples with recurrent miscarriage: a case-control study. Hum Reprod 2002;17:446–51.
8. Doubilet PM, Benson CB, Bourne T, et al. Diagnostic criteria for nonviable pregnancy early in the first trimester. Society of Radiologists in Ultrasound Multispecialty Panel on Early First Trimester Diagnosis of Miscarriage and Exclusion of a Viable Intrauterine Pregnancy. N Engl J Med 2013;369:1443–51.
9. Practice Committee of American Society for Reproductive Medicine. Medical treatment of ectopic pregnancy: a committee opinion. Fertil Steril 2013;100:638–44.
10. Callen PW, Norton ME, Scoutt LM, et al. Callen's Ultrasonography in Obstetrics and Gynecology. Sixth edition. Philadelphia: Elsevier; 2017.
11. Jeve Y, Rana R, Bhide A, et al. Accuracy of first trimester ultrasound in the diagnosis of early embryonic demise: a systematic review. Ultrasound Obstet Gynecol 2011;38:489–96.
12. Pexsters A, Luts J, van Schoubroeck D, et al. Clinical implications of intra- and interobserver reproducibility of transvaginal sonographic measurements of gestational sac and crown-rump length at 6–9 weeks' gestation. Ultrasound Obstet Gynecol 2011;38(5):510–5.
13. American College of Obstetricians and Gynecologists. Tubal ectopic pregnancy. ACOG Practice Bulletin No. 193. Obstet Gynecol 2018;131:e91–103.
14. Hoover KW, Tao G, Kent CK. Trends in the diagnosis and treatment of ectopic pregnancy in the United States. Obstet Gynecol 2010;115:495–502.
15. Chukus A, Tirada N, Restrepo R, et al. Uncommon implantation sites of ectopic pregnancy: thinking beyond the complex adnexal mass. Radiographics 2015;35(3):946–59.
16. Mukul LV, Teal SB. Current management of ectopic pregnancy. Obstet Gynecol Clin North Am 2007;34(3):403–19.
17. Ong C, Su LL, Chia D, et al. Sonographic diagnosis and successful medical management of an intramural ectopic pregnancy. J Clin Ultrasound 2010;38(6):320–4.

18. Barnhar KT. Ectopic pregnancy. N Engl J Med 2009;361:379–87.
19. Lee GS, Hur SY, Kown I, et al. Diagnosis of early intramural ectopic pregnancy. J Clin Ultrasound 2005;33(4):190–2.
20. Senapati S, Barnhart KT. Biomarkers for ectopic pregnancy and pregnancy of unknown location. Fertil Steril 2013;99(4):1107–16.
21. Barnhart K, Mennuti MT, Benjamin I, et al. Prompt diagnosis of ectopic pregnancy in an emergency department setting. Obstet Gynecol 1994;84:1010–5.
22. Condous G, Okaro E, Khalid A, et al. The accuracy of transvaginal ultrasonography for the diagnosis of ectopic pregnancy prior to surgery. Hum Reprod 2005; 20(5):1404.
23. Timor-Tritsch IE, Monteagudo MC, Matera C, et al. Sonographic evolution of cornual pregnancies treated without surgery. Obstet Gynecol 1992;79(6):1044.
24. Wang J, Xie X. Sonographic diagnosis of intramural pregnancy. J Ultrasound Med 2013;32(12):2215–7.
25. Tanaka Y, Mimura K, Kanagawa T, et al. Three-dimensional sonography in the differential diagnosis of interstitial, angular, and intrauterine pregnancies in a septate uterus. J Ultrasound Med 2014;33(11):2013–5.
26. Seeber BE, Barnhart KT. Suspected ectopic pregnancy. Obstet Gynecol 2006; 107:399–413.
27. Maymon R, Shulman A. Controversies and problems in the current management of tubal pregnancy. Hum Reprod Update 1996;2:541–51.
28. Mol BW, van der Veen F, Bossuyt PM. Symptom-free women at increased risk of ectopic pregnancy: should we screen? Acta Obstet Gynecol Scand 2002;81: 661–72.
29. Van Mello NM, Mol F, Verhoeve HR, et al. Methotrexate or expectant management in women with an ectopic pregnancy or pregnancy of unknown location and low serum β-hCG concentrations? A randomized comparison. Hum Reprod 2013; 28:60–7.

# Cesarean Scar Pregnancy

## Diagnosis and Pathogenesis

Ilan E. Timor-Tritsch, MD[a,*], Ana Monteagudo, MD[b], Giuseppe Calì, MD[c,1], Francesco D'Antonio, MD[d], Andrea Kaelin Agten, MD[e]

**KEYWORDS**

- Cesarean scar pregnancy • Ultrasound • Cesarean delivery • Diagnosis
- Placenta accreta spectrum

**KEY POINTS**

- Cesarean scar pregnancy (CSP) is a potentially dangerous, man-made consequence of a previous cesarean delivery (CD).
- CSP and placenta accreta spectrum (PAS) share the same histologic picture. CSP is a precursor of PAS.
- Most patients with a CSP diagnosed in the first trimester that reach the third trimester of pregnancy have the potential to deliver a liveborn infant via repeat CD, almost all have different degrees of PAS, and in most cases will have hysterectomy.
- The best diagnostic tool is transvaginal ultrasound.
- An international CSP registry was created www.csp-registry.com. The authors encourage its use to upload cases.

## INTRODUCTION

Cesarean scar pregnancy (CSP) is a potentially dangerous consequence of a previous cesarean delivery (CD). If unrecognized and inadequately managed, it can lead to untoward complications throughout all three trimesters of the pregnancy. It's rate of occurrence parallels the mounting rate of cesarean sections. The late consequences

Nothing to declare.
[a] Department of Obstetrics and Gynecology, NYU School of Medicine, NYU Langone Health, 550 1st Avenue, New York, NY 10016, USA; [b] Department of Obstetrics, Gynecology, and Reproductive Science, Icahn School of Medicine at Mount Sinai, New York, NY, USA; [c] Department of Obstetrics and Gynecology, Arnas Civico Hospital, Palermo, Italy; [d] Fetal Medicine Unit, Department of Obstetrics and Gynecology, University of Foggia, Foggia, Italy; [e] Nottingham University Hospitals NHS, Queens Medical Centre, Derby Road, Nottingham, NG7 2UH, UK
[1] Present address: viale Acacie 26, Casteldaccia, Palermo 90014, Italia.
* Corresponding author.
*E-mail address:* ilan.timor@nyumc.org

Obstet Gynecol Clin N Am 46 (2019) 797–811
https://doi.org/10.1016/j.ogc.2019.07.009
obgyn.theclinics.com

of CD, such as placenta previa and placenta accrete, were known for a long time. However, it took more than a decade for the obstetric community to make the connection between CSP and the placenta accreta spectrum (PAS). The authors discuss the pathogenesis and diagnosis in this article.

## NOMENCLATURE AND TERMS

Various terms were and are still used for CSP, such as "cesarean ectopic pregnancy," "cesarean scar ectopic," "ectopic," "isthmocele," and "cesarean delivery scar pregnancy." Here we use the term cesarean scar pregnancy. The two main reasons are: CSP is not an ectopic gestation because, if left to continue, it expands/morphs into an intrauterine pregnancy; and treatments usually used for what are considered "real" ectopic pregnancies (tubal, cornual, interstitial, and cervical) cannot be applied in their customary form for CSP.

There has been a change in nomenclature in recent years. In different countries and by different professional societies pathologically adherent placentae were referred to as morbidly adherent placenta, abnormally implanted placenta, placenta adherence disorder, or simply by the generalized term placenta accreta referring to all the three of their known severities. In the first part of 2019 FIGO introduced the term placenta accreta spectrum suggesting an all-inclusive term for the disease.[1]

## BACKGROUND

The occurrence of CSP is closely related to a previous CD. In the United States the rate of CD estimated in 2017 was 32.0%.[2] The cesarean section rate is lower today. The Centers for Disease Control and Prevention reveals that the overall rate of cesarean section births have stopped increasing and steadied at 32% from 2009 to 2011.[3]

## INCIDENCE

The true incidence of CSP is unknown. Almost all articles and related articles quote the only available estimates that the range is from 1/1800 to 1/2500 of all CD performed.[4,5] One can expect an increase of the reported incidence caused by increased awareness and the more accurate diagnosis of this entity.

## RISK FACTORS FOR CESAREAN SCAR PREGNANCY

The only risk factor for CSP is one or more previous CDs.

## PATHOGENESIS

During a normal pregnancy the trophoblast penetrates the myometrium and remodels the vascular bed to enable a low-resistance/high-velocity blood flow to the conceptus. This physiologic "invasion" is stopped by the Nitabuch fibrinoid layer, a layer of fibrin (fibrinoid material) between the boundary zone of compact endometrium and the cytotrophoblastic shell in the placenta. This layer is naturally present between the endometrium in normally attached placentae. Previous uterine surgery or uterine interventions lead to thin or absent decidua basalis in scarred areas of the lower uterine segment leading to an unopposed penetration of the trophoblast thought to create placental accretism. Tantbirojn and colleagues[6] take this phenomenon a step further writing: "We conclude that the pathogenesis of placenta accreta is multi-dimensional, involving increased, but incomplete trophoblast invasion in a background of absent decidua. We further propose that placenta increta and percreta are not caused by a further invasion of extravillous trophoblast in the uterine wall, rather they likely arise secondary to dehiscence of a scar, leading to the presence of *chorionic villi* deep within the uterine wall, and thus give extravillous trophoblast greater access to the deep myometrium."

## WHAT IS THE CESAREAN SCAR PREGNANCY?

CSP occurs when a blastocyst implants in a microscopic or macroscopic tract on the uterine scar or in the "niche" (or dehiscence) left behind by an incision site of the previous CD. The mechanism is the same after uterine surgery (curettage, myomectomy, endometrial ablation, manual removal of placenta, or any intrauterine surgical manipulation) with one significant difference: the latter causes are extremely rare (**Fig. 1**A, B).

The difference between the "on the scar" and "in the niche" implantation is that in the first variety there is a measurable myometrial thickness between the placenta/gestational sac and the anterior uterine surface or the bladder, whereas in the second form the placenta/gestational sac complex is at close proximity to the bladder or the anterior uterine surface (see **Fig. 1**A, B). It seems that there is a difference in outcome between the two forms of implantation if the decision is to continue the pregnancy.[7]

## WHAT IS A NICHE OF A PREVIOUS CESAREAN SECTION?

The niche or dehiscence is a discontinuity of the low anterior uterine wall seen after the healing process of a previous CD. At times a thick scar forms without leaving behind a defect, other times a usually triangular defect is visible either on an unenhanced ultrasound (US) or highlighted by a saline infusion US examination.[8,9]

It should be realized that regardless of the size or measurements of the niche on the sagittal uterine sections, a transverse/coronal section may reveal the actual size of the defect because the uterine incision is usually made in a transverse fashion. This is easily seen if a three-dimensional US image of the uterus is sought.

Risk factors for development of niches could be classified into four categories: those related (1) to closure technique, (2) to development of the lower uterine segment or location of the incision, (3) to wound healing, and (4) to miscellaneous factors. Probable other risk factors are single-layer myometrium closure, multiple cesarean sections, and uterine retroflexion. However, there is no single causative factor

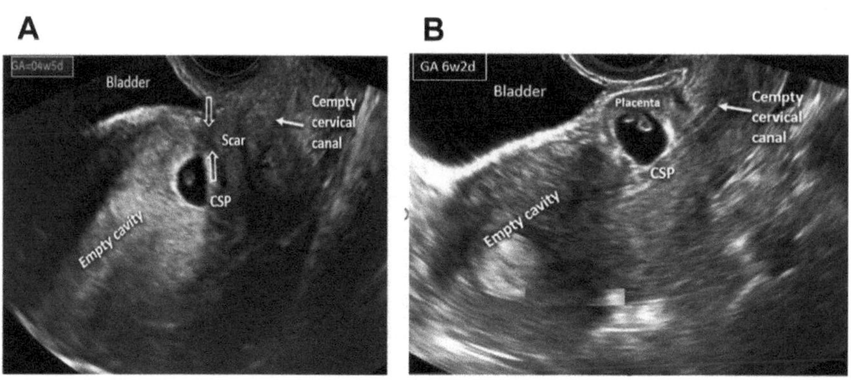


**Fig. 1.** The two implantation modes of CSP. (*A*) "On the scar" with measurable (usually ≥2–3 mm) myometrial thickness between placenta/gestational sac and bladder. (*B*) "In the niche" with <2 mm or no measurable myometrium between placenta/gestational sac and bladder.

convincingly proven. Because uterine retroversion was touched on, it has to be mentioned that the detection of a retroverted uterus in a patient presenting with a subsequent pregnancy with a history of a previous CD is a good reason to perform a detailed scan to rule out a CSP.[10]

## CLINICAL PRESENTATION OF CESAREAN SCAR PREGNANCY

As in every intrauterine pregnancy vaginal bleeding of different degrees may be the first sign of a CSP. Pain is usually not a typical presenting symptom. Patients may be asymptomatic and only become aware of a CSP when detected by US. The initial and early US between 5 and 7 weeks is critical because many CSPs are misdiagnosed as threatened abortion, miscarriage, or simply intrauterine pregnancies. Misdiagnoses may lead to curettage for a presumed failed pregnancy causing profuse bleeding and emergency surgical interventions and can end with hysterectomy. The history of a previous CD and a low, anterior gestational sac (at times in an anteverted retroflexed uterus) with or without heart activity should be considered a CSP unless proven otherwise before any surgical intervention.

## DIAGNOSIS OF CESAREAN SCAR PREGNANCY

Every woman who presents in the first trimester to the obstetrics/gynecology practitioner with a positive pregnancy test and a history of a previous CD should be considered a CSP until proven otherwise.

The best and first-line imaging modality to diagnose a CSP is transvaginal US (TVUS). It presents a clear advantage over the transabdominal imaging. In some articles the authors used MRI for the diagnosis. Our view is that TVUS provides the precise diagnosis in almost all cases without the need of additional imaging modalities. In addition, MRI is more expensive, time consuming, and often delays the diagnosis. We diagnose CSP based on a positive pregnancy test in addition to the sonographic criteria shown in **Figs. 2–8**:

1. An empty uterine cavity and closed, empty endocervical canal.
2. Detection of an early gestational sac and/or placenta in close proximity of the hysterotomy scar/niche with fetal or embryonic pole and/or yolk sac with or without heartbeat (depending on the gestational age). Before 7 weeks the gestational sac may mold or morph into the shape of the niche in which it implants.
3. An absent or thin-appearing myometrial layer between the gestational sac and the anterior uterine wall or the bladder wall.
4. Abundant blood flow around the gestational sac determined by Doppler interrogation. The detection of subjectively estimated rich peritrophoblastic blood flow. This is best achieved if the Doppler region of interest is restricted to the area of the gestational sac and using the most sensitive Doppler settings (ie, a low pulse repetition frequency). An anteflexed/retroverted uterus strengthens the diagnosis.

A timely diagnosis of a CSP presents clear advantage when their management is considered. However, it is never too late in pregnancy to diagnose a CSP. If in the second trimester a low, anterior placenta or frank previa was diagnosed in a patient with a previous CD, one should make every effort to find a first trimester US picture and retroactively re-evaluate for the sonographic criteria of CSP.

It cannot be emphasized enough that after 7 weeks in continuing pregnancies the chorionic/gestational sac "moves" toward the fundus populating the uterine cavity (see **Fig. 3**). Despite a good history of a previous CD and the sighting of an anteflexed/retroverted uterus with a sac in the cavity, clinicians are often mislead thinking

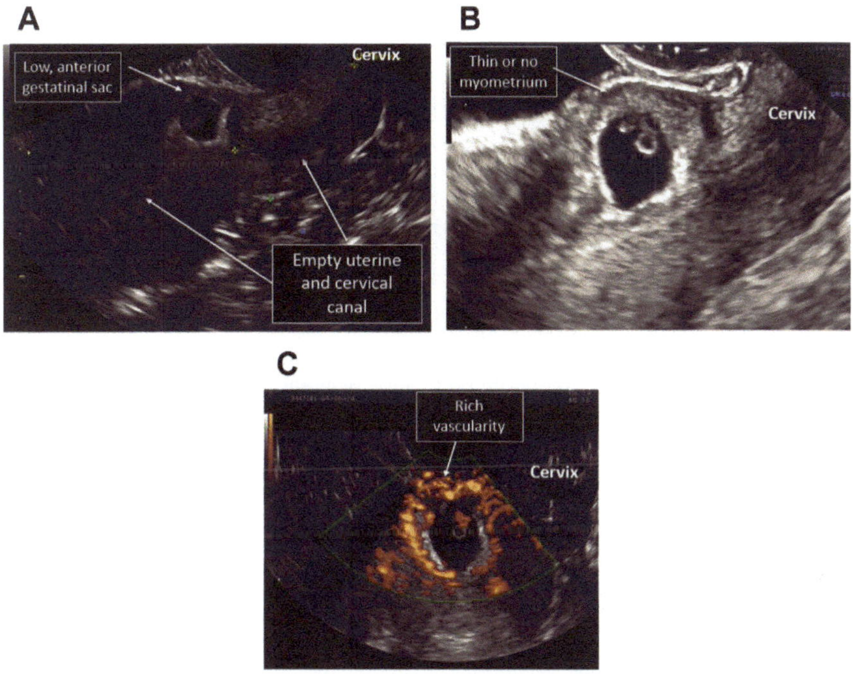


**Fig. 2.** Sonographic criteria for the diagnosis of CSP. (*A*) Low, anterior position of the placenta/gestational sac; empty uterine cavity; empty cervical canal. (*B*) Thin or no detectable myometrium between the placenta/gestational sac and the bladder. (*C*) Unusually increased vascularity between the placenta/sac and the bladder or internal cervical os.

it is a normal intrauterine pregnancy. The mistake is made by disregarding the real pathognomonic sign of a CSP, namely the low anterior location of the placenta, the increased vascularity at the placental/bladder interface, and the usually present placenta previa. It should repeatedly be emphasized that, while the sac and its embryo/fetus "moves up" into the uterine cavity, the placenta with its vascularity remains anchored in its incipient site of implantation fulfilling the diagnostic criteria of a CSP, and thus a placenta accreta. This basic and extremely important concept is shown in **Fig. 3**.

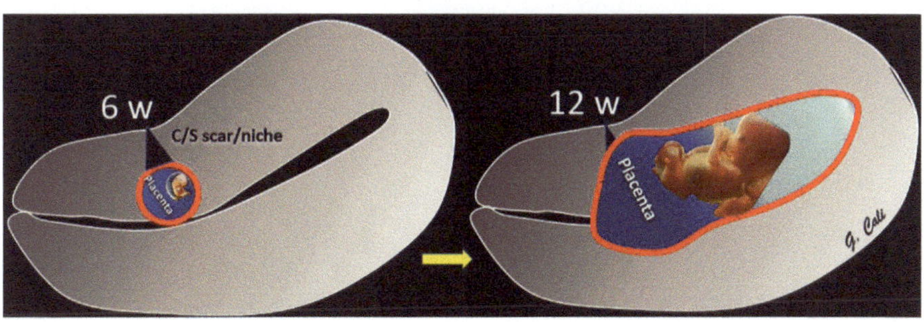


**Fig. 3.** Schematic demonstration of the gradual increase in size of the gestational sac in a continuing pregnancy. The sac with the fetus is moving up into the uterine cavity leaving behind the placenta with its vascularity. This may lead to misdiagnosing a CSP as a normal intrauterine pregnancy leading to complications. (*Courtesy of* G. Cali, MD, Palermo, Italy.)

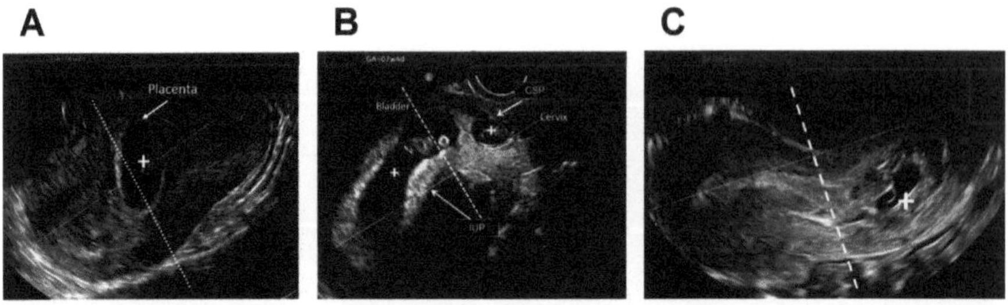


**Fig. 4.** Easy protocol for the diagnosis and differential diagnosis of CSP, intrauterine pregnancy, and cervical pregnancy on a sagittal, longitudinal US image of the uterus. (*A*) The center of the sac (*plus sign*) is below the plotted half line (ie, closer to the cervix), hence a CSP. (*B*) On this heterotopic, intrauterine, and CSP, the center of the upper sac is above the half line and marks an intrauterine pregnancy, whereas the center of the other lower sac is below that line indicating a CSP. (*C*) Although the center of this sac is below the half line, the sac is within the posterior lip of the cervix and is, therefore, a cervical pregnancy. IUP, intrauterine pregnancy.

## DIFFERENTIAL DIAGNOSIS OF CESAREAN SCAR PREGNANCY

The differential diagnoses of CSP are: cervical pregnancy and a miscarriage in progress "caught" in transition, close to the internal os or the cervical canal. It should be stressed that cervical pregnancies are rare and most importantly usually do not occur in patients with previous CDs. Miscarriages on their way to be expelled from the uterus do not have an actively beating heart. In the case of a sac on its way out, the exerting pressure on the uterus with the vaginal probe results in sliding of the sac toward the cervical canal and back when the pressure is released. A true CSP does not move away if pushed with the probe. Unfortunately missed diagnoses of CSP reported in the literature are exceedingly high. Of 751 cases of CSP 107 (13.6%) were missed or misdiagnosed resulting in a large number of complications, some as severe to require hysterectomy and thus a loss of fertility.[11]

Ballas and colleagues performed a retrospective review examining first trimester US images of surgically proven cases of placenta accrete and percreta confirming the suspicion that sonographic markers of CSP were present in all 10 cases in question.

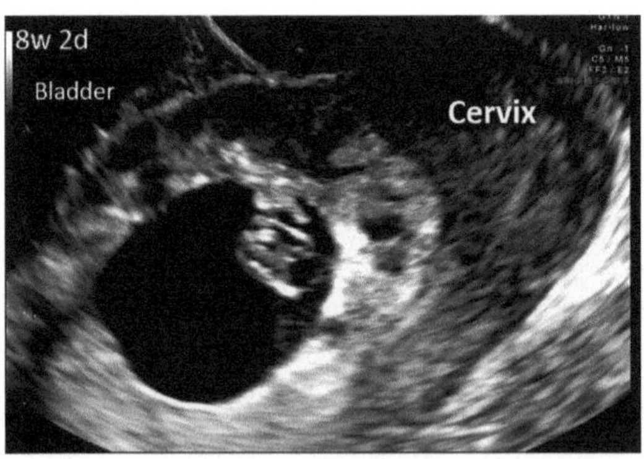


**Fig. 5.** Sonographic criteria of CSP. Partial or complete placenta previa. In this image, the placenta is covering the internal os at 8 weeks, 2 days. It is also a good example of lacunae in the placenta.

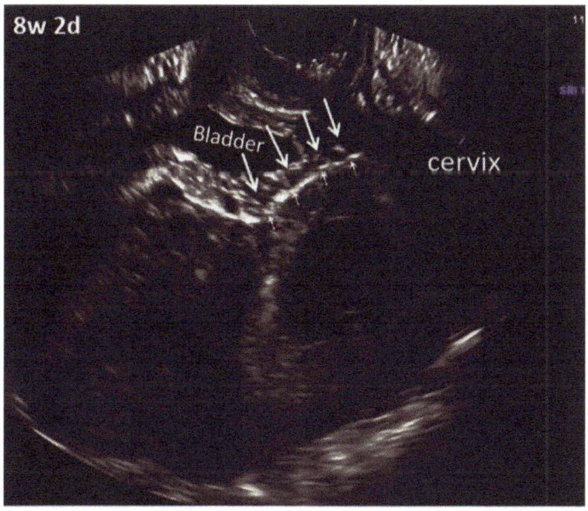


**Fig. 6.** Sonographic criteria of CSP. Close proximity of the deeply implanted pregnancy in the niche of the previous CD with no measurable myometrium or clear space between the gestational sac and bladder (*arrows*).

We published an article specifically targeting the obstetric and gynecologic community who are at the front line of encountering patients with early pregnancies.[12] We advise practitioners to draw a line perpendicular to the anteroposterior, longitudinal axis of the uterus on the US picture. If the center of the gestational sac is seen below that line, closer to the cervix, it is almost sure that it is a scar pregnancy (or in rare cases a cervical pregnancy). If the center of the sac is above that line, closer to the uterine fundus, it is a normal intrauterine pregnancy. This algorithm performs best before 8 weeks (see **Fig. 4**).

## IS THERE A PLACENTA ACCRETA SPECTRUM IN THE FIRST TRIMESTER OF PREGNANCY?

Several articles suspected that there is pathologically implanted placenta in the first trimester. However, the first reliable publication on the subject was Comstock and

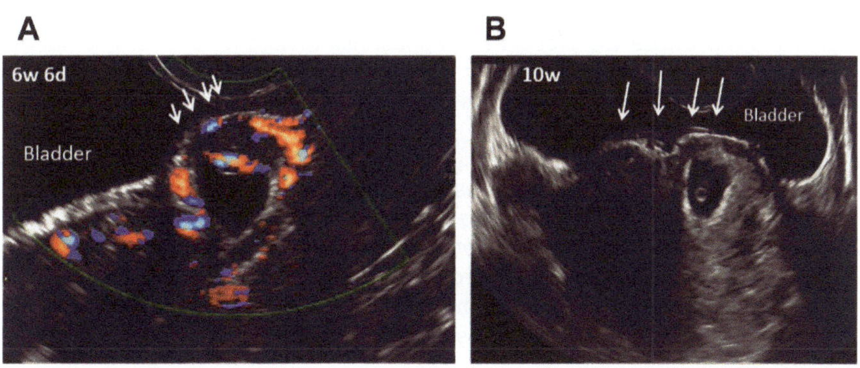


**Fig. 7.** Sonographic criteria of CSP. Interrupted or deformed bladder line. (*A*) Six weeks, 6 days CSP bulging (*arrow*) into the comfortably full bladder (cca 300 mL) disturbing the otherwise smooth bladder line. (*B*) Ten weeks CSP causing more distortion of the bladder line.

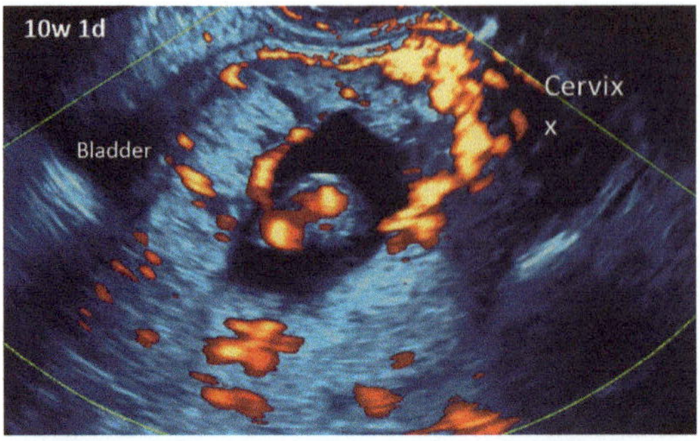


**Fig. 8.** Sonographic criteria of CSP. Color Doppler image of a CSP at 10 weeks, 1 day. The myometrium under the bladder is extremely thin and there is increased vascularity at the site of implantation.

colleagues.[13] More than a decade later articles by Rac and colleagues,[14] D'Antonio and colleagues,[15] and Cali and colleagues[16] (three articles) reported that there are sonographic markers of PAS in the first trimester and they can be recognized at different gestational ages.

The following is a list of the sonographic identifiers of an early PAS:

1. *Previous CD*. This is not a sonographic entity; however, it is a sine qua non ingredient to establish the diagnosis.
2. *Anteverted/retroflexed uterus*. Coupled with the history of previous CD and a low-positioned gestational sac it supports the diagnosis.
3. *Low anterior gestational sac in the uterus* (see **Figs. 1–3**). This was discussed previously and is the most reliable first trimester predictor of a potential placental adherence disorder. It is present in 100% between 5 and 7 weeks. It should be mentioned that it is present only in 23% of the CSPs at 11 to 14 weeks.[16]
4. *Placenta previa or low anterior placenta* (see **Fig. 5**). Combining the history of a previous CD with the presence of a first trimester placenta previa is probably the best two predictors of PAS in the first trimester. The question arises if a first trimester placenta previa should be reported or not. If clinical information does not require reporting its presence, many US sites do not draw the attention of obstetricians to it during the first trimester. Our view is that because the combination of placenta previa and previous CD present the highest risk factors for a PAS, it is not only logical and reasonable to include it in the report, but we believe it should be mandatory. Reporting it may lead to its timely diagnosis and proper steps to its management.[17]
5. *Placental lacunae* (see **Fig. 5**). In early first trimester (5–7 weeks) it is rarely present; however, after 7 weeks it is progressively seen at a rate of 78% to 81%, mostly if the placenta is low anterior covering the cervix.[16]
6. *Thin/no myometrium between placenta and bladder interphase* (see **Figs. 1**B and **6**). Between 5 and 7 weeks it is hard to detect and measure; however, after that time it is increasingly present and measurable. Between 11 and 14 weeks it was found to be present in 92% of cases of PAS.[16]

Several authors attempted to use the myometrial thickness between the sac/placenta as a valuable marker of PAS. Comstock and Bronsteen[18] mention: "Low lying: versus–surrounded by myometrium." Twickler and colleagues[19] make measurement reporting that: "<1 mm predicted morbidly adherent placenta (MAP)." Naji and colleagues[20] are somewhat complex attributing the sac as being: "away from scar, close to scar, crossing the scar or inside the CSP scar." Finally, Rac and colleagues[14] came to the conclusion that: "smallest anterior myometrial thickness on 1st Δ sonography significantly improved detection of morbidly adherent placenta. Our data showed that a myometrial thickness less than 3 mm was associated with poor outcome."

We measured the myometrial thickness between the placenta and the anterior uterine surface or bladder and found a difference in the rate of PAS and the resulting rate of hysterectomies as a function of this distance[7]:

1. *Irregular or disrupted bladder line* (see **Fig. 7**). Similarly to some of the previous markers, disturbance of the usually smooth bladder line (provided the bladder is not overdistended) is sporadically seen before 8 weeks. However, depending on the closeness of the gestational sac to the bladder, it is progressively apparent and may be seen in almost 90% of cases.[16]
2. *Increased vascularity at bladder/placenta interphase* (see **Fig. 8**). One of the important but rather subjective and hardly quantifiable US markers of CSP (and therefore also for PAS) is the degree of vascularization of the placenta/myometrium or placenta/cervix interphase. It is progressively seen as the pregnancy progresses. Although present even before 7 weeks, it is well documented to be obvious after that time and it is seen almost 90% of the time between 11 and 14 weeks.

Cali and colleagues[16] reviewed the literature to ascertain whether US signs suggestive of PAS are present in the first trimester and to test the strength of association and the predictive accuracy of such signs in detecting PAS in the first trimester. Nine studies with 578 pregnancies at risk for PAS were included. Their evaluation revealed that at least one US sign suggestive of PAS was detected in 83.7% (95% confidence interval [CI], 61.3–97.5) of cases with the confirmed diagnosis. They concluded that US signs of PAS are already present during the first trimester of pregnancy, especially before 11 weeks of gestation, which are those typical of a CSP. Low implantation of the gestational sac was the most common US sign associated with PAS in the first trimester of pregnancy.

**Fig. 9** demonstrates the progression of a 10-week 2-days CSP into a 36-weeks placenta accreta using color Doppler evaluation of the subplacental blood vessels.

## NATURAL HISTORY OF CESAREAN SCAR PREGNANCY

It is to be expected that several early, first trimester CSPs spontaneously demise much like some intrauterine gestations, of which approximately 15% do so. However, the exact number of spontaneously failing CSPs is unknown. A reasonable speculation is that this may be at least the rate of those in utero considering that the implantation site may not be the most favorable environment for a scar pregnancy. Some patients may elect termination of the pregnancy after evidence-based counseling to avoid possible complications in the second and third trimesters.

If the pregnancy is continued and placenta accreta or percreta develop, these pregnancies may lead to disastrous outcomes, such as vaginal or intra-abdominal bleeding, uterine rupture, and shock, requiring lifesaving surgical procedures. The authors reported findings of 42 articles containing descriptions of 47 cases of MAP, which was treated in the first and second trimesters. Thirty-two had one to three previous CDs. Spontaneous uterine rupture occurred in 15 of the 47 cases (32%), mostly

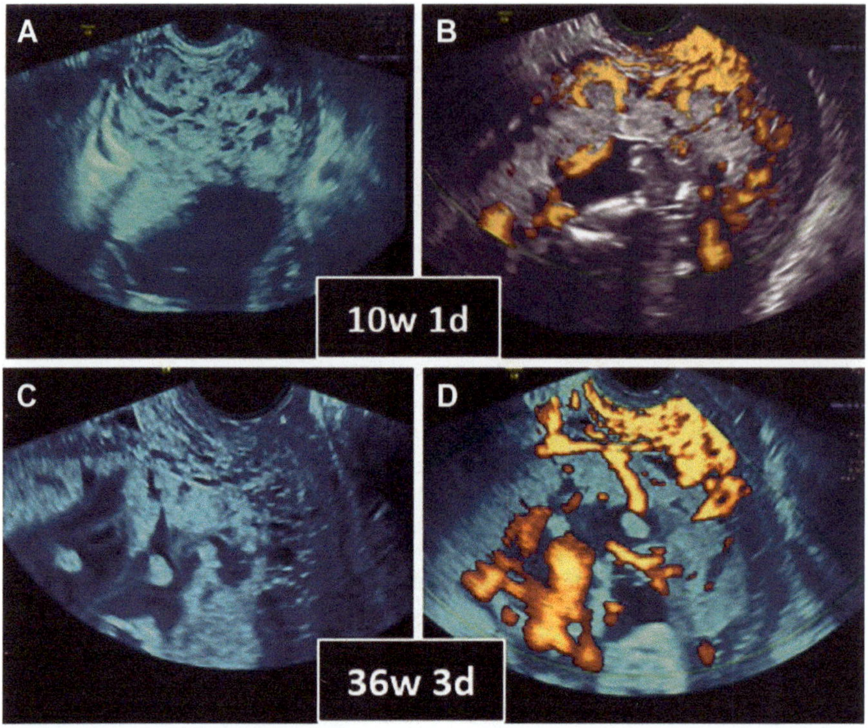


**Fig. 9.** (*A, B*) Side by side gray scale and power Doppler images of a CSP at 10 weeks and 1 day and (*C, D*) as a full blown placenta accreta at 36 weeks and 3 days.

silent ruptures with bleeding, shock, and hemoperitoneum leading to laparotomy, uterine artery embolization, and/or hysterectomy. Mean gestational age at rupture was 18.1 weeks (range, 6–28 weeks). Five patients (10.6%) had uterine artery embolizations, whereas 37 (78.7%) had laparotomies and 35 (74.4%) had hysterectomies. One patient had an arteriovenous malformation after the dilation and curettage with subsequent embolization requiring a hysterectomy.[11] By reviewing these articles we surmised that those patients with a history of previous CDs most certainly had a first trimester CSP. We certainly use this information in our counseling sessions of women that have CSP with positive fetal heart activity.

Until recently not much was known about the fate of a continuing CSP. The question was whether the first trimester CSP and the second and third trimester PAS are the same disease with different clinical appearances, or are they different entities? Our hypothesis was based on the previously mentioned observation of Comstock and colleagues.[13]

The authors asked two pathologists who were blinded to the diagnosis to evaluate histologic slides of early placenta accreta and of CSP. They attested that the various degrees of myometrial and/or scar tissue invasion by placental villi were consistent with the classic definition of PAS. Therefore, our conclusion was that the early placenta accreta and placental implantation in CSP are histopathologically identicle.[21,22]

Ballas and colleagues[22] performed a retrospective review of 10 cases with women undergoing CD for MAP followed by hysterectomy where the histology showed placenta accreta. At gestational ages between 8 and 14 weeks the pregnancies fulfilled the diagnostic criteria of CSP. These women went on to deliver live offspring at the expense of hysterectomy because of PAS.

Our group reported on a collaborative study in which 10 patients diagnosed with CSPs opted to continue the pregnancy.[23] We wanted to provide additional sonographic, clinical, and histologic proof that if left alone, CSP can result in a live offspring but the pregnancy will be complicated by third trimester PAS that may lead to hysterectomy. Nine of the 10 patients included delivered live-born neonates between 32 and 37 weeks. However, all 10 patients underwent hysterectomy at the time of CD, with total blood loss ranging from 300 to 6000 mL. In all 10 cases placenta percreta was the histopathologic diagnosis.

The authors proved the hypothesis that CSP is a precursor of PAS, both sharing the same histopathology. Several consecutive articles were published to describe the natural history of the undisturbed CSP.[15,16,24,25]

## DOES THE DISTANCE BETWEEN THE GESTATIONAL SAC AND THE ANTERIOR UTERINE SURFACE/BLADDER PREDICT OUTCOME?

In the last few years based on clinical impression and increasing experience, clinicians started to evaluate if a deeply embedded gestational sac and placenta "in the niche" or dehiscence results in a more ominous outcome than if it is implanted "on the scar" (discussed previously).

## RECURRENT, HETEROTOPIC, AND MULTIPLE CESAREAN SCAR PREGNANCIES

Reviewing the pertinent literature published through 2011 we identified seven recurrent cases of CSP.[11] Ben Nagi reported a 5% rate of recurrent CSP among 21 pregnancies after prior conservatively managed CSP.[26]

Bennett and colleagues[27] and our group reported of a single patient with five recurrent CSPs. After the first four live CSPs were injected with local intragestational methotrexate, the last delivered near term with repeat CD and total abdominal hysterectomy for MAP.

Sadeghi and coworkers[28] published 59 (81%) subsequent pregnancies among 73 women with prior CSP. Fifteen (25%) had recurrent CSP.

Wang and colleagues[29] report on 15.6% recurrence rate in 32 patients. Patients treated in the first trimester CSP should not be reassured that this may not happen again in a future pregnancy. Rarely, but possibly, two gestational sacs with two embryos are present as a twin CSP (see **Figs. 4**B and **9**).

Heterotopic pregnancies were also reported and merit special attention because the intrauterine pregnancy can result in live offspring. There were several articles reporting on such heterotopic pregnancies.[5,28,30–40] The best review containing detailed information is by Ugurlucan and colleagues.[35] Sadeghi and colleagues[28] reported on six heterotopic CSPs.

The possibility of heterotopic CSP after CS should be considered, especially when a pregnancy is the result of assisted reproductive technology. This is the rarest form of heterotopic pregnancy with one embryo/fetus in the scar of a previous CD and the other in the uterine cavity. Most treatments rely on US guide to place needles and reduce the scar pregnancy by intragestational injection of KCl. The best treatment is still unclear. Fortunately, most intrauterine pregnancies are preserved after treatment (**Fig. 10**).

There was also a triplet CSP published.[40]

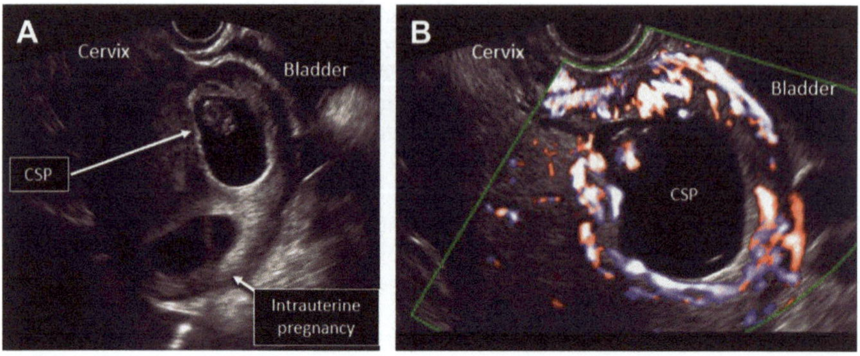


**Fig. 10.** Heterotopic cesarean scar and intrauterine pregnancies at 5 weeks, 2 days. The pregnancy was continued until 30 weeks at which time a CD resulted in the live birth of both fetuses. One had severe intrauterine growth restriction and a hysterectomy was performed for placenta accreta. (*A*) CSP on grey-scale image. (*B*) CSP with increased vascularity on Color Doppler.

## PREGNANCY FOLLOWING TREATMENT OF CESAREAN SCAR PREGNANCY

There are no reliable articles dealing with this issue. However, compiling the clinical information on the 751 cases of CSP we found descriptions of 64 intrauterine pregnancies after first trimester treatment of CSPs.[11] Pregnancies and deliveries after CSPs may be underreported. Wang and colleagues[41] reviewed 32 cases of CSP. Seven had subsequent pregnancies.

Ben Nagi and coworkers[42] published probably the largest series of reproductive performance of women after a history of CSP. They followed 40 women with CSP. The uterus was conserved in 38 of 40 cases. Follow-up data were available in 29 of 38 (76%) women, 24 out of 29 (83%) attempted to become pregnant, and 21 out of 24 (88%; 95% CI, 75–100) women conceived spontaneously. Twenty out of 21 (95%; 95% CI, 86–100) pregnancies were intrauterine and one woman (5%; 95% CI, 0–14) had a recurrent CSP. Thirteen out of 20 (65%; 95% CI, 44–86) intrauterine pregnancies seemed normal, 9 of 13 (69%) were delivered by CD, and 7 of 20 (35%; 95% CI, 14–56) intrauterine pregnancies ended in spontaneous abortions. Their conclusion was that reproductive outcomes following treatment of CSP are favorable. The risk of complications including recurrent scar implantation seems to be low. Yamaguchi and colleagues[43] successfully treated eight CSP cases with local methotrexate injection with TVUS guidance. Four of the five patients desiring subsequent pregnancies had uneventful deliveries and recurrent CSP was diagnosed in one patient.

Additional reports in the literature resulting in live births from subsequent pregnancies attest to the success of planning for another pregnancy. In such cases the importance of a very early (possibly between 5 and 7 weeks) TVUS examination should be explained to the patient, because in our view the recurrence rate of CSP is significant.

## SHORT CESAREAN-TO-PREGNANCY INTERVAL: IS IT A RISK FACTOR FOR SUBSEQUENT CESAREAN SCAR PREGNANCY

Only indirect information is available in the literature. It was suggested that short pregnancy intervals contribute to development of placenta accreta. A case-control study of uterine scar failures among laboring patients with previous low transverse CD was published with special attention to their interpregnancy interval (IPI). An IPI of less than 6 months was significantly more prevalent among case patients with uterine scar failure ($P$ = .02). Mean IPI interval was less in all cases of uterine scar failure ($P$ = .06). They concluded that the IPI was inversely associated with likelihood of uterine scar failure during subsequent labor.[44] Based on the previously mentioned information one can only infer that it may be applicable for CSP.[44]

## SUMMARY

1. CSP is a complication-ridden, potentially dangerous clinical entity. Its occurrence rate is closely related to that of CDs.
2. The best diagnostic tool is TVUS. Grayscale and color Doppler US provide satisfactory diagnostic information. MRI is not necessary for making an accurate diagnosis. Every patient with previous CD should be screened for CSP. A patient with previous CD and low anterior gestation is CSP unless proven otherwise.[17]
3. CSP and PAS share the same histologic picture. CSP is a precursor of PAS.
4. Most patients with CSP diagnosed in the first trimester that reached the third trimester of pregnancy deliver via repeat CD, almost all have different degrees of PAS, and in most cases have hysterectomy.
5. The obstetric/gynecologic community is in urgent need of standardized diagnostic and management protocols. An international CSP registry was created www.csp-registry.com. We encourage its use to upload cases.

## REFERENCES


1. Jauniaux E, Bhide A, Kennedy A, et al. FIGO consensus guidelines on placenta accreta spectrum disorders: prenatal diagnosis and screening. Int J Gynaecol Obstet 2018;140:274–80.
2. Martin JA, Hamilton BE, Osterman MJK, et al. Births: final data for 2017. NVSS 2017;67(8):1–50. Available at: https://www.cdc.gov/nchs/data/nvsr/nvsr67/nvsr67_08-508.pdf.
3. Hamilton BE, Martin JA, Ventura SJ. Births: preliminary data for 2012. Natl Vital Stat Rep 2013;62:1–20.
4. Jauniaux E, Jurkovic D. Placenta accreta: pathogenesis of a 20th century iatrogenic uterine disease. Placenta 2012;33:244–51.
5. Jurkovic D, Hillaby K, Woelfer B, et al. Cesarean scar pregnancy. Ultrasound Obstet Gynecol 2003;21:310.
6. Tantbirojn P, Crum CP, Parast MM. Pathophysiology of placenta creta: the role of decidua and extravillous trophoblast. Placenta 2008;29:639–45.
7. Kaelin Agten A, Cali G, Monteagudo A, et al. The clinical outcome of cesarean scar pregnancies implanted "on the scar" versus "in the niche". Am J Obstet Gynecol 2017;216:510.e1-6.
8. Monteagudo A, Carreno C, Timor-Tritsch IE. Saline infusion sonohysterography in nonpregnant women with previous cesarean delivery: the "niche" in the scar. J Ultrasound Med 2001;20:1105–15.
9. Jordans IPM, de Leeuw RA, Stegwee SI, et al. Sonographic examination of uterine niche in non-pregnant women: a modified Delphi procedure. Ultrasound Obstet Gynecol 2019;53:107–15.
10. Kaelin Agten A, Honart A, Monteagudo A, et al. Cesarean delivery changes the natural position of the uterus on transvaginal ultrasonography. J Ultrasound Med 2018;37:1179–83.

11. Timor-Tritsch IE, Monteagudo A. Unforeseen consequences of the increasing rate of cesarean deliveries: early placenta accreta and cesarean scar pregnancy. A review. Am J Obstet Gynecol 2012;207:14–29.
12. Timor-Tritsch IE, Haynes MC, Monteagudo A, et al. Ultrasound diagnosis and management of acquired uterine enhanced myometrial vascularity/arteriovenous malformations. Am J Obstet Gynecol 2016;214(6):731.e1-10.
13. Comstock CH, Lee W, Vettraino IM, et al. The early sonographic appearance of placenta accreta. J Ultrasound Med 2003;22:19–23 [quiz: 4–6].
14. Rac MW, Moschos E, Wells CE, et al. Sonographic findings of morbidly adherent placenta in the first trimester. J Ultrasound Med 2016;35:263–9.
15. D'Antonio F, Timor-Tritsch IE, Palacios-Jaraquemada J, et al. First-trimester detection of abnormally invasive placenta in high-risk women: systematic review and meta-analysis. Ultrasound Obstet Gynecol 2018;51:176–83.
16. Cali G, Timor-Trisch IE, Palacios-Jaraquemada J, et al. Changes in ultrasonography indicators of abnormally invasive placenta during pregnancy. Int J Gynaecol Obstet 2018;140:319–25.
17. Timor-Tritsch IE, D'Antonio F, Cali G, et al. Early first-trimester transvaginal ultrasound is indicated in pregnancy after previous cesarean delivery: should it be mandatory? Ultrasound Obstet Gynecol 2019;54(2):156–63.
18. Comstock CH, Bronsteen RA. The antenatal diagnosis of placenta accreta. BJOG 2014;121:171–81 [discussion: 81–2].
19. Twickler DM, Lucas MJ, Balis AB, et al. Color flow mapping for myometrial invasion in women with a prior cesarean delivery. J Matern Fetal Med 2000;9:330–5.
20. Naji O, Wynants L, Smith A, et al. Does the presence of a Caesarean section scar affect implantation site and early pregnancy outcome in women attending an early pregnancy assessment unit? Hum Reprod 2013;28:1489–96.
21. Timor-Tritsch IE, Monteagudo A, Cali G, et al. Cesarean scar pregnancy and early placenta accreta share common histology. Ultrasound Obstet Gynecol 2014;43: 383–95.
22. Ballas J, Pretorius D, Hull AD, et al. Identifying sonographic markers for placenta accreta in the first trimester. J Ultrasound Med 2012;31:1835–41.
23. Timor-Tritsch IE, Monteagudo A, Cali G, et al. Cesarean scar pregnancy is a precursor of morbidly adherent placenta. Ultrasound Obstet Gynecol 2014;44: 346–53.
24. Cali G, Forlani F, Timor-Tritsch IE, et al. Natural history of Cesarean scar pregnancy on prenatal ultrasound: the crossover sign. Ultrasound Obstet Gynecol 2017;50:100–4.
25. Cali G, Forlani F, Minneci G, et al. First-trimester prediction of surgical outcome in abnormally invasive placenta using the cross-over sign. Ultrasound Obstet Gynecol 2018;51:184–8.
26. Ben Nagi J, Ofili-Yebovi D, Sawyer E, et al. Successful treatment of a recurrent Cesarean scar ectopic pregnancy by surgical repair of the uterine defect. Ultrasound Obstet Gynecol 2006;28:855–6.
27. Bennett TA, Morgan J, Timor-Tritsch IE, et al. Fifth recurrent Cesarean scar pregnancy: observations of a case and historical perspective. Ultrasound Obstet Gynecol 2017;50:658–60.
28. Sadeghi H, Rutherford T, Rackow BW, et al. Cesarean scar ectopic pregnancy: case series and review of the literature. Am J Perinatol 2010;27:111–20.
29. Wang Q, Peng HL, He L, et al. Reproductive outcomes after previous cesarean scar pregnancy: follow up of 189 women. Taiwan J Obstet Gynecol 2015;54: 551–3.

30. Demirel LC, Bodur H, Selam B, et al. Laparoscopic management of heterotopic cesarean scar pregnancy with preservation of intrauterine gestation and delivery at term: case report. Fertil Steril 2009;91:1293.e5-7.
31. Duenas-Garcia OF, Young C. Heterotopic cesarean scar pregnancy associated with a levonorgestrel-releasing intrauterine device. Int J Gynaecol Obstet 2011; 114:153–4.
32. Hsieh BC, Hwang JL, Pan HS, et al. Heterotopic Caesarean scar pregnancy combined with intrauterine pregnancy successfully treated with embryo aspiration for selective embryo reduction: case report. Hum Reprod 2004;19:285–7.
33. Salomon LJ, Fernandez H, Chauveaud A, et al. Successful management of a heterotopic Caesarean scar pregnancy: potassium chloride injection with preservation of the intrauterine gestation: case report. Hum Reprod 2003;18:189–91.
34. Taskin S, Taskin EA, Ciftci TT. Heterotopic cesarean scar pregnancy: how should it be managed? Obstet Gynecol Surv 2009;64:690–5 [quiz: 7].
35. Ugurlucan FG, Bastu E, Dogan M, et al. Management of cesarean heterotopic pregnancy with transvaginal ultrasound-guided potassium chloride injection and gestational sac aspiration, and review of the literature. J Minim Invasive Gynecol 2012;19:671–3.
36. Uysal F, Uysal A. Spontaneous heterotopic cesarean scar pregnancy: conservative management by transvaginal sonographic guidance and successful pregnancy outcome. J Ultrasound Med 2013;32:547–8.
37. Wang CJ, Tsai F, Chen C, et al. Hysteroscopic management of heterotopic cesarean scar pregnancy. Fertil Steril 2010;94:1529.e15-8.
38. Wang CN, Chen CK, Wang HS, et al. Successful management of heterotopic cesarean scar pregnancy combined with intrauterine pregnancy after in vitro fertilization-embryo transfer. Fertil Steril 2007;88:706.e13-6.
39. Yazicioglu HF, Turgut S, Madazli R, et al. An unusual case of heterotopic twin pregnancy managed successfully with selective feticide. Ultrasound Obstet Gynecol 2004;23:626–7.
40. Litwicka K, Greco E, Prefumo F, et al. Successful management of a triplet heterotopic caesarean scar pregnancy after in vitro fertilization-embryo transfer. Fertil Steril 2011;95:291.e1-3.
41. Wang YL, Su TH, Chen HS. Laparoscopic management of an ectopic pregnancy in a lower segment cesarean section scar: a review and case report. J Minim Invasive Gynecol 2005;12:73–9.
42. Ben Nagi J, Helmy S, Ofili-Yebovi D, et al. Reproductive outcomes of women with a previous history of Caesarean scar ectopic pregnancies. Hum Reprod 2007;22: 2012–5.
43. Yamaguchi M, Honda R, Uchino K, et al. Transvaginal methotrexate injection for the treatment of cesarean scar pregnancy: efficacy and subsequent fecundity. J Minim Invasive Gynecol 2014;21:877–83.
44. Esposito MA, Menihan CA, Malee MP. Association of interpregnancy interval with uterine scar failure in labor: a case-control study. Am J Obstet Gynecol 2000;183: 1180–3.

# Cesarean Scar Pregnancy

## Patient Counseling and Management

Ilan E. Timor-Tritsch, MD[a,*], Ana Monteagudo, MD[b], Giuseppe Calì, MD[c,1], Francesco D'Antonio, MD[d], Andrea Kaelin Agten, MD[e]

**KEYWORDS**

- Cesarean scar pregnancy • Ultrasound • Cesarean delivery • Treatment
- Placenta accreta spectrum

**KEY POINTS**

- There is no universally agreed upon and adopted management protocol for cesarean scar pregnancy (CSP) supported by professional societies in the United States or around the world.
- After the diagnosis, evidence-based counseling should follow, resulting in a clear decision of the patient as to the management.
- A live CSP requires immediate and time-sensitive action before further growth of the embryo/fetus and its exponentially growing vascularity.
- Patients diagnosed as well as those suspected for a CSP should be referred to a facility experienced in managing such cases and where there is a possibility to respond to possible emergency situations.
- A wide variety of different treatment protocols to terminate a CSP are available. Treatments are usually selected by the caregiver's experience, availability of treatment means, and facilities, taking into consideration possible complications and their emergent solutions.
- Methotrexate, injected as a single dose systemically, is usually ineffective and delays the final treatment, however, as an adjuvant to other treatments that have a proven efficiency.
- Sharp curetting and uterine artery embolization (UAE) *alone* should not be first line treatments. UAE is effective as an adjunct procedure and in cases of emergency owing to sustained hemorrhage.

*Continued*

[a] Department of Obstetrics and Gynecology, NYU School of Medicine, NYU Langone Health, 550 1st Avenue, New York, NY 10016, USA; [b] Department of Obstetrics, Gynecology, and Reproductive Science, Icahn School of Medicine at Mount Sinai, New York, NY, USA; [c] Department of Obstetrics and Gynaecology, Arnas Civico Hospital, Palermo, Italy; [d] Fetal Medicine Unit, Department of Obstetrics and Gynecology, University of Foggia, Foggia, Italy; [e] Nottingham University Hospitals NHS, Queens Medical Centre, Derby Road, Nottingham, NG7 2UH, UK

[1] Present address: Viale Acacie 26 Casteldaccia, Palermo 90014, Italia.

* Corresponding author.

*E-mail address:* ilan.timor@nyumc.org

Obstet Gynecol Clin N Am 46 (2019) 813–828
https://doi.org/10.1016/j.ogc.2019.07.010
0889-8545/19/
obgyn.theclinics.com

*Continued*

- Insertion and inflation of a single Foley balloon catheter or even more so double cervical ripening catheters are effective to prevent or treat bleeding following any local treatment of CSP.
- An International CSP Registry was created (www.csp-registry.com). The authors encourage its use to upload cases.

## INTRODUCTION

There is no universally agreed upon and adopted management protocol supported by professional societies in the United States or around the world for the treatment of cesarean scar pregnancy (CSP). There is a wide range of management options in the literature, and many of them can to lead to severe bleeding complications, which can result in loss of fertility or even maternal death. If inadequately managed, it can lead to untoward complications throughout all 3 trimesters of the pregnancy.[1–3]

This article discusses patient counseling and management options for CSP based on review of the literature and the authors' clinical experience. Diagnosis and pathogenesis of CSP can be found in the Ilan E. Timor-Tritsch and collegaues' article, "Cesarean Scar Pregnancy: Diagnosis and Pathogenesis," in this issue of *Obstetrics and Gynecology Clinics of North America*.

## COUNSELING PATIENTS WITH A FIRST-TRIMESTER CESAREAN SCAR PREGNANCY

After the diagnosis of CSP has been made, patient counseling follows. However, one must first determine viability. If *no yolk sac and/or embryo and/or heartbeat* are seen, the patient should be reexamined every 2 to 3 days. If by reasonably good dating, or after 1 week of ultrasound (US) examinations, there is no heart activity and no yolk sac and/or embryo are detected, the management should be restricted to sonographic and biochemical follow-up.

The explanation for this approach lies in the fact that reliable dating heart activity is detectable by TVS as early as 6 weeks to 6 weeks and 2 days. Therefore, the patient without an embryonic heartbeat at 5 to 6 weeks should be checked every 2 to 3 days to ascertain a live embryo or a pregnancy failure. Only after this time should the pregnancy be considered live or a pregnancy failure. If the pregnancy failed, it should be assigned for weekly follow-up until the human chorionic gonadotropin (hCG) is zero and the sac with its vascularity recedes completely. Some practitioners start administering MTX even if no heart activity was seen to assure early effect of the drug. This approach may not be unreasonable; however, both the patient and the doctor *must* be sure that there is no desire to continue to wait, recognizing it still may be possible for the pregnancy to be viable albeit with potential consequences and risks.

If *positive heart activity* was seen, the counseling should describe the 2 main diametrically opposite clinical management options that need to be decided on as early as possible, which is (a) to terminate or (b) to continue the pregnancy. Expectant management of *CSP with positive embryonic/fetal heart activity* is associated with a high burden of maternal morbidity, such as severe hemorrhage, early uterine rupture (**Fig. 1**), severe placental adherence spectrum (PAS), and hysterectomy. Despite this, a significant proportion of pregnancies complicated by CSP may progress to, or close

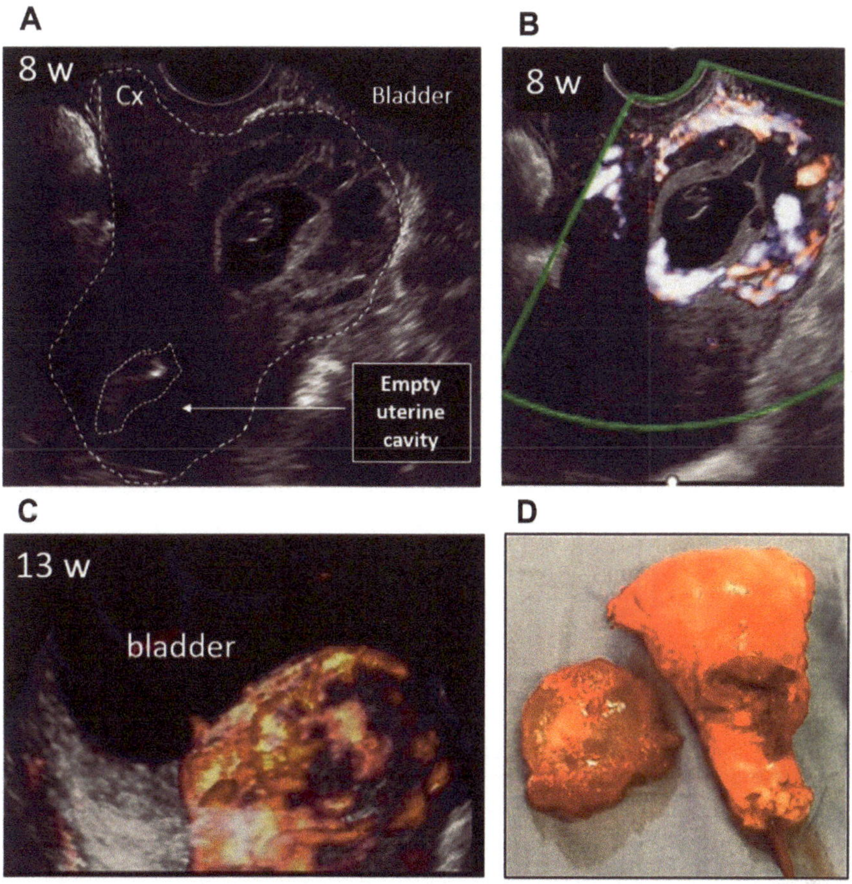


**Fig. 1.** Outcome of a CSP diagnosed in the first trimester with emphasis on the first-trimester parameters of CSP as (*A* and *B*) low anterior implantation, placenta previa, placental lacunae and vascularity, and empty uterine cavity at 8 weeks and (*C*) at 13 weeks depicting rich vascularity and (*D*) the ruptured uterus.

to term, thus questioning whether TOP should be the only therapeutic option offered to these women.[4]

A live CSP requires immediate and time-sensitive action before further growth of the embryo/fetus and its exponentially growing vascularity. Counseling of patients with a first-trimester CSP changed in the last several years owing to knowledge acquired about its natural history. In the last few years, almost all clinicians were leaning toward immediate termination of the CSP. Today, because of the information about the natural history of CSP and the possibility of delivering a live-born offspring, counseling has changed. Although the patient has the possibility of delivering a live offspring, she must be informed that a placenta accreta or PAS may occur, often leading to hysterectomy. Management and treatment should be individualized based on the patient's age, number of previous cesarean deliveries (CDs), number of children, and the expertise of her providers managing her care. The authors' guidelines in counseling a patient with CSP demonstrating heart activity is shown in **Fig. 2**.

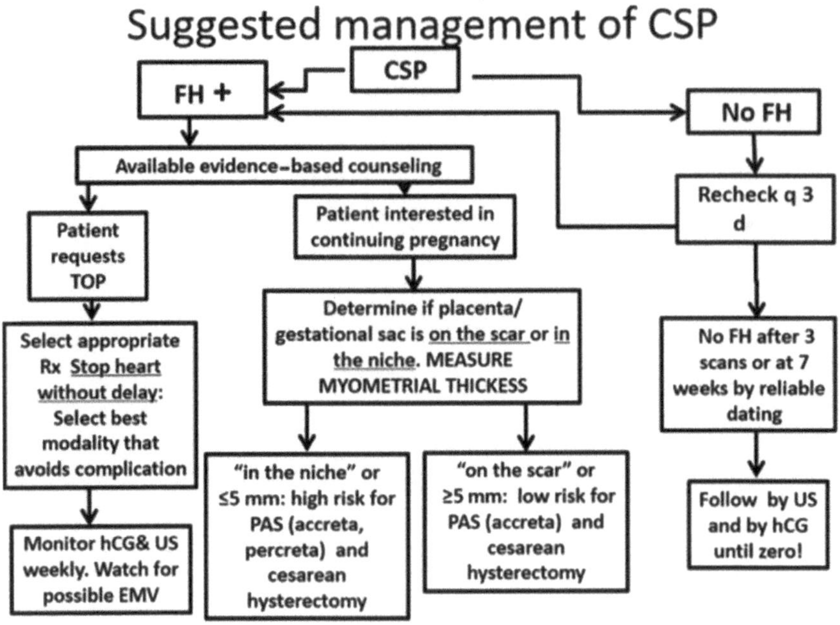


**Fig. 2.** The management protocol of CSP adopted by the authors' ultrasound division. TOP, termination of pregnancy.

Because the causative connection between CSP and PAS has been sufficiently proven, the authors embarked on a "mission" to raise the awareness of an early US scan in pregnancies following a CD. In a recent opinion article, the authors assembled compelling arguments for why early first-trimester screening at 5 to 8 weeks for pregnancies following previous CDs would prove to be beneficial.[5]

The authors reviewed several articles to emphasize the perils of undiagnosed or misdiagnosed CSPs, leading to multiple surgeries, uterine artery embolization (UAE), loss of fertility, and in rare cases, documented deaths.[6–22]

The authors evoked the well-documented histopathologic connection between CSP and PAS suggesting that CSP is a precursor to PAS. The authors also argued that the US markers to recognize scar pregnancies are already present in the first trimester. Finally, they stress that early 5- to 7-week US screening for CSP is strongly indicated (if not mandated) in any patient with a previous cesarean section and that this screening can be easily implemented alongside several other proven first-trimester screening studies. It is clear to us, nonetheless, that the economic and medical policy issues have to be resolved by the professional governing bodies before widespread adaptation.

## MANAGEMENT OF CESAREAN SCAR PREGNANCY

It is the authors' firm opinion that patients diagnosed as well as those suspected for a CSP should be referred to the following:

1. A facility experienced in managing such cases and
2. A facility where there is a possibility to respond to possible emergency situations.

Such facilities should also have readily available interventional radiology services for their operating rooms. A well-staffed blood bank is essential because bleeding complications are more frequent than often anticipated. Most management schemes can be classified by one of the following:

A. Major surgery (requiring general anesthesia)
   a. Laparotomy (hysterectomy or local excision)
   b. Excision by laparoscopy, hysteroscopy, or transvaginal approach
   c. Dilatation of the cervix followed by sharp or blunt curetting
   d. Suction aspiration without dilatation of the cervix

   The last 2 can be guided by continuous real-time transabdominal US.

B. Minimally invasive procedures
   a. Minimally invasive procedures without general anesthesia, such as local injection of methotrexate (MTX) or potassium chloride (KCl) with or without vasopressin.
C. Systemic medication single- or multidose intramuscular or intravenous administration of MTX
D. UAE
E. Combination of the above treatments
   a. Several articles reported on combining treatments in a planned, simultaneous, or sequential fashion
   b. Treatments may also change after the first-line therapy failed
F. Local pressure by inflatable balloons
   a. Most recently placing and inflating a single Foley balloon or a double cervical ripening Cook balloon to prevent and/or control cervical or uterine bleeding following local treatments, such as aspiration, curettage, and/or local intragestational injection have also been reported.[23]

## PRIMARY TREATMENT OPTIONS OF CESAREAN SCAR PREGNANCY

Because of its relative rarity, diverse and sometime extreme treatments and their complications are described in the literature. The publications reflect relatively small case series or often only a single case. There is no conventional treatment protocol available. Surgeons generally use dilation and curettage (D&C), laparoscopy, and hysteroscopy or laparotomy. Obstetricians, radiologists, and in vitro fertilization specialists seem to favor systemic, parenteral administration of MTX or US-guided local intragestational sac MTX (or KCl). On occasion, the help of an interventional radiologist is requested to embolize the CSP. A list of the treatments, their efficacy, and complications ending in the year 2012 has been reviewed.[3] Since then, numerous additional treatment protocols and combinations were reported. As an example, the article by Yin and colleagues[24] describes a single-center treatment of 90 patients with CSP applying at least 3 different kinds of treatment modalities did not conclude with a suggested treatment plan with minimal complications. The single cases and their results are insufficient to draw a clear conclusion as to which treatment was most effective, resulting in minimal or no complications.

Because there is no consensus in treating CSP,[25] it is clear to us that an international registry is needed to arrive at the most efficient treatments or management with the least complications while retaining fertility when desired. In fact, a registry was started at the end of 2018, and cases can be uploaded creating a username. The site can be reached at www.csp-registry.com. The authors encourage participation in this effort to find a common denominator between the diagnosis and treatment of CSP.

## THE MOST FREQUENTLY USED TREATMENT MODALITIES

In general, before any other treatment or the correct diagnosis is established, systemic administration of MTX is indicated. Methotrexate is probably the only treatment an inexperienced clinician with CSP is able to give a patient short of the more involved treatment protocols. Almost all patients referred to the authors from other offices already had "on-board" MTX in the hopes that it will stop heartbeats. If it does, it is extremely hard to attribute the cessation of the embryonic heartbeats to MTX because at least 10% of early pregnancy results in miscarriage *without* administration of MTX. Observing cessation of heartbeats after systemic MTX most probably influenced the general view that an intramuscular dose of MTX is an appropriate treatment of CSP. As a result, the "generalists" usually wait and hope that the patient and scar pregnancy will respond. This approach will cost the patient precious days during which the gestation, embryo, and its vascularization progress will grow, presenting the referral center with a greater challenge as to the secondary treatment. All in all, a first systemic injection at the first diagnosis is not contraindicated; however, the patient should be referred immediately and without delay to a center that will render the patient more effective, minimal complications and less involved treatment. In addition, MTX has to be administered after careful evaluation of the uterus especially in cases where the pregnancy is the result of an assisted reproductive technology because the danger of an unrecognized, much desired pregnancy will be terminated.

### *Systemic, Single-Dose Methotrexate*

The usual protocols suggest a dose of 1 mg/kg of body weight or 50 mg/m$^2$ of body surface area. This treatment was associated with a complication rate of 62.1%, mostly because it required a second treatment when the fetal heartbeat did not cease after several days.[3] This unusually high complication rate was challenged[26] and prompted a reevaluation of the reported data; however, after an even more rigorous reevaluation of the data, the results suggested an even higher complication rate of 66.1%. It should be said that several days after injection of the drug it seemed that the drug "worked." This observation most probably influenced the general view that an intramuscular dose of MTX is an appropriate treatment of CSP. However, in reality, it is difficult to attribute the cessation of the heartbeats to MTX because at least 15% of early pregnancies result in miscarriage *without* administration of MTX. The high failure rate with systemic MTX may be caused by its slow action and questionable ability to stop cardiac activity and placental invasion. Results can take days, and during all this waiting time, the gestational sac, the embryo or fetus, and its vascularity are slowly but clearly growing. After the failure, secondary treatments have to deal with a larger gestation and its more abundant vascularization. The concerns of the slow action of systemic MTX treatment are also suggested by Yin and colleagues.[24]

In China, Jiang and colleagues[27] treated 33 patients with CSP. Of 13 patients treated with intravenous MTX alone, 3 of the 13 required hysterectomy for profuse bleeding.

### *Systemic, Multidose, Sequential Methotrexate*

The doses of MTX injected are similar to the dose for the single-dose regimen. However, 2 to 3 intramuscular injections (1 mg/kg of body weight or 50 mg/mm$^2$ of surface area) are given at an interval of 2 or 3 days over 1 week. Thus, the total amount is higher than in the single-dose regimen. One should be aware of the cumulative effects of this drug on the liver and bone marrow and the overall failure rate.[28]

It is hard to assess the rate of complications associated with the multidose approach because it was often used with or after "first-line" or "follow-up" treatment. Generally speaking, it is clear that careful administration MTX can successfully be administered as an adjunct and combined with other mostly nonsurgical treatments.

### *Suction Aspiration or Dilation and Curettage, Alone or in Combination*

This treatment requires general anesthesia. The 305 cases involving this treatment had a mean complication rate of about 62% (range: 29%-86%).[3] This approach led to the greatest number of unanticipated bleeding complications at times needing an emergent second- or third-line surgical treatment. Frequently hysterectomy could not be avoided.

The most plausible explanation for the bleeding complication is that following a normal delivery or spontaneous abortion: the multilayered myometrial grid of the myometrium constricts blood vessels after placental separation. During curettage, vessels are exposed, and in the cervix, there is less or insufficient muscle grid to constrict and contain the bleeding. If D&C or suction aspiration is still planned, blood products and a Foley balloon catheter should be readily available.[29] Reports of using a Foley balloon catheter as a backup after significant bleeding occurred following curettage have been published.[27,30] In one of the reviews, CSPs with D&C was associated with a 28% risk of hemorrhage.[23]

Kiyokawa and colleagues[31] recently reported on a CSP treated first with intragestational sac injection of MTX and KCl as well as with systemic MTX. However, because the sac and serum hCG persisted, D&C was performed. Severe hemorrhage occurred and continued during the procedure, requiring emergent UAE. As other similar cases, it demonstrates the perils of a sharp curettage for CSPs.

US-guided D&C may be the first choice for treating CSP if the cesarean scar is greater than 2- or 3-mm thick, blood flow is not abundant, and the maximum diameter of the gestational sac is less than 30 mm and the gestational age is greater than 7 weeks.[32,33]

Backup of UAE seems to mitigate the risk of bleeding, and although D&C was associated with a 28% risk of hemorrhage, that risk dropped to 4% when combined with UAE.[23]

Cali and colleagues successfully used the following sequential treatment approach in 8 of their patients. Once admitted to the hospital, the patient undergoes UAE, and after 5 days, a gentle suction aspiration under continuous real-time US is performed followed by immediate insertion and inflation of a Foley balloon catheter for bleeding prevention and control.[29] Several recent articles advocate the safe and uncomplicated use of sac aspiration; however, all were followed or preceded by other treatment methods.[34]

### *Uterine Artery Embolization, Alone or in Combination*

Uterine artery embolization, alone or in combination, requires general anesthesia. The complication rate was 47% among the 64 cases described in a review of 751 cases of CSP. It seems that UAE is not the best first-line treatment if administered alone as a single-agent therapy, because it has a relatively delayed effect, which allows the gestation to progress and the vascularity to increase. This delayed action was the reason that Cali and colleagues (personal communication) waited 5 days after UAE of their patients with CSP before a suction aspiration was undertaken.

If UAE fails, the clinician must contend with a larger gestation applying a secondary treatment. UAE appeared to work better combined with other noninvasive and invasive (suction aspiration) treatments.[35] In the report of Gao and colleagues,[36] UAE combined with D&C within 24 hours was an effective uterine preservation treatment of CSP and was associated with less blood loss and a shorter hospital stay than administration of MTX followed by D&C.

However, it is hard to evaluate its actual complication rates, because some articles have insufficient data. In the authors' 60 cases of CSP, UAE was used in 4 patients with persistent vaginal bleeding or development of AVM. One of the patients with UAE continued to bleed, and a hysterectomy was performed.[37]

### *Excision by Laparotomy, Alone or in Combination with Hysteroscopy*

General anesthesia is required. The overall complication rate for 108 cases was 13.8%.[3] However, if hysteroscopy was combined with transabdominal US guidance, no complications were noted. If hysteroscopy was combined with mifepristone, the complication rate was 17%. It appears that when performed by an experienced clinician with US guidance, hysteroscopy may be a reasonable operative solution to CSP.[38–47]

The authors speculate that if hysteroscopic excision is selected, the adjuvant use of an inflatable Foley balloon catheter for prevention or treatment of eventual bleeding from the operative site should be considered.

### *Intragestational Sac Injection of Methotrexate or Potassium Chloride, with Continuous, Real-Time Ultrasound Guidance*

When this approach is used, no anesthesia is required. This approach (**Fig. 3**) had the fewest and least-involved complications. Of the 83 cases, only 9 (10.8%) involved complications. Cases performed with transabdominal sonography guidance had a slightly higher complication rate (15%) than those using transvaginal sonography (TVS) guidance.[3,37]

Since the publication of the authors' review, a handful of articles reported on the successful use of the local, intragestational sac injection. Yin and colleagues[24] treated 20 of 34 patients with CSP by local MTX, TVS-guided intragestational sac injection of MTX without complications. Yamaguchi and colleagues[48] successfully treated 8 CSP cases with local MTX injection with TVS guidance. Two patients needed additional MTX therapy via local injection or systemic administration. Four of the 5 patients had subsequent pregnancies and uneventful deliveries. Recurrent CSP was diagnosed in 1 patient. Pang and colleagues[49] successfully treated 3 patients with local injection.

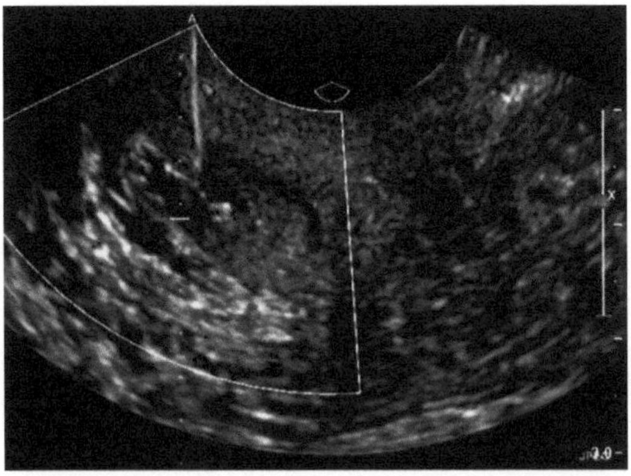

**Fig. 3.** Treatment of CSP. Transvaginal US-guided, real-time US controlled local, intragestational sac injection of MTX or KCl. The needle is imaged entering the gestational sac containing the embryo.

Because local injections do not require general anesthesia providing final treatment, it appears to be one of the most effective and simple treatment performed by transabdominal US or TVS guidance when future fertility is desired.

### *Use of a Foley Balloon Catheter to Treat and Control Bleeding*

Inserting a Foley balloon catheter and inflating it at the site of the CSP is a relatively new approach.[27,50,51] The authors used this approach as an adjuvant to treatments of CSP.[29] The Foley catheters have balloons of different capacity, and they can be used alone (usually in gestations of 5–7 weeks by placing pressure on the small gestational sac). This approach has almost always been used in conjunction with another treatment or as backup if bleeding occurs. The authors suggest 12-French size with 10-mL silicone balloon catheter, although the authors have also used a 14-French catheter with a 30-mL balloon capacity successfully in an 8-week CSP case (**Fig. 4**). There are no data indicating the length of time the catheter should be kept in place. In the authors' experience, 24 to 48 hours is the preferred duration, with the outer end of the catheter fastened to the patient's thigh. The authors also provide antibiotic coverage and reevaluate the effect in 2 days or as needed. General anesthesia is not required.

### *The Modified Use of a Cervical Ripening Double Balloon*

Based on the authors' experience of the successful use of single Foley balloons in treating CSP and encouraged by the publication of 1 case treated with a double balloon catheter,[52] the authors started to use a special cervical ripening double Cook catheter.[53]

Patients with live cervical pregnancy and CSP between 6 and 8 weeks' gestation were considered for the office-based treatment. Three live cervical pregnancies and 7 live cesarean scar pregnancies ranging from 6 1/7 to 7 4/7 weeks were successfully treated. Paracervical block was administered in 3 patients for pain control. Insertion of the catheter and inflation of the upper balloon were done under transabdominal US guidance. The lower (pressure) balloon was inflated opposite the gestational sac under transvaginal US guidance. After an hour, the area of the sac was scanned. When fetal cardiac activity was absent (usually 1–3 hours) and no bleeding was noted, patients were discharged. After 2 to 3 days, a follow-up appointment was scheduled for possible catheter removal. Serial US and serum hCG were followed weekly or as needed.

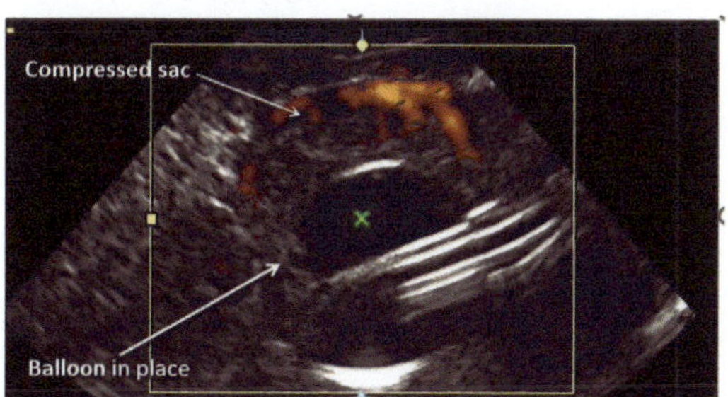


**Fig. 4.** Treatment of CSP. US-guided insertion of a single Foley balloon catheter inflating it opposite the gestational sac to compress it, stopping the heart activity. It can be used after a previous local, intragestational injection of MTX or KCl to prevent bleeding. The X marks the center of the inflated balloon.

The authors' experience suggests that the double balloon is a successful, minimally invasive, and well-tolerated single treatment for cervical pregnancy (**Fig. 5**) and CSP (**Fig. 6**). This simple treatment method has 4 main advantages: it effectively stops embryonic cardiac activity, it prevents bleeding complications, it does not usually require any additional invasive therapies, and it is familiar to obstetricians-gynecologists who use the same cervical ripening catheters for labor induction. Its wider application, however, has to be validated on a larger patient population.

The authors followed up their observations by supplementing it by sharing their experience in a follow-up article.[54] The authors stressed to carefully control the inflation of the balloons. This treatment was administered to 38 patients by several centers contributing to its validation. There was only 1 hysterectomy because of late occurring bleeding in a patient who did not follow postprocedure instructions.[55] The authors continue to use this treatment method as their main approach and will continue to upload their results in the International Registry of CSP. As the data accumulate, the authors hope it will prove to be the treatment regimen of choice in scar pregnancies at or before 8 weeks.

### *Transvaginal Surgical Excision*

There is 1 article describing a transvaginal surgical approach excising the gestational sac after elevating the bladder, followed by curetting the area, and finally, closing using a continuous suture.[34] The investigators described 49 cases with only 18% minor complications, thus describing this approach as easy and safe. Three patients had intrauterine pregnancy, one after 6 months and two after 12 months postoperatively. One patient had a recurrent CSP postoperatively and a transvaginal surgical management; another patient had an intrauterine pregnancy 5 months postoperatively, and D&C was performed to prevent uterine rupture. Again, although interesting, many more cases are needed to fully assess the risks and benefits of this approach.

## ENHANCED MYOMETRIAL VASCULARITY/ANTERIOVENOUS MALFORMATIONS IN CESAREAN SCAR PREGNANCIES

During pregnancy, the uterine vascular bed beneath the placenta is remodeled, providing the conceptus with blood through dilated, low-resistance, high-velocity

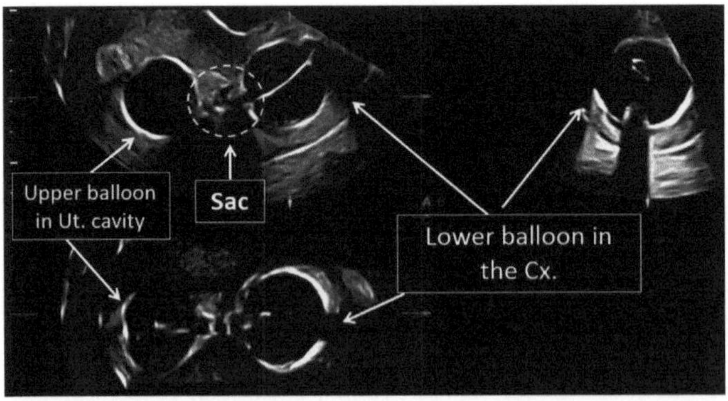


**Fig. 5.** Treatment of cervical pregnancy. Example of the use of a cervical ripening double balloon catheter in a 7 weeks' cervical pregnancy scanned using 3-dimensional US showing the relationship of the 2 balloons by the orthogonal planes.

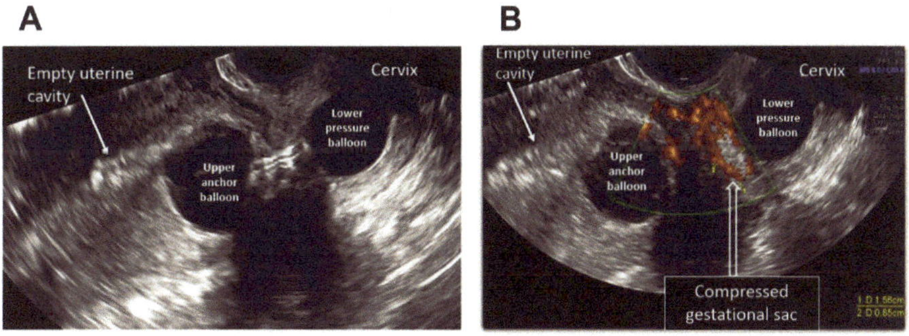


**Fig. 6.** Example of the use of a cervical ripening double balloon catheter in a 7 weeks and 2 days' CSP. (*A*) The transabdominal US-guided and inflated upper (anchor) balloon and the transvaginal US-guided and inflated lower "treatment" or "pressure" balloons are shown. (*B*) The compressed gestational sac with the embryo between the inflated balloons is also imaged.

blood vessels. After a miscarriage, a D&C, or a treated CSP, the return of normal vascularity is slow and often complicated by a high-velocity AVM/EMV.[56–58]

Usually treated or miscarried CSPs regress without intervention. Treatments leaving retained products of conception are more frequently complicated by EMV. In the extreme, an EMV may require complex treatment (eg, UAE and/or Total abdominal hysterectomy).

In general, EMV/AVM is a pathologic "short circuit" of the bloodstream between an organ's arterial and venous supply. In the case of a uterine EMV, the blood flow assumes an unusually high velocity, rendering the vessels into a vascular fistula. Although uncommon when they do occur, they may cause life-threatening hemorrhage, because of the thin wall of the abnormal blood vessels, which are disrupted after menstruation or instrumentation.[59] Acquired uterine EMVs can be spontaneous after a miscarried CCP but are usually traumatic, resulting from prior D&C, medical abortion, treatments such as D&C, local injection, or single- or double-balloon treatments. They are detected at the first US scans when the patient presents for vaginal bleeding[60] or at follow-up US scans after the above-mentioned treatments[59,61–63] (**Fig. 7**).

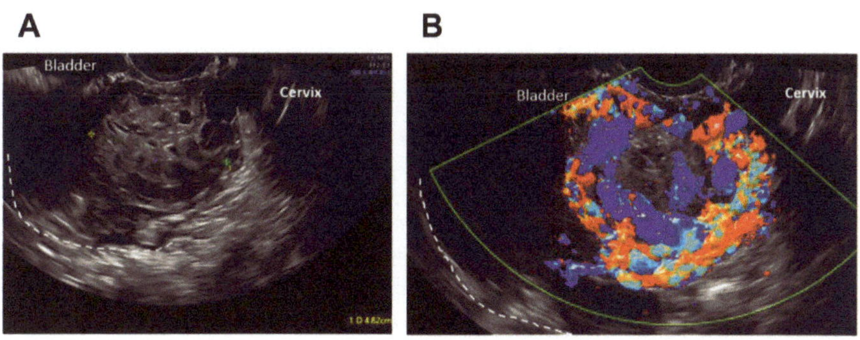


**Fig. 7.** Complication of a treated CSP. (*A*) Gray-scale and (*B*) color Doppler images of the uterus approximately 5 weeks after a treated CSP that developed into an EMV or, in other words, an arteriovenous fistulous lesion. The peak systolic velocity of the blood rushing through it was greater than 80 cm/s. It was successfully treated by UAE, and the uterus returned to its normal shape and function in 3 months.

In the 751 cases of CSP reviewed by the authors, there were 8 cases with descriptions of AVM detected in the scar pregnancies. Some of these were diagnosed before interventions; others were detected as a result of treatment. The primary management of 3 was by UAE, and the other 5 was with hysterectomies.[3] In the authors' series of 60 CSPs, they diagnosed 5 patients with AVM.[37] One presented almost 67 days after D&C of a misdiagnosed CSP and had unsuccessful UAE followed by hysterectomy. One presented with vaginal bleeding to the emergency department and was immediately embolized. Two patients developed AVM after local intragestational sac injection of MTX and underwent successful UAE. One patient had intractable bleeding without any intervention of a CSP and was embolized because the blood vessels demonstrated increasingly high-velocity and high-diastolic blood flow on Doppler testing.

Kiyokawa and colleagues[31] published a case of what they called "pseudoaneurysm" following focal injection of MTX and KCl with systemic MTX treatment. Because the serum hCG and the gestational sac were still persistent, D&C was performed with interventional radiologists on standby. Severe hemorrhage occurred and continued during the procedure, which necessitated emergent UAE.

As previously stated, US presents a valuable tool for the diagnosis of AVM and guidelines for their treatment.[64]

## SUMMARY

1. Counseling a patient with CSP must be evidence based (see **Fig. 2**).
2. If termination of a CSP with positive heart activity is chosen, it should be done without delay.
3. If pregnancy continues, a CSP can result in a live offspring.
4. The overwhelming majority of patients with a CSP diagnosed in the first trimester that reached the third trimester of pregnancy will deliver via repeat CD; almost all have different degrees of PAS, and in most cases, will require a hysterectomy.
5. Despite a large number of modalities to terminate a CSP, there is no clear consensus about the best way to achieve it. Because there is no single best treatment, one should choose the one with the least complications and gain experience with that approach.
6. MTX, injected as a single dose systemically is usually ineffective and delays the final treatment; however, it can be used as an adjuvant to other treatments that have a proven efficiency. Treatment with low complications is US-guided local, intragestational sac injection of MTX/KCl as well as hysteroscopic excision.
7. Sharp curetting and UAE *alone* should not be first-line treatments. UAE is effective as an adjunct procedure, and in cases of emergency owing to sustained hemorrhage.
8. Insertion and inflation of a single Foley balloon catheter or even more so double cervical ripening catheters are effective to prevent or treat bleeding following any local treatment of CSP.
9. The obstetric/gynecologic community is in urgent need of standardized diagnostic and management protocols. An International CSP Registry was created (www.csp-registry.com). The authors encourage its use to upload cases.

In closing, the authors recommend following the pertinent literature because it is constantly being updated with new information about CSP and PAS.

## REFERENCES

1. Larsen JV, Solomon MH. Pregnancy in a uterine scar sacculus–an unusual cause of postabortal haemorrhage. A case report. S Afr Med J 1978;53:142–3.

2. Vial Y, Petignat P, Hohlfeld P. Pregnancy in a cesarean scar. Ultrasound Obstet Gynecol 2000;16:592–3.
3. Timor-Tritsch IE, Monteagudo A. Unforeseen consequences of the increasing rate of cesarean deliveries: early placenta accreta and cesarean scar pregnancy. A review. Am J Obstet Gynecol 2012;207:14–29.
4. D'Antonio F, Timor-Tritsch IE, Palacios-Jaraquemada J, et al. First-trimester detection of abnormally invasive placenta in high-risk women: systematic review and meta-analysis. Ultrasound Obstet Gynecol 2018;51:176–83.
5. Timor-Tritsch IE, D'Antonio F, Cali G, et al. Early first-trimester transvaginal ultrasound is indicated in pregnancy after previous cesarean delivery: should it be mandatory? Ultrasound Obstet Gynecol 2019;54(2):156–63.
6. Abbas F, Talati J, Wasti S, et al. Placenta percreta with bladder invasion as a cause of life threatening hemorrhage. J Urol 2000;164:1270–4.
7. Berhie SH, Molina RL, Davis MR, et al. Beware the scar: laparoscopic hysterectomy for 7-week cesarean delivery scar implantation pregnancy. Am J Obstet Gynecol 2015;212:247.e1-2.
8. Ecker JL, Sorem KA, Soodak L, et al. Placenta increta complicating a first-trimester abortion. A case report. J Reprod Med 1992;37:893–5.
9. Gherman RB, McBrayer S, Tichenor J, et al. Placenta increta complicating first-trimester D&C. Obstet Gynecol 1999;93:845.
10. Hamid H, Zulida R, Norhafizah M. Massive haemorrhage secondary to placenta percreta in the first trimester: a case report. Clin Exp Obstet Gynecol 2015;42:101–3.
11. Hopker M, Fleckenstein G, Heyl W, et al. Placenta percreta in week 10 of pregnancy with consecutive hysterectomy: case report. Hum Reprod 2002;17:817–20.
12. Izabela UW, Krzysztof N, Ryszard P, et al. Placenta praevia increta with caesarean section scar invasion. Ginekol Pol 2011;82:471–3.
13. Lazarus EJ. Early rupture of the gravid uterus. Am J Obstet Gynecol 1978;132:224.
14. Liao CY, Huang HW, Tsui WH. Unusual imaging findings of placenta accreta resulting in early hysterectomy in first trimester–two case reports. Taiwan J Obstet Gynecol 2016;55:910–2.
15. Marcus S, Cheng E, Goff B. Extrauterine pregnancy resulting from early uterine rupture. Obstet Gynecol 1999;94:804–5.
16. Nonaka M, Toyoki H, Imai A. Cesarean section scar pregnancy may be the cause of serious hemorrhage after first-trimester abortion by dilatation and curettage. Int J Gynaecol Obstet 2006;95:50–1.
17. Overcash RT, Khackician ZH. Late-first-trimester cesarean section scar ectopic pregnancy with placenta increta: a case report. J Reprod Med 2012;57:61–4.
18. Reyftmann L, Vernhet H, Boulot P. Management of massive uterine bleeding in a cesarean scar pregnancy. Int J Gynaecol Obstet 2005;89:154–5.
19. Smith A, Ash A, Maxwell D. Sonographic diagnosis of cesarean scar pregnancy at 16 weeks. J Clin Ultrasound 2007;35:212–5.
20. Wong HS, Zuccollo J, Tait J, et al. Placenta accreta in the first trimester of pregnancy: sonographic findings. J Clin Ultrasound 2009;37:100–3.
21. Woolcott RJ, Nicholl M, Gibson JS. A case of placenta percreta presenting in the first trimester of pregnancy. Aust N Z J Obstet Gynaecol 1987;27:258–60.
22. Yang JI, Kim HY, Kim HS, et al. Diagnosis in the first trimester of placenta accreta with previous Cesarean section. Ultrasound Obstet Gynecol 2009;34:116–8.

23. Maheux-Lacroix S, Li F, Bujold E, et al. Cesarean scar pregnancies: a systematic review of treatment options. J Minim Invasive Gynecol 2017;24:915–25.
24. Yin XH, Yang SZ, Wang ZQ, et al. Injection of MTX for the treatment of cesarean scar pregnancy: comparison between different methods. Int J Clin Exp Med 2014;7:1867–72.
25. Litwicka K, Greco E. Caesarean scar pregnancy: a review of management options. Curr Opin Obstet Gynecol 2013;25:456–61.
26. Timor-Tritsch IE, Monteagudo A. Reply. Am J Obstet Gynecol 2014;210:380–1.
27. Jiang T, Liu G, Huang L, et al. Methotrexate therapy followed by suction curettage followed by Foley tamponade for caesarean scar pregnancy. Eur J Obstet Gynecol Reprod Biol 2011;156:209–11.
28. Kutuk MS, Uysal G, Dolanbay M, et al. Successful medical treatment of cesarean scar ectopic pregnancies with systemic multidose methotrexate: single-center experience. J Obstet Gynaecol Res 2014;40:1700–6.
29. Timor-Tritsch IE, Cali G, Monteagudo A, et al. Foley balloon catheter to prevent or manage bleeding during treatment for cervical and Cesarean scar pregnancy. Ultrasound Obstet Gynecol 2015;46:118–23.
30. Yu XL, Zhang N, Zuo WL. Cesarean scar pregnancy: an analysis of 100 cases. Zhonghua Yi Xue Za Zhi 2011;91:3186–9 [in Chinese].
31. Kiyokawa S, Chiyoda T, Ueno K, et al. Development of pseudoaneurysm in cesarean section scar pregnancy: a case report and literature review. J Med Ultrason (2001) 2018;45:357–62.
32. Liu S, Sun J, Cai B, et al. Management of cesarean scar pregnancy using ultrasound-guided dilation and curettage. J Minim Invasive Gynecol 2016;23: 707–11.
33. Polat I, Ekiz A, Acar DK, et al. Suction curettage as first line treatment in cases with cesarean scar pregnancy: feasibility and effectiveness in early pregnancy. J Matern Fetal Neonatal Med 2016;29:1066–71.
34. Li JB, Kong LZ, Fan L, et al. Transvaginal surgical management of cesarean scar pregnancy: analysis of 49 cases from one tertiary care center. Eur J Obstet Gynecol Reprod Biol 2014;182:102–6.
35. Cao S, Zhu L, Jin L, et al. Uterine artery embolization in cesarean scar pregnancy: safe and effective intervention. Chin Med J (Engl) 2014;127:2322–6.
36. Gao L, Huang Z, Gao J, et al. Uterine artery embolization followed by dilation and curettage within 24 hours compared with systemic methotrexate for cesarean scar pregnancy. Int J Gynaecol Obstet 2014;127:147–51.
37. Timor-Tritsch IE, Khatib N, Monteagudo A, et al. Cesarean scar pregnancies: experience of 60 cases. J Ultrasound Med 2015;34:601–10.
38. Chang Y, Kay N, Chen YH, et al. Resectoscopic treatment of ectopic pregnancy in previous cesarean delivery scar defect with vasopressin injection. Fertil Steril 2011;96:e80–2.
39. Chao A, Wang TH, Wang CJ, et al. Hysteroscopic management of cesarean scar pregnancy after unsuccessful methotrexate treatment. J Minim Invasive Gynecol 2005;12:374–6.
40. Chen ZY, Zhang XM, Xu H, et al. Management of cesarean scar pregnancy by hysteroscopy combined with uterine artery embolism. Zhonghua Fu Chan Ke Za Zhi 2011;46:591–4 [in Chinese].
41. Deans R, Abbott J. Hysteroscopic management of cesarean scar ectopic pregnancy. Fertil Steril 2010;93:1735–40.

42. Gubbini G, Centini G, Nascetti D, et al. Surgical hysteroscopic treatment of cesarean-induced isthmocele in restoring fertility: prospective study. J Minim Invasive Gynecol 2011;18:234–7.
43. Li H, Guo HY, Han JS, et al. Endoscopic treatment of ectopic pregnancy in a cesarean scar. J Minim Invasive Gynecol 2011;18:31–5.
44. Lyu J, Fu X, Wang H. Therapeutic effect of hysteroscopic surgery in treatment of small mass of caesarean scar pregnancy. Zhonghua Fu Chan Ke Za Zhi 2014;49: 14–7 [in Chinese].
45. Ozkan S, Caliskan E, Ozeren S, et al. Three-dimensional ultrasonographic diagnosis and hysteroscopic management of a viable cesarean scar ectopic pregnancy. J Obstet Gynaecol Res 2007;33:873–7.
46. Robinson JK, Dayal MB, Gindoff P, et al. A novel surgical treatment for cesarean scar pregnancy: laparoscopically assisted operative hysteroscopy. Fertil Steril 2009;92:1497 e13–6.
47. Wang CJ, Chao AS, Yuen LT, et al. Endoscopic management of cesarean scar pregnancy. Fertil Steril 2006;85:494.e1-4.
48. Yamaguchi M, Honda R, Uchino K, et al. Transvaginal methotrexate injection for the treatment of cesarean scar pregnancy: efficacy and subsequent fecundity. J Minim Invasive Gynecol 2014;21:877–83.
49. Pang YP, Tan WC, Yong TT, et al. Caesarean section scar pregnancy: a case series at a single tertiary centre. Singapore Med J 2012;53:638–42.
50. Atilgan R, Aslan K, Can B, et al. Successful management of pelvic bleeding after caesarean hysterectomy by means of Foley catheter-condom balloon tamponade. BMJ Case Rep 2014;2014 [pii:bcr2014204770].
51. Shao HJ, Ma JT, Yang XE, et al. Diagnosis and treatment of cesarean scar pregnancy. Zhonghua Yi Xue Za Zhi 2010;90:2616–9 [in Chinese].
52. Tsui KH, Lin LT, Yu KJ, et al. Double-balloon cervical ripening catheter works well as an intrauterine balloon tamponade in post-abortion massive hemorrhage. Taiwan J Obstet Gynecol 2012;51:426–9.
53. Timor-Tritsch IE, Monteagudo A, Bennett TA, et al. A new minimally invasive treatment for cesarean scar pregnancy and cervical pregnancy. Am J Obstet Gynecol 2016;215:351 e1–8.
54. Timor-Tritsch IE, Monteagudo A, Kaelin Agten A. Recap-minimally invasive treatment for cesarean scar pregnancy using a double-balloon catheter: additional suggestions to the technique. Am J Obstet Gynecol 2017;217:496–7.
55. Monteagudo A, Cali G, Rebarber A, et al. Minimally invasive treatment of cesarean scar and cervical pregnancies using a cervical ripening double balloon catheter: expanding the clinical series. J Ultrasound Med 2019;38:785–93.
56. Van den Bosch T, Van Schoubroeck D, Timmerman D. Maximum peak systolic velocity and management of highly vascularized retained products of conception. J Ultrasound Med 2015;34:1577–82.
57. Timor-Tritsch IE, Haynes MC, Monteagudo A, et al. Ultrasound diagnosis and management of acquired uterine enhanced myometrial vascularity/arteriovenous malformations. Am J Obstet Gynecol 2016;214:731.e1-10.
58. Kaelin Agten A, Ringel N, Ramos J, et al. Standardization of peak systolic velocity measurement in enhanced myometrial vascularity. Am J Obstet Gynecol 2016; 215:802–3.
59. Polat P, Suma S, Kantarcy M, et al. Color Doppler US in the evaluation of uterine vascular abnormalities. Radiographics 2002;22:47–53.

60. Mou Y, Xu Y, Hu Y, et al. Giant uterine artery pseudoaneurysm after a missed miscarriage termination in a cesarean scar pregnancy. BMC Womens Health 2014;14:89.
61. Chou MM, Hwang JI, Tseng JJ, et al. Cesarean scar pregnancy: quantitative assessment of uterine neovascularization with 3-dimensional color power Doppler imaging and successful treatment with uterine artery embolization. Am J Obstet Gynecol 2004;190:866–8.
62. Rygh AB, Greve OJ, Fjetland L, et al. Arteriovenous malformation as a consequence of a scar pregnancy. Acta Obstet Gynecol Scand 2009;88:853–5.
63. Akbayir O, Gedikbasi A, Akyol A, et al. Cesarean scar pregnancy: a rare cause of uterine arteriovenous malformation. J Clin Ultrasound 2011;39:534–8.
64. Timmerman D, Wauters J, Van Calenbergh S, et al. Color Doppler imaging is a valuable tool for the diagnosis and management of uterine vascular malformations. Ultrasound Obstet Gynecol 2003;21:570–7.

# First-Trimester Ultrasound

Jenny Y. Mei, MD[a], Yalda Afshar, MD, PhD[b,*], Lawrence D. Platt, MD[c,d]

**KEYWORDS**

- First trimester • Ultrasound • Early anatomy • Anatomic assessment
- Prenatal screening

**KEY POINTS**

- In the past several decades, major advancements in high-resolution transvaginal ultrasound transducers have allowed the first-trimester ultrasound examination to evolve beyond aneuploidy screening and include early fetal anatomy.
- Many studies through the years have shown the ability to visualize key anatomic landmarks as well as major abnormalities.
- The detection rate of fetal anomalies is highest when combining both transvaginal and transabdominal approach as compared with either approach alone.
- Despite the increase in and convenience of cell-free DNA via noninvasive prenatal testing (NIPT), a comprehensive first-trimester ultrasound provides valuable clinical information that cannot be detected with NIPT alone.
- Lack of experience in provider and sonographer training, increasing maternal obesity, and underdevelopment of certain anatomic structures at earlier gestational ages limit evaluation of certain abnormalities on early anatomic assessment.

## INTRODUCTION

In the late 1980s, ultrasound (US) evaluation of the fetus at less than 16 weeks' gestational age (GA) was significantly improved by the development of high-resolution transvaginal ultrasound (TVUS) transducers.[1–5] Such advancements allowed new ability to assess both normal and abnormal anatomy of the fetal brain, heart, kidneys, and other organs. Soon thereafter, nuchal translucency (NT) was established as a US

The authors have nothing to disclose.

[a] Department of Obstetrics and Gynecology, University of California, Los Angeles, 10833 Le Conte Avenue, Room 27-139 CHS, Los Angeles, CA 90095, USA; [b] Division of Maternal-Fetal Medicine, Department of Obstetrics and Gynecology, University of California, 10833 Le Conte Avenue, Room 27-139 CHS, Los Angeles, CA 90095, USA; [c] Division of Maternal-Fetal Medicine, Department of Obstetrics and Gynecology, University of California, Los Angeles, 6310 San Vicente Boulevard, Suite 520, Los Angeles, CA 90048, USA; [d] Center for Fetal Medicine and Women's Ultrasound, 6310 San Vicente Boulevard, Suite 520, Los Angeles, CA 90048, USA
* Corresponding author.
*E-mail address:* yafshar@mednet.ucla.edu
twitter: @yafshar (Y.A.); @Ctr4Fetalmed (L.D.P.)

Obstet Gynecol Clin N Am 46 (2019) 829–852
https://doi.org/10.1016/j.ogc.2019.07.011

screening tool for aneuploidy.[6–9] Over the past 2 decades, the first-trimester US examination has evolved beyond viability and aneuploidy screening.

Today, indications for the first-trimester US in pregnancy include those listed in **Box 1**. If a transabdominal (TA) examination is not definitive, a transvaginal (TV) or transperineal scan should be performed whenever possible.

In recent years, more emphasis has been placed on including assessment of fetal anatomy in early gestation. In 2012, the International Society of Ultrasound in Obstetrics and Gynecology (ISUOG) stated that the purpose of the first-trimester fetal US includes "not only the chorionicity and amnionicity in number of fetuses" but also "to detect gross fetal malformation."[10] The assessment should be performed between 11 and 14 weeks of gestation and should include "the head, neck, face, spine, chest, heart, abdomen, abdominal wall, extremities, placenta, and cord." The theory behind such statements is that if an organ is or was developed at that stage of pregnancy, it can be seen; furthermore, if there is a major malformation, it should be seen. Led by the American Institute of Ultrasound in Medicine, an imaging consortium in the United States is currently redrafting new guidelines for first-trimester US assessment (**Figs. 1** and **2**).

## GUIDELINES TO FETAL IMAGING

Today, offering NT screening and biochemical testing at 11 to 14 weeks' GA is considered standard of care.[11] US at NT screening is an important juncture to assess both basic anatomy and perform aneuploidy screening. Of note, having the introduction of cell-free DNA via noninvasive prenatal testing (NIPT) has seen a decrease in the use of first-trimester combined screening.[12,13]

The NT is the sonographic appearance of the fluid collection under the skin behind the fetal neck and back at 11 to 13 + 6/7 weeks' GA.[14] There are standardized criteria

**Box 1**
**Indications for the first-trimester ultrasound**

Confirm of the presence of an intrauterine pregnancy

Confirmation of cardiac activity

Estimation of GA

Diagnose or evaluate multiple gestations, including determination of chorionicity/amnionicity

Evaluation of suspected ectopic pregnancy

Evaluation of the cause of vaginal bleeding

Evaluation of pelvic pain

Evaluation of suspected gestational trophoblastic disease

Assessment for gross fetal anomalies

Measurement of the NT when part of a screening program for fetal aneuploidy

Imaging as an adjunct to chorionic villus sampling, embryo transfer, and localization and removal of an intrauterine device

Evaluation of maternal pelvic masses and/or uterine abnormalities

*Adapted from* AIUM-ACR-ACOG-SMFM-SRU Practice parameter for the performance of standard diagnostic obstetric ultrasound examinations. J Ultrasound Med 2018;37(11):E13-E24; with permission.

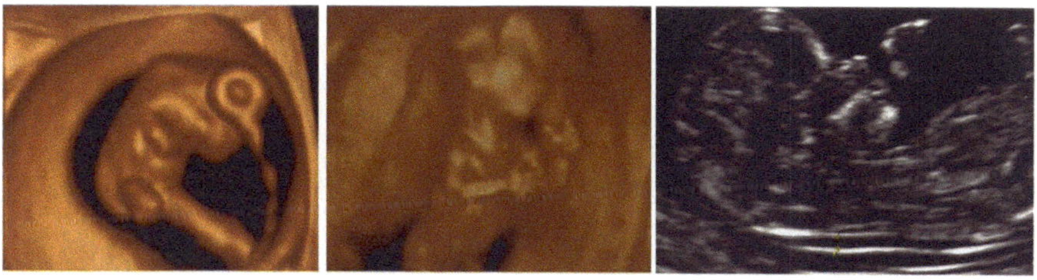

**Fig. 1.** Two-dimensional and 3D US illustrate what can be seen on fetal anatomy between 8 and 11 weeks of gestation.

for measurement of the NT according to the UK Fetal Medicine Foundation and Nuchal Translucency Quality Review Program in the United States.[15–17] Those criteria are listed in **Box 2** (**Figs. 3** and **4**).

Per ISUOG guidelines, the minimal required biometric measurements in the first trimester include crown-rump length (CRL), biparietal diameter (BPD), head circumference (HC), abdominal circumference (AC), and femur length (FL).[10]

The main advantages of an early anatomic assessment at the time were exclusion of major anomalies, earlier genetic diagnosis, and potential pregnancy planning. Limitations included taking into account the later development of many anatomic structures and pathologic conditions as well. There is also a general lack of familiarity and experience with first-trimester anatomic assessments, and some raise concerns regarding potentially rising costs, overburdening of US laboratories, and disputable outcomes.

## TECHNICAL ASPECTS IN MEASUREMENT STANDARDIZATION

In assessing early fetal gestation, the midsagittal view should yield the fetal profile, nasal bone, NT, spine with overlying skin, posterior fossa, and extremities. The axial view is best for viewing head, neck, heart, lungs, abdomen, cord insertion, kidneys, and bladder. Through the sagittal view and 5 transverse views and sweeps, the following measurements should be obtained: fetal heart rate, CRL, NT, posterior fossa, and cardiac axis (**Figs. 5** and **6**).

When operating the US during a first-trimester assessment, there are several modes that come into play. The B-mode, or "Brightness mode," is basic 2-dimensional (2D) imaging that includes any form of gray-scale display. B-mode contains the least amount of sonographic energy. M-mode, or "Motion mode," is used to assess the motion of fetal cardiac chambers and valves to document cardiac activity.

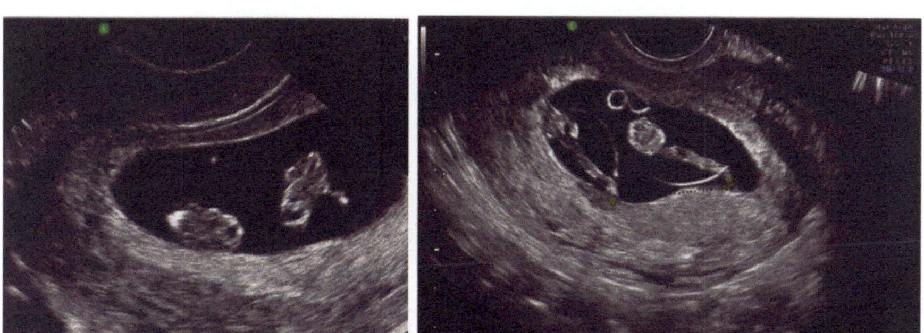

**Fig. 2.** Monochorionic diamniotic twins with cord insertions far apart from each other.

**Box 2**
**Guidelines for nuchal translucency measurement**

The margins of the NT edges must be clear with the angle of insonation perpendicular to the NT line.

The fetus must be in the midsagittal plane. The tip of the nose, palate, and diencephalon should be seen.

The image must be magnified so that it is filled by the fetal head, neck, and upper thorax.

The fetal neck must be in a neutral position, with the head in line with the spine, not flexed and not hyperextended.

The amnion must be seen as separate from the NT line.

The (+) calipers on the US screen must be used to perform the NT measurement.

Electronic calipers must be placed on the inner borders of the nuchal line with none of the horizontal crossbar itself protruding into the space.

The calipers must be placed perpendicular to the long axis of the fetus.

The measurements must be obtained at the widest space of the NT.

*Adapted from* AIUM-ACR-ACOG-SMFM-SRU Practice parameter for the performance of standard diagnostic obstetric ultrasound examinations. J Ultrasound Med 2018;37(11):E13-E24; with permission.

M-mode is a single-beam, high-pulse repetition frequency and is the preferred method for documentation of cardiac activity because it contains less energy than spectral Doppler. The spectral (or pulsed) Doppler detects apparent variation in frequency of a sound wave as the source approaches or moves away; the change in frequency is proportional to the speed of movement of the sound emitting or reflecting objects, that is, red blood cells within a vessel. Spectral Doppler has greater energy output and thus more potential bioeffects on the developing fetus.

Regarding the bioeffects of US in early gestation, the various modes vary in safety profile. The acoustic outputs of B-mode and M-mode are not high enough to produce deleterious effects and thus are deemed safe for all stages of pregnancy.[18] Spectral Doppler, however, focuses US beam energy on small anatomic targets and thus

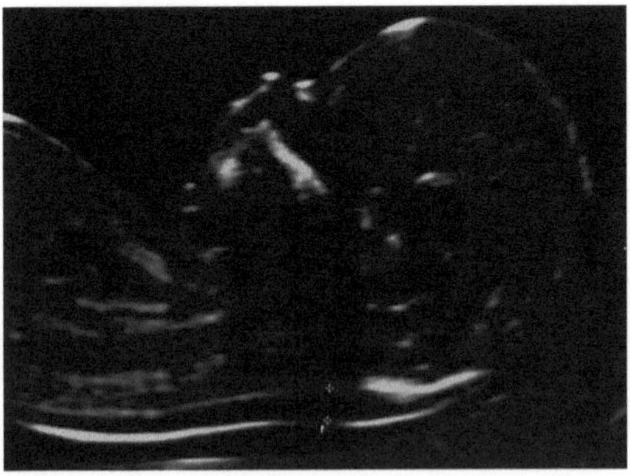

**Fig. 3.** NT measurement.

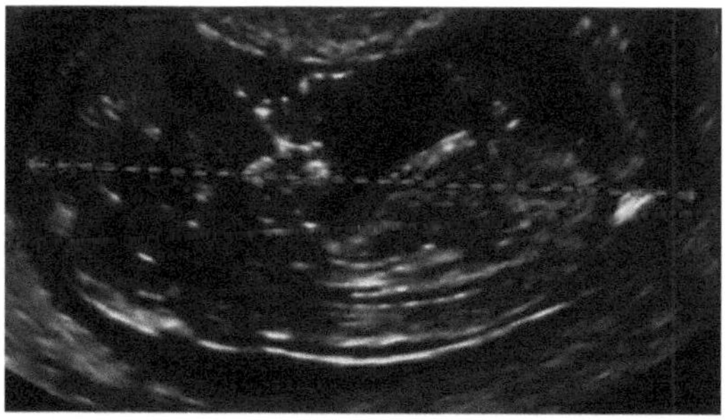

**Fig. 4.** Standardized measurement of CRL.

should not be used routinely in first-trimester US.[19] Use of 3-dimensional (3D) and 4-dimensional US is considered as safe as B-mode.[20] In general, the as low as reasonably achievable (ALARA) principle is upheld with sonographic imaging: using a power output, ALARA, so fetal exposure time is limited.[21]

## FIRST-TRIMESTER PREGNANCY DATING

Biometric measurements for first-trimester dating include mean gestational sac diameter (MSD), CRL, and fetal BPD, and HC if greater than 11-weeks' GA. Of these, the most used is CRL.

MSD can be used to confirm an intrauterine pregnancy but not viability. In general, a gestational sac without an embryo suggests approximately 5 to 6 weeks' GA. It is not recommended to rely solely on MSD for an estimated due date.

CRL has proven to be a more precise dating method and is the preferred choice. It is assessed via the longest straight-line distance from the top of the head to the rump of the embryo or fetus. A mean of 3 discrete measurements is used. For an accurate CRL per ISUOG guidelines, the fetus must be in neutral position and fluid must be visible between the chin and chest. The ideal time for assessment is 8 + 0 to 13 6/7 weeks' gestation, and CRL is accurate to within ±5 days in 95% of cases within this timeframe.[16]

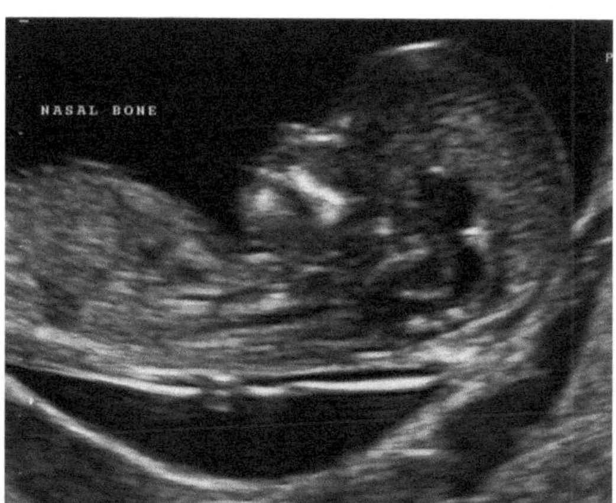


**Fig. 5.** Normal posterior fossa.

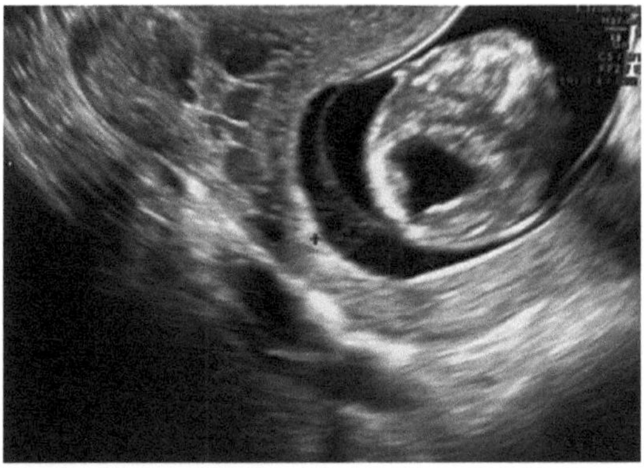

Fig. 6. Abnormal posterior fossa (Dandy-Walker malformation).

Fetal biometry must be used for dating beyond the limits set above for CRL. Starting at 14 weeks' GA, BPD, HC, AC, and FL are used for dating. For head measurements at 10 weeks, the midline third ventricle, interhemispheric fissure, and choroid plexus are good landmarks to use. By 13 weeks, the thalamus and third ventricle are landmarks for BPD and HC. De Basio and colleagues[21] found that between 10 and 14 weeks, one can measure the humerus, ulna, femur, tibia, and foot in more than 95% of cases (**Figs. 7–9**, **Table 1**).

## THE DETAILED FIRST-TRIMESTER ULTRASOUND EXAMINATION

Advances in US technology in recent years have allowed fetal anatomic assessment, and in turn, congenital diagnoses to be made earlier in pregnancy. With the advent of both TA and TV high-frequency transducers, the opportunity to make the diagnosis of major congenital anomalies in the first trimester has now become commonplace. An important question that now lays before those performing first-trimester US is whether performing a US assessment of the fetal anatomy in the first trimester is one of choice or of obligation.

Major fetal abnormalities that can be easily identified on first-trimester US include hydrops, neural tube defects, anencephaly, alobar holoprosencephaly, body stalk anomaly, limb abnormalities, ectopia cordis, large omphalocele, large gastroschisis, megacystis, conjoined twins, and molar placenta. Furthermore, certain markers of aneuploidy can be quickly assessed as well. For example, evaluating for hypoplastic nasal bone, abnormal flow in ductus venosus, or tricuspid regurgitation can aid in the assessment of aneuploidy risk and counseling.

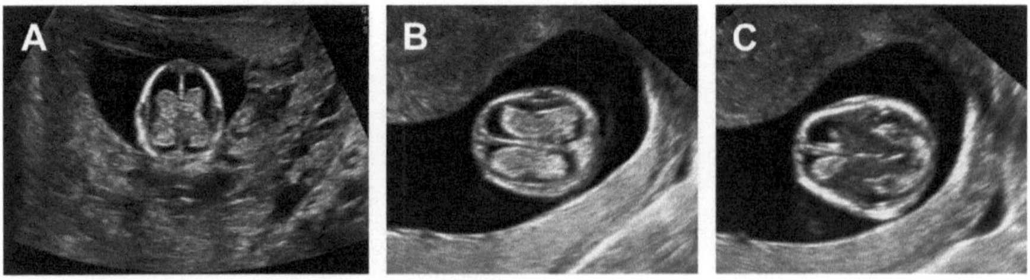


Fig. 7. (*A–C*) Normal central nervous system.

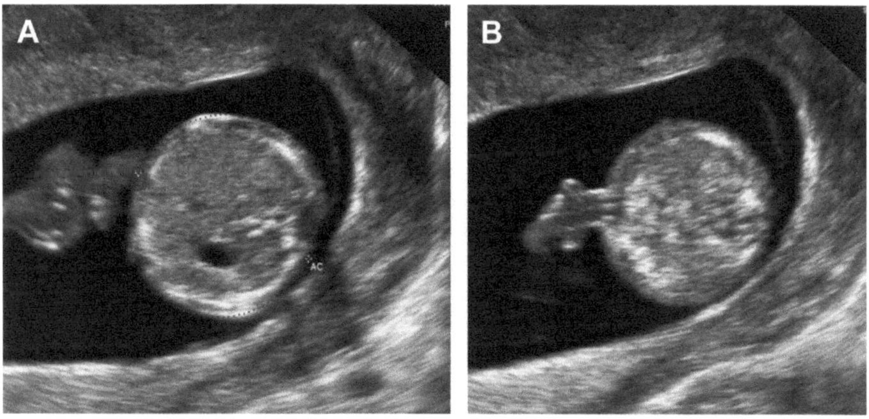


**Fig. 8.** Normal abdomen at 12 weeks with (*A*) stomach and (*B*) cord insertion.

Setbacks include lack of experience in providers and sonographers as well as the fact that not all anatomic structures are well formed, and thus, certain pathologic conditions have yet to develop. Major structures of the central nervous system, for example, corpus callosum, are not expected to be well formed until 22 weeks of

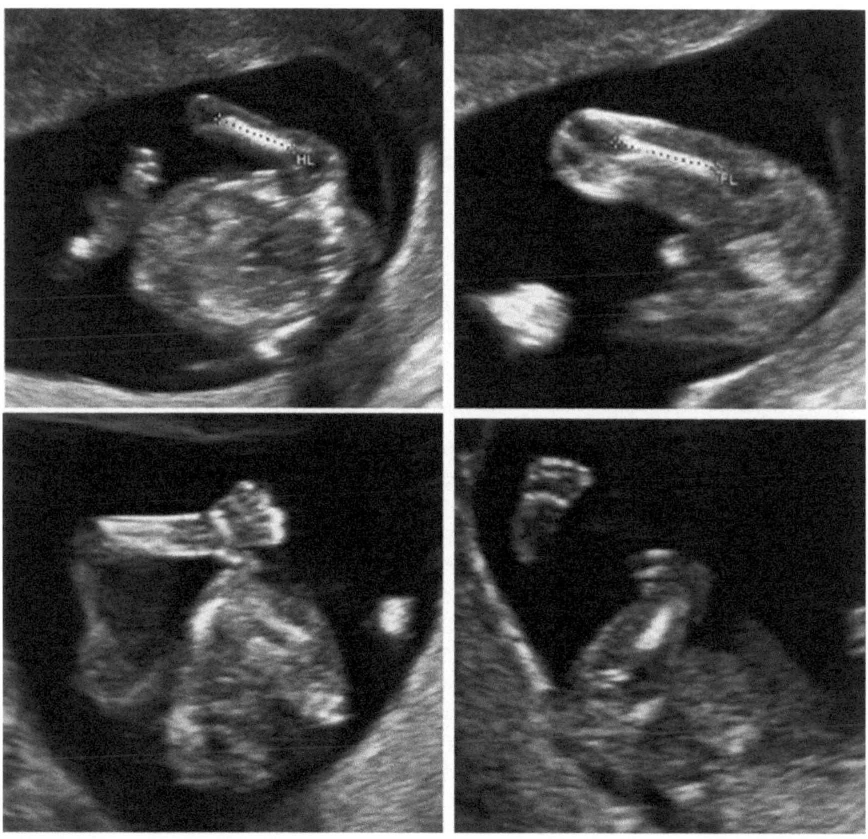

**Fig. 9.** Fetal limbs seen at 12 weeks of gestation.

**Table 1**
**Visualization rate of landmarks between 10 and 14 weeks**

| Structure | Measurable (%) |
|---|---|
| Humerus | 97.9 |
| Ulna | 97.7 |
| Femur | 97.7 |
| Tibia | 97.9 |
| Foot | 93.2 |

*Adapted from* De Biasio P, Prefumo F, Lantieri PB, et al. Reference values for fetal limb biometry at 10-14 weeks of gestation. Ultrasound Obstet Gynecol 2002;19(6):590.

gestation. Certain pathologic conditions, such as congenital heart malformations or skeletal dysplasias, are very subtle and can be difficult to recognize in the first trimester. Other pathologic conditions, such as diaphragmatic hernias, will not be demonstrable until later in the pregnancy as well.

## THE BEGINNINGS OF FIRST-TRIMESTER ANATOMIC ULTRASOUND

The earliest studies assessing fetal anatomy in the first trimester began in the 1990s. Achiron and Tadmor[1] conducted a 12-month study of 800 pregnant women between 9 and 13 weeks' gestation assessing fetal anatomy via TA followed by TV US. On first-trimester TVUS, 8 cases of fetal abnormality were detected, including anencephaly, myelomeningoceles, and cystic hygromas. All normal first-trimester US were then rescreened in midtrimester by TAUS at which point 5 additional cases were detected, including hydrocephaly, agenesis of corpus callosum, bilateral ureteropelvic obstruction, hypoplastic right heart, and tetralogy of Fallot. One case of ventricular septal defect and coarctation of the aorta was not detected on either scan. The study's conclusion was that TVUS was more sensitive than TAUS in the detection of first-trimester anomalies; however, a follow-up, standard TAUS was recommended in the second trimester. This study conducted almost 30 years ago was a sound predictor of where the future of first-trimester US would go.

## WHAT CAN BE SEEN?

Per ISUOG guidelines, **Table 2** lists an expected anatomic assessment between 11 and 13 6/7 weeks' gestation.

A study by Whitlow and Economides[22] in 1998 found using TVUS and TAUS together yielded a visualization success rate of greater than 98% in all categories by 13 weeks' GA (**Table 3**). Furthermore, Huggon and colleagues[23] suggested that up to 72% of major malformations can be identified before 14 weeks' gestation.

Pitalis and colleagues[24] conducted an evaluation of a 2-step US screening protocol for the detection of major fetal structural defects. The retrospective study of 3902 pregnancies evaluated US first between 11 and 14 weeks and the second between 20 and 24 weeks. Sixty-one (1.56%) fetuses with structural defects were detected in total, with 26 (42.6%) diagnosed in the first trimester, 29 (47.5%) in the second trimester, and 6 (9.9%) in the third trimester; the overall detection rate was 90.2%. In particular, the conclusion of value was the finding that approximately 40% of major structural defects were detected in the first trimester between 11 and 14 weeks.

**Table 2**
**First-trimester ultrasound anatomy**

| Organ/Anatomic Area | Present and/or Normal? |
|---|---|
| Head | Present<br>Cranial bones<br>Midline falx<br>Choroid plexus–filled ventricles |
| Neck | Normal appearance<br>NT thickness |
| Face | Eyes with lens<br>Nasal bone<br>Normal profile/mandible<br>Intact lips |
| Spine | Vertebrae (longitudinal and axial)<br>Intact overlying skin |
| Chest | Symmetric lung fields<br>No effusions or masses |
| Heart | Cardiac regular activity<br>Four symmetric chambers |
| Abdomen | Stomach present in left upper quadrant<br>Bladder<br>Kidneys |
| Abdominal wall | Normal cord insertion<br>No umbilical defects |
| Extremities | Four limbs each with 3 segments<br>Hands and feet with normal orientation |
| Placenta | Size and texture |
| Cord | Three-vessel cord |

*Adapted from* Salomon LJ, Alfirevic Z, Bilardo CM, et al. ISUOG practice guidelines: performance of first-trimester fetal ultrasound scan. Ultrasound Obstet Gynecol 2013;41(1):106; with permission.

**Table 3**
**Percent success rate of visualization of structures using transvaginal and transabdominal ultrasound in combination**

| Structures | 11 wk (%) | 12 wk (%) | 13 wk (%) | 14 wk (%) |
|---|---|---|---|---|
| Brain | 90 | 99 | 100 | 100 |
| Spine | 92 | 99 | 100 | 100 |
| Face | 95 | 99 | 100 | 100 |
| Lungs | 96 | 99 | 99 | 100 |
| Heart | 83 | 96 | 98 | 98 |
| Abdomen | 99 | 100 | 100 | 100 |
| Gastrointestinal | 97 | 99 | 99 | 100 |
| Kidneys | 86 | 97 | 99 | 99 |
| Limbs | 99 | 100 | 100 | 100 |

*Adapted from* Whitlow BJ, Economides DL. The optimal gestational age to examine fetal anatomy and measure nuchal translucency in the first trimester. Ultrasound Obstet Gynecol 1998;11(4):260; with permission.

Several studies have investigated the ability to visualize heart views during the first trimester, a notably more challenging feat. Haak and van Vugt[25] found that the 4-chamber view could be visualized between 10 and 13 6/7 weeks with nearly 100% detection rate (>98%) by 13 + 6 weeks. These findings echoed those of Gembruch and colleagues[26] in 1993 and were repeated in 2000,[27] which also found that by 13 6/7 weeks, 100% of the 4-chamber view and outflow tracts can be seen. These results were of note in contrast to Johnson and colleagues[28] in 1992, who demonstrated an inability to see most of the 4-chamber view and outflow tracking combination (**Tables 4** and **5**).

Vimpelli and colleagues[29] also found slightly lower detection rates when evaluating cardiac views in first-trimester imaging; out of an unselected study population looking at the 4-chamber view, the outflow tracts, the 3-vessel view, aortic arch, and ductal arch, all views could be seen in 62% of patients between 11 to 13 and 6 weeks. There was an almost 74% detection rate of the 4-chamber view at the GA whereby the views were in the highest (**Fig. 10**).

In the early 2000s, feasibility studies were performed to evaluate the implementation of anatomic evaluation of fetuses in the first trimester given that in the United States, most scans were done by sonographers and not physicians like in Europe and other parts of the world. Timor-Tritsch and colleagues[30] analyzed a study population of 223 patients with 7 sonographers divided into 2 groups evaluating studies at 11 to 12 weeks versus at 13 to 14 weeks. Both TV and TA scanning were performed, and 37 structures in total were evaluated. Overall, time spent per scan was 20 to 23 minutes. The detection rates are noted in the corresponding **Table 6**. Of note, the lowest detection rates were seen for 4-chamber heart view, aortic arch, ductal arch, left ventricular outflow tract (LVOT), right ventricular outflow tract (RVOT), and genitalia. There was a significantly more difficult time obtaining the 4-chamber view at 11 to 12 weeks (detected 27% of the time vs 41% at 13–14 weeks). RVOT was visualized at 61% at 13 to 14 weeks; LVOT at 58%. All other structures were identified more than 90% of the time. Overall, despite these numbers, the anatomy scans were feasible at 11 to 14 weeks, albeit with detection rates slightly lower than expected. The study concluded that an early fetal anatomy scan can effectively be done by well-trained, experienced sonographers, and a 13- to 14-week scan is more effective than an 11- to 12-week scan. TV scanning was significantly more useful than TA as well.

Souka and colleagues[31] found very similar results in their feasibility study examining cardiac and noncardiac anatomy in a low-risk population of 1144 patients. Noncardiac anatomy was successfully seen in 86% of patients, specifically in 84% of patients

**Table 4**
**Visualization rate of 4-chamber heart by gestational age**

| Author | 10 – 10 + 6 | 11 – 11 + 6 | 12 + 12 + 6 | 13 – 13 + 6 |
|---|---|---|---|---|
| Dolkart,[48] 1991 | 0 | 30 | 90 | 100 |
| Johnson et al,[28] 1992 | 27 | 58 | 71 | 74 |
| Bronshtein & Blumenfeld,[2] 1992 | NE | 17 | 36 | 100 |
| Gembruch et al,[26] 1993 | NE | 80 | 93 | 100 |
| Gembruch,[49] 2000 | 56 | 88 | 93 | 100 |
| Haak & van Vugt,[25] 2003 | NE | 85 | 97 | 98 |

*Abbreviation:* NE, not evaluated.

*Adapted from* Haak MC, van Vugt JMG. Echocardiography in early pregnancy: review of literature. J Ultrasound Med 2003;22:274; with permission.

**Table 5**
**Visualization rate of 4-chamber view and outflow tracts by gestational age**

| Authors | 10 – 10 + 6 | 11 – 11 + 6 | 12 – 12 + 6 | 13 – 13 + 6 |
|---|---|---|---|---|
| Johnson et al,[28] 1992 | 0 | 0 | 31 | 43 |
| Gembruch et al,[26] 1993 | NE | 67 | 80 | 100 |
| Gembruch et al,[27] 2000 | 44 | 75 | 93 | 100 |
| Haak & van Vugt,[25] 2003 | NE | 20 | 60 | 92 |

*Adapted from* Haak MC, van Vugt JMG. Echocardiography in early pregnancy: review of literature. J Ultrasound Med 2003;22:275; with permission.

when CRL was 45 to 54 mm and in 96% when CRL was greater than 65 mm. The 4-chamber view was seen in 93% at 13 weeks and 97% at 14 weeks. The investigators concluded that fetal anatomy examination is feasible during the routine 11- to 14-weeks scan, although the optimal time to examine cardiac and noncardiac anatomy is at 12 weeks to the end of the 13th week. TV approach is undoubtedly important to incorporate.

More specifically, just obtaining a first-trimester cardiac axis is a useful screen for fetal congenital heart defect in early gestation.[32] A case-control study of 197 fetuses demonstrated that an abnormal cardiac axis was able to detect two-thirds of fetuses with congenital heart disease and recommend the addition of cardiac axis to the first-trimester US assessment.

Later studies found more consistently high success rates evaluating fetal anatomy in the first trimester. A randomized, prospective trial of first-trimester screening by Timor-Tritsch and colleagues[33] showed that when one uses a trained sonographer or sonologist using high-frequency TVUS and TAUS, 37 anatomic structures can be successfully visualized in most cases. They concluded that there was an urgent need to evaluate first-trimester anatomy and determine what role it would ultimately play in the current standard of practice.

Similarly, Luchi and colleagues[34] performed an observational study to evaluate the feasibility of a detailed anatomy scan in assessing fetal organs, structures, and systems in the first trimester. They divided 977 singletons undergoing first-trimester screening for aneuploidies into 3 groups by GA and CRL. Of note, the scans were performed by a single operator and targeted 26 fetal anatomic structures. The overall detection rate was 96% at 11 weeks and reached 100% at 12 and 13 weeks, with a significant standard deviation between 11 and 12/13 weeks for most anatomic structures. They concluded that evaluation of fetal structures in the first trimester is feasible with high accuracy, and furthermore, visualization of most fetal organs improves from 11 to 13 weeks.

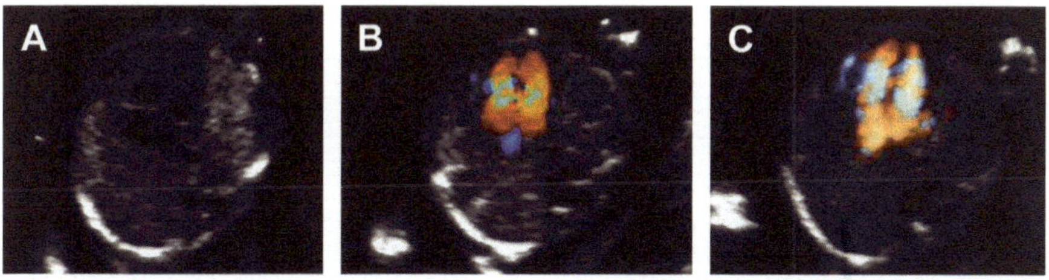


**Fig. 10.** Cardiac axis with 4-chamber view. (*A*) 2D US. (*B*) 2D + color Doppler. (*C*) 2D + HD, color Doppler.

**Table 6**
**Visualization rates by structures and gestational age (% visualized)**

| Structures Visualized | 11–12 wk GA | 13–14 wk GA |
|---|---|---|
| Head-intracranial anatomy | 95 | 95 |
| Choroid plexus | 95 | 95 |
| Cerebellum | 52 | 69 |
| Calvarium | 99 | 98 |
| Lateral ventricles | 99 | 92 |
| Face | 74 | 83 |
| Lenses | 88 | 89 |
| NT | 96 | 93 |
| Profile | 91 | 89 |
| Nose/lips | 71 | 79 |
| Spine, cervical | 80 | 89 |
| Thoracic | 81 | 87 |
| Lumbar | 71 | 77 |
| Sacral | 35 | 48 |
| Heart, axis | 71 | 73 |
| Four-chamber view | 27 | 41 |
| Aortic arch | 18 | 30 |
| Ductal arch | 15 | 24 |
| LVOT | 39 | 58 |
| RVOT | 37 | 61 |
| Chest and abdomen | | |
| Lungs | 64 | 77 |
| Diaphragm | 87 | 92 |
| Kidneys | 81 | 91 |
| Bladder | 93 | 96 |
| Stomach | 98 | 98 |
| Genitalia | 32 | 50 |
| Cord vessels | 84 | 90 |
| Abdominal wall | 97 | 96 |
| Bowel | 77 | 88 |
| Extremities | | |
| Humerus | 98 | 97 |
| Radius/ulna | 95 | 98 |
| Hands | 98 | 98 |
| Fingers | 86 | 93 |
| Femur | 98 | 97 |
| Tibia/fibula | 93 | 94 |
| Feet | 98 | 93 |
| Placental location | 100 | 100 |
| Time spent for scan | 20 ± 11′ | 23 ± 11′ |

*Adapted from* Timor-Tritsch IE, Bashiri A, Monteagudo A, et al. Qualified and trained sonographers in the US can perform early fetal anatomy scans between 11 and 14 weeks. Am J Obstet Gynecol 2004;191(4):1249; with permission.

A systematic review by Rossi and Prefumo[35] analyzed the accuracy and efficacy of early US in identifying fetal anomalies between 11 and 14 weeks of gestation. Nineteen articles were included with a total of 78,002 fetuses that underwent US at 11 to 14 weeks. In total, 996 malformations were present; 472 (51%) were detected. Neck anomalies yielded the highest detection rate (92%); limbs (34%), face (34%), and genitourinary anomalies (34%) yielded the lowest. Fetal echocardiograms performed at less than 14 weeks detected 53% of congenital heart disease. Overall, the detection rate was highest when combining both the TA and the TV approach (63%) as compared with TA (51%) or TV (34%) alone.

A more recent systematic review by Karim and colleagues[36] analyzed 30 studies to assess the diagnostic accuracy of US in the detection of congenital fetal anomalies before 14 weeks' gestation. The pooled estimate for detection of major abnormalities in low-risk populations (19 studies, 115,731 fetuses) was 46.1%; the detection for all abnormalities in this group was 32.35%. In high-risk populations (6 studies, 2841 fetuses), the overall detection rate was 61.18%. The study also found that the use of a standardized anatomic protocol improved the sensitivity of first-trimester US screening for all anomalies and major anomalies; the investigators recommended that such a protocol should be undertaken to optimize first-trimester anomaly detection.

Kenkhuis and colleagues[37] looked at 5534 patients who underwent a 12- to 13-week gestation scan in addition to the usual 20-week anomaly scan. Out of 85 total anomalies detected prenatally, 54 (63.5%) were detected on the early scan, including 100% of all severe anomalies (neural tube defect, omphalocele, megacystis, severe congenital and severe skeletal anomalies). Thus, an early scan by a competent sonographer can detect about half of the prenatally detectable structural anomalies and 100% of those expected to be seen at this stage.

Petousis and colleagues[38] recently conducted a prospective observational study on routine scans at 11 to 13 + 6 weeks with similar findings. First-trimester findings were compared with those of the anomaly scan at 20 to 23 + 6 weeks and the postnatal examination. After excluding 17 chromosomal abnormalities, major fetal structural defects were seen in 57 (1.7%) of 3361 cases; of these, 27 (47.3%) were seen at 11 to 13 + 6 weeks, including all cases of acrania, exomphalos, megacystis, and body stalk anomaly. In addition, 36.4% (4/11) of major cardiac defects, 38% (6/16) of limb defects, and 100% (2/2) of facial clefts were seen. In conclusion, targeted US examination may identify 100% of the "always" detectable major abnormalities and a portion of the "sometimes" detectable anomalies in the first trimester.

## WHAT DOES THIS MEAN FOR SECOND-TRIMESTER ULTRASOUNDS?

With the advent of first-trimester anatomy US evaluation, some raised the question of what role the second-trimester scan served and how its role could potentially be altered. In 1 study specifically looking at early fetal anomaly scanning in a population at increased risk for abnormalities, 101 fetuses were scanned at 11 to 14 weeks of gestation by both TVUS and TAUS.[39] Additional scans were performed at 18 to 21 and 30 to 32 weeks. Overall, 11% of anomalies were found; 9 of the 11 were found at 11 to 14 weeks. When the 11- to 14- and 18- to 21-week scans were combined, 91% of all malformations were detected. The investigators concluded that although late first-trimester US can diagnose most anomalies in an at-risk population, the addition of an 18- to 22-week scan is essential.

A 5-year prospective study by Ebrashy and colleagues[40] had similar findings. TA scans were performed on 2876 patients at 13 to 14 weeks; if a full fetal anatomic survey was not achieved, a TVUS was performed as well. In total, 1350 TVUS were performed. A midtrimester fetal anatomy scan was then performed in patients who had not dropped out, miscarried, or undergone pregnancy termination. TVUS was significantly better in visualizing the cranium, spine, stomach, kidneys, bladder, and upper and lower limbs as compared with TAUS. Complete fetal anatomy surveys were achieved in 64% of TA scans and 82% of TV scans. However, heart and kidneys were not properly visualized in 42% of TAUS and 27% of TVUS at 13 weeks. In comparison, they were not fully visualized in only 1.6% of TAUS and 0% of TVUS in the second-trimester scans. In total, 31 anomalies were detected across both trimesters. In the first trimester, 21 were detected, and 14 resulted in termination of the pregnancy. In the second trimester, there were 10 new anomalous cases detected. Thus, although earlier scanning has great potential for visualizing with fetal anatomy with accuracy and TVUS can be used to complement TAUS, second-trimester scans remain crucial for detailed fetal anatomic survey.

## FIRST-TRIMESTER ULTRASOUND AND MATERNAL OBESITY

Increasing maternal obesity has significantly impacted US visualization in this growing patient subgroup, especially in TA imaging. Maternal obesity increases the rate of subvisualization of fetal cardiac and craniospinal structures and may require visualization of the structures after 18 to 22 weeks using the TA approach.[41] Tsai and colleagues[42] in 2010 assessed that complete visualization was achieved in at least 7 to 8 markers, but the changes demonstrated that completion rates for US screening and detection of aneuploidy were inversely related to maternal obesity. Obese women end up by and large being underscreened, especially if they were not able to obtain a fetal anatomic survey until the second trimester (**Figs. 11** and **12**, **Tables 7** and **8**).

## FIRST-TRIMESTER ULTRASOUND AND ANEUPLOIDY SCREENING

First-trimester US plays a large role in aneuploidy screening. Traditionally, the first-trimester risk assessment incorporated NT with maternal serum analytes for aneuploidy screening. In a recent study, Grande and colleagues[43] sought to assess the sensitivity of first-trimester US for diagnosing different structural anomalies in chromosomally normal pregnancies. Out of 13,723 first-trimester scans, 439 (3.2%) fetuses with structural anomalies were identified (194 major, 245 minor). Of the major structural anomalies, 49% were detected in the first trimester. Of those, 69% of skeletal and 57% of cardiac anomalies were associated with an increased NT (38%) or abnormal ductus venosus flow (52%). Interestingly, they did not find that an absent nasal bone was associated with any structural defects. Traditionally, hypoplastic or not ossified nasal bones are associated with trisomy 21 and other aneuploidies.

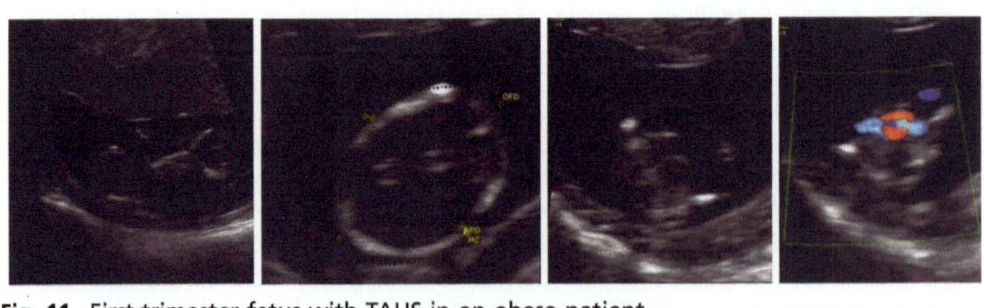

**Fig. 11.** First-trimester fetus with TAUS in an obese patient.

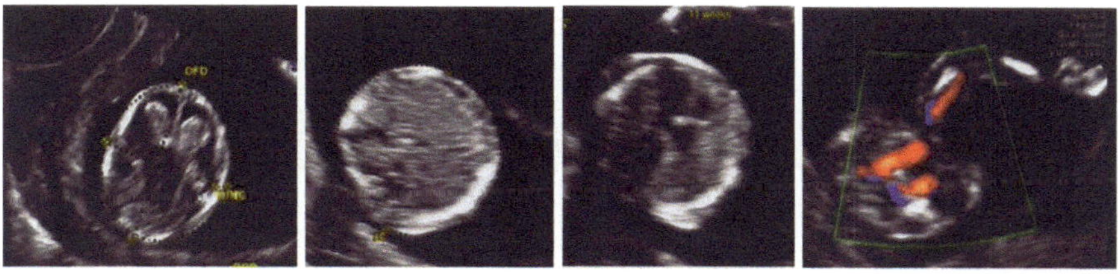

**Fig. 12.** First-trimester fetus with TVUS in an obese patient.

Overall, Grande and colleagues' study results suggested about 50% of major structural abnormalities can be diagnosed in the first trimester and having an increased NT or abnormal ductus venosus is associated with cardiac and skeletal defects. This study established a role for aneuploidy markers in the detection of abnormalities, which may facilitate early detection (**Fig. 13**).

Becker and colleagues[44] also recently reviewed 6879 consecutive fetuses in which 6565 had a "normal" NT (≤95%ile) and 314 had an increased NT (>95%ile). All fetuses received a first-trimester TAUS and a fetal echocardiogram. The prevalence of major anomalies in fetuses with a "normal" NT was 1.7%, of which 87.4% of these diagnoses were made prenatally. Furthermore, 29.8% of chromosomal abnormalities were in the "normal" NT group, and 77% of the major anomalies accompanied by a normal karyotype were found in this group as well. Overall, a relevant number of major anomalies is seen in fetuses with a "normal" NT, and of those, more than half can be detected by first-trimester scans. Thus, fetuses with "normal" NT should still be offered detailed anatomic scanning in the second trimester.

Iliescu and colleagues[45] proposed using an extended US examination protocol in their prospective study of 5472 women at 12 to 13 + 6 weeks' gestation. All women were examined using an extended US protocol that involved a color Doppler cardiac sweep and identification of early contingent markers for major abnormalities. The prevalence of lethal and severe malformations was 1.39%. Of these, the first-trimester scans detected 40.6% of the cases overall and 76.3% of major structural defects. Ninety percent of major congenital heart disease and 69.5% of major central nervous system anomalies were detected. Furthermore, the detection rate for major anomalies in fetuses with increased NT was 96%; in fetuses with normal NT, it was 66.7%. Most cases (67.1%) with major abnormalities presented with normal NT.

**Table 7**
**The impact of maternal obesity on midtrimester sonographic visualization of fetal cardiac and craniospinal structures**

| Group | Category | BMI (kg/m²) | % SUV-Cardiac | % SUV-Craniospinal |
|---|---|---|---|---|
| I | Nonobese | <30 | 19 | 29 |
| II | Class I obesity | 30–34 | 30 | 37 |
| III | Class II obesity | 35–39 | 39 | 43 |
| IV | Class III obesity | >40 | 49 | 53 |

*Abbreviations:* BMI, body mass index; SUV, sonographic visualization.

*Modified from* Hendler I, Blackwell SC, Bujold E, et al. The impact of maternal obesity on midtrimester sonographic visualization of fetal cardiac and craniospinal structures. Int J Obes Relat Metab Disord 2004;28(12):1610.

**Table 8**
**Ultrasound screening for fetal aneuploidy in the overweight and obese gravida**

| | Normal (%) | Overweight (%) | Obese: Class I (%) | Obese: Class II (%) | Obese: Class III (%) | *P* Value |
|---|---|---|---|---|---|---|
| Completion rates | 64 | 64 | 61 | 55 | 47 | <.001 |
| Screen positive rates (≥1 marker) | 16 | 13 | 15 | 12 | 10 | <.02 |

Conclusion: Completion rates for US aneuploidy screening are inversely related to maternal obesity. Obese women are underscreened as a whole.

*Adapted from* Tsai LJ, Ho M, Pressman EK, et al. Ultrasound screening for fetal aneuploidy using soft markers in the overweight and obese gravida. Perinat Diagn 2010;30(9):823; with permission.

In recent years, the advent of using cell-free DNA via NIPT has been increasingly incorporated into practice as an adjunct to traditional aneuploidy screening. Rao and colleagues[46] performed a retrospective review of the utility of first-trimester US in the setting of NIPT incorporation into practice. Out of 1906 patients who underwent first-trimester scans, 959 (50%) also had NIPT performed. Although the US detected 42 fetal (2.2%), 286 gynecologic (15.0%), and 317 placental (16.6%) findings, NIPT results were discordant with US findings in 18/42 (42%) cases. Subgroup analysis revealed that cell-free DNA as the sole method of prenatal screening in the first trimester would miss 95% of the fetal findings detected with US. Thus, a comprehensive first-trimester US provides valuable clinical information about fetal and maternal anatomy that cannot be detected with NIPT alone and should remain an important clinical tool in prenatal diagnosis despite the convenience of NIPT.

## FIRST-TRIMESTER ULTRASOUND ANOMALIES

In light of these study findings, **Figs. 14–28** demonstrate various examples of first-trimester US scans and various findings visualized using high-frequency vaginal transducers.

## THE ADVANTAGES OF EARLY SCANS AND DETECTION

Many benefits can arise from early scanning and detection of possible anomalies. In general, earlier recognition of normal anatomy, when present, aids in decreasing patient anxiety. More importantly, when malformations are encountered, the patient's

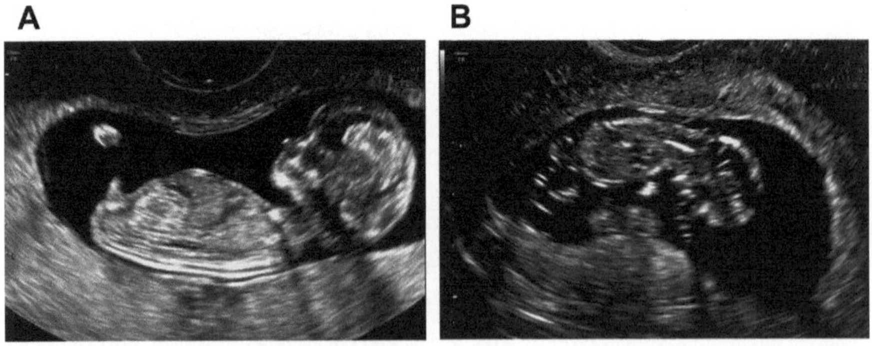

**Fig. 13.** (*A*) Nasal bone with (*B*) increased NT.

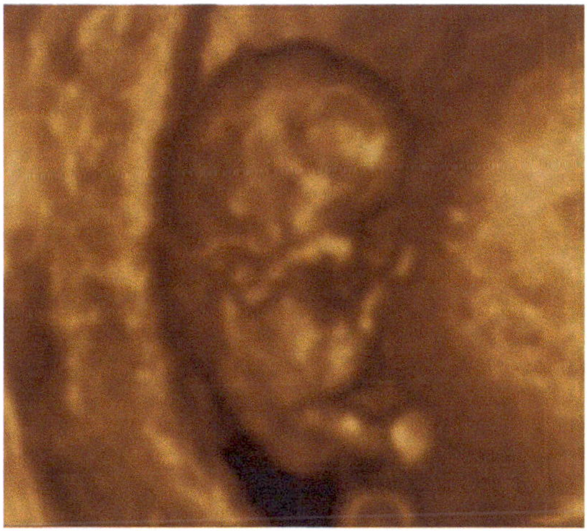

**Fig. 14.** Midgut herniation.

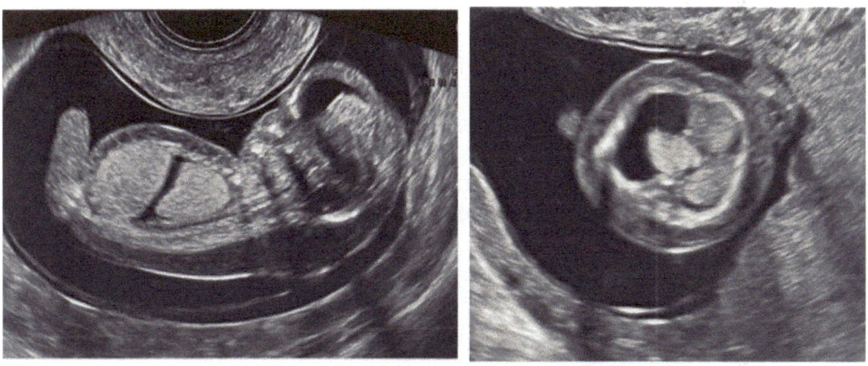

**Fig. 15.** Fetus at 12 weeks of gestation with increased NT and hydrops.

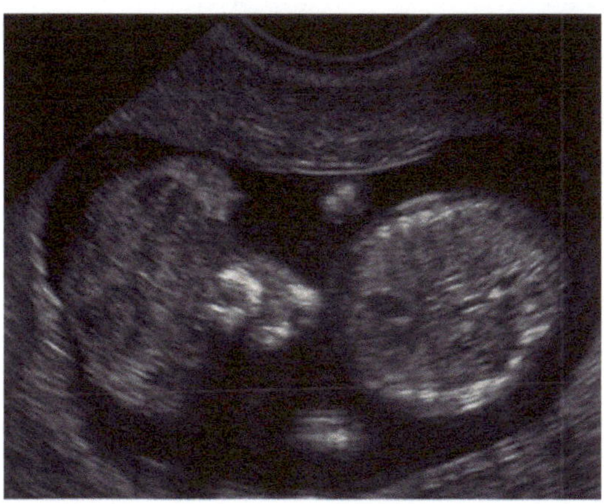

**Fig. 16.** Anencephaly.

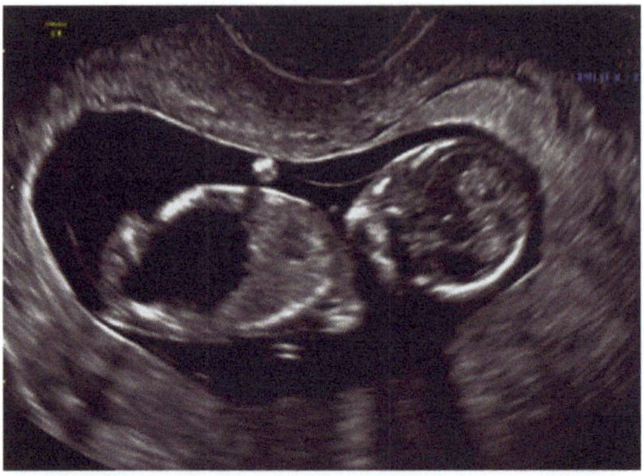

Fig. 17. Fetus at 12 weeks and 4 days of gestation with bladder obstruction with posterior urethral valves.

choice of termination remains. In Kenkhuis and colleagues'[37] study, after first- or second-trimester diagnosis of an anomaly, parents elected for termination of pregnancy in 83.3% and 25.8% of cases, respectively.

Earlier termination, when necessary, is safer, psychologically easier for the patient, and more commonly available in the community. Second-trimester terminations are more difficult to perform, and there are significantly fewer trained individuals nationwide, due in part to recent political discourse regarding reproductive rights. Studies from the Centers for Disease Control and Prevention have shown that complications were less common in first-trimester terminations.[47] Overall, a dilation-and-curettage abortion procedure at 11 to 12 weeks has a death rate of 1.1 per 100,000, as compared with a dilation-and-evacuation procedure at 16 to

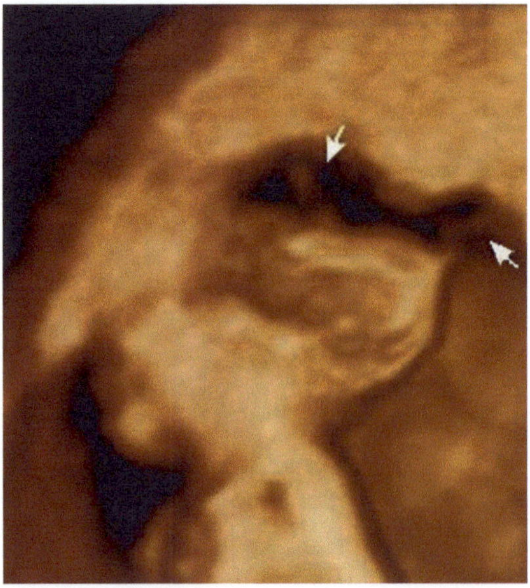

Fig. 18. Amniotic band syndrome (*arrows*) seen on 3D US.

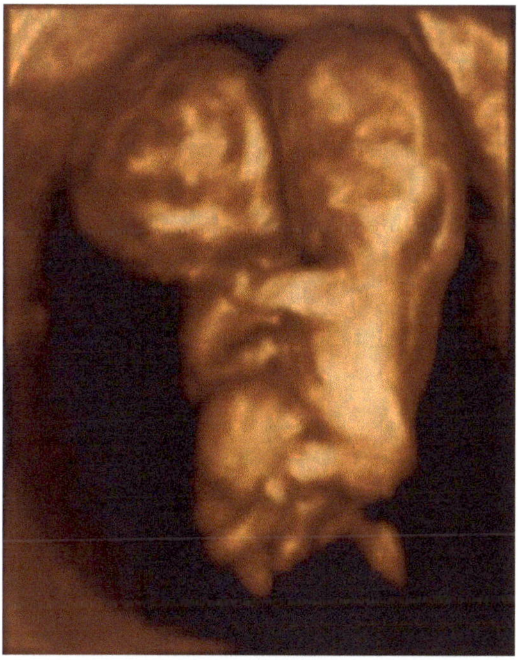

Fig. 19. Thoracopagus seen at 10 weeks of gestation.

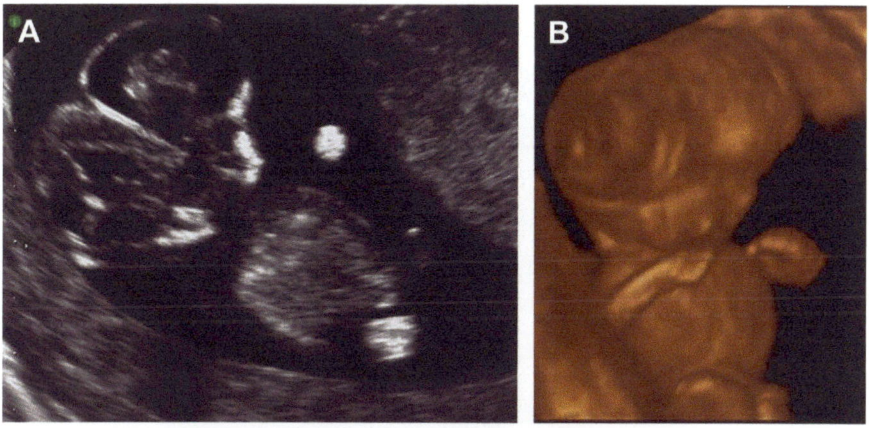


Fig. 20. (*A*, *B*) Dicephalus diagnosed at 10 weeks of gestation.

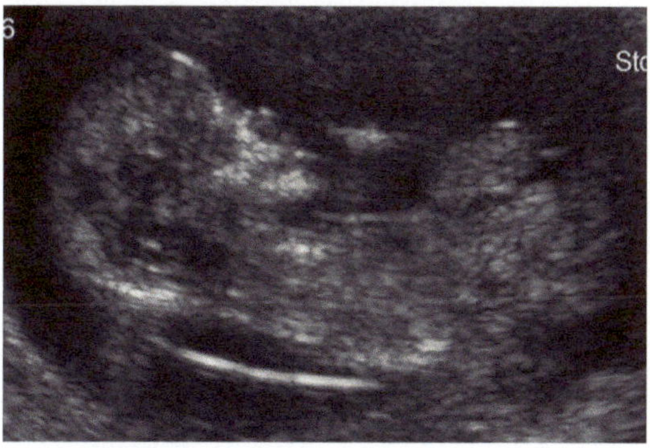

Fig. 21. Limb-body-wall complex at 12 weeks.

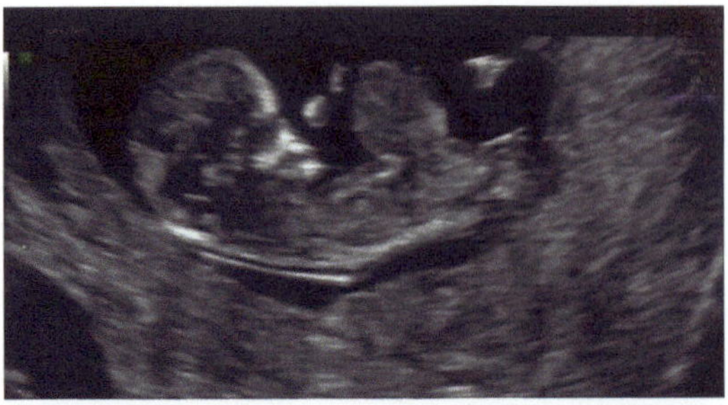

**Fig. 22.** Omphalocele diagnosed at 11 weeks of gestation as well as neural tube defect.

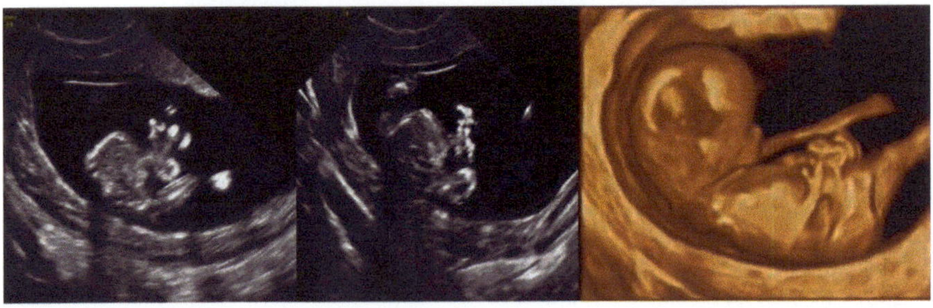

**Fig. 23.** Gastroschisis.

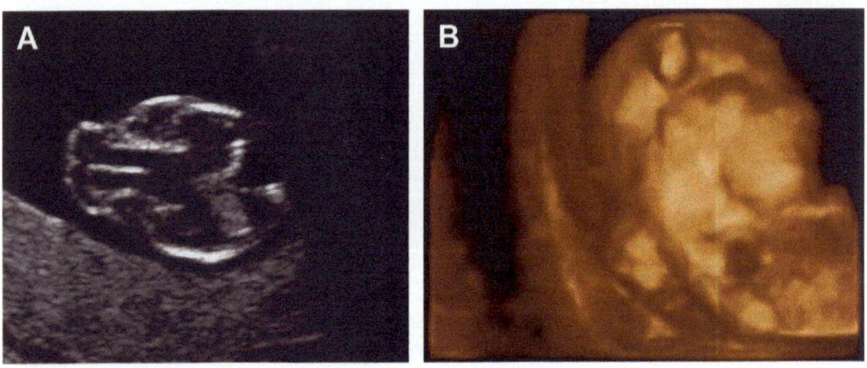


**Fig. 24.** (*A*, *B*) Neural tube defect.

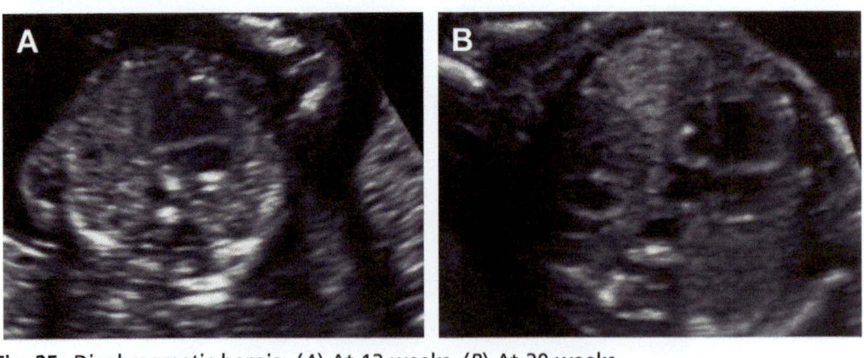


**Fig. 25.** Diaphragmatic hernia. (*A*) At 13 weeks. (*B*) At 20 weeks.

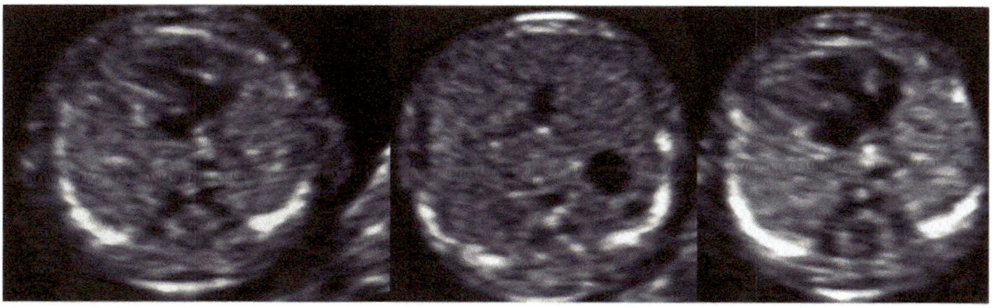

Fig. 26. Abnormal situs.

20 weeks, at which point the rate increases to 6.5 per 100,000. Earlier detection of major anomalies provides the patient with the benefit of more information to make an informed decision.

## WHAT IS NEXT

With continued improvement of US technology and more frequent use of TV imaging, more fetal anatomy can be seen at earlier GAs than ever before. Guidelines for imaging parameters in the first trimester, as noted earlier, are evolving, and the expectations for a more detailed anatomic survey will be suggested.

However, given that certain structures are still not fully developed at earlier GAs, the need for a second-trimester scan is still very relevant.

At this time, limitations lie in the evaluation of certain organ structures, although high-frequency transducers make the task easier. If the organ is or was developed at that stage of pregnancy, it can be seen. If there is a major malformation, it too should be seen. Achieving these goals may require a review of embryology to understand what is normal and abnormal as well as better training programs to teach essentials of scanning in the first trimester. Although there is a gap in training and expertise at this point, one will never reach the detection rate that is possible unless one begins to look. The experience of the quality assurance programs put in place for NT monitoring reveals the possibility of improvement in scanning over time with epidemiologic monitoring. It thus seems possible to expect an ever-higher level of performance in the detection of fetal abnormalities in the first trimester.

Based on current literature, it is clear that fetal anatomy is recognizable on a first-trimester scan. In the new era of prenatal diagnosis with cell-free DNA, the need to enhance imaging capabilities is evr increasingly upon us. Including a thorough anatomic scan on first-trimester US is the next frontier in providing standard of care.

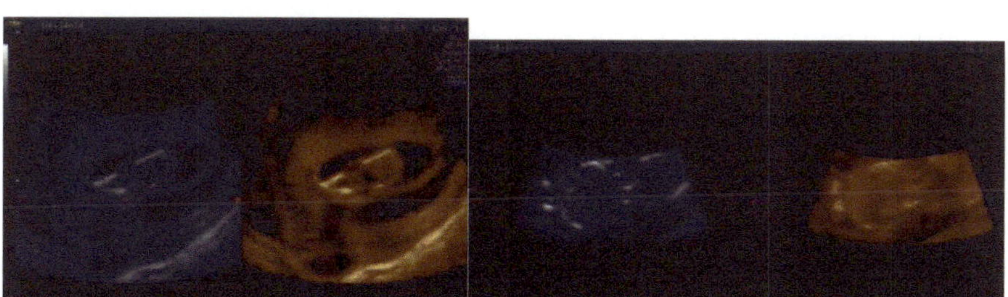

Fig. 27. Sirenomelia, otherwise known as sacral agenesis.

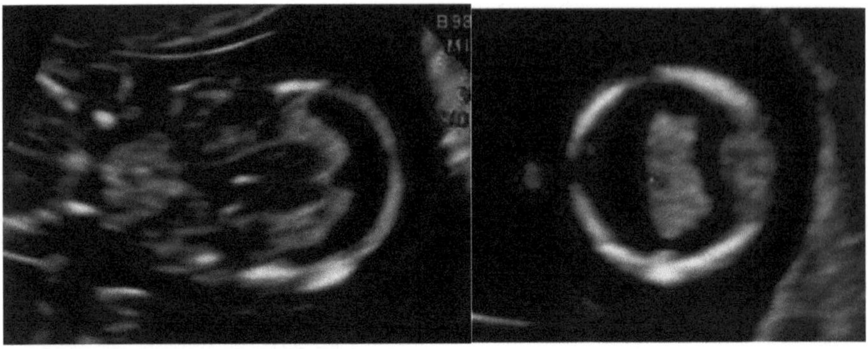

**Fig. 28.** Alobar holoprosencephaly.

## REFERENCES


1. Achiron R, Tadmor O. Screening for fetal anomalies during the first trimester of pregnancy: transvaginal versus transabdominal sonography. Ultrasound Obstet Gynecol 1991;1:186–91.
2. Bronshtein M, Blumenfeld Z. Transvaginal sonography-detection of findings suggestive of fetal chromosomal anomalies in the first and early second trimester. Prenat Diagn 1992;12:587–93.
3. Bronshten M, Siegler E, Eshcoli Z, et al. Transvaginal ultrasound measurements of the fetal heart at 11 to 17 weeks of gestation. Am J Perinatol 1992;9:38–42.
4. Gembruch U, Knopfle G, Chatterjee M, et al. First-trimester diagnosis of fetal congenital heart disease by transvaginal two-dimensional and Doppler echocardiography. Obstet Gynecol 1990;75:496–8.
5. Rottem S, Bronshtein M. Transvaginal sonographic diagnosis of congenital anomalies between 9 weeks and 16 weeks, menstrual age. J Clin Ultrasound 1990;18: 307–14.
6. Szabo J, Gellen J. Nuchal fluid accumulation in trisomy-21 detected by vaginosonography in first trimester. Lancet 1990;336:1133.
7. Schulte-Vallentin M, Schindler H. Non-echogenic nuchal oedema as a marker in trisomy 21 screening. Lancet 1992;339:1053.
8. Nicolaides KH, Azar G, Byrne D, et al. Fetal nuchal translucency: ultrasound screening for chromosomal defects in first trimester of pregnancy. BMJ (Clin Res Ed) 1992;304:867–9.
9. Afshar Y, Gutkin R, Krakow D, et al. First-trimester abdominal circumference (versus crown rump length) improves precision in inter- and intraobserver variability. J Ultrasound Med 2018. https://doi.org/10.1002/jum.14913.
10. Salomon LJ, Alfirevic Z, Bilardo CM, et al. ISUOG practice guidelines: performance of first-trimester fetal ultrasound scan. Ultrasound Obstet Gynecol 2013; 41:102–13.
11. ACOG Practice Bulletin No. 163: screening for fetal aneuploidy. Obstet Gynecol 2016;127:e123–37.
12. Shah FT, French KS, Osann KE, et al. Impact of cell-free fetal DNA screening on patients' choice of invasive procedures after a positive California prenatal screen result. J Clin Med 2014;3:849–64.

13. Lambert-Messerlian G, Palomaki GE. Fewer women aged 35 and older choose serum screening for Down's syndrome: impact and implications. J Med Screen 2018. https://doi.org/10.1177/0969141318797961.
14. Nicolaides KH. Screening for fetal aneuploidies at 11 to 13 weeks. Prenat Diagn 2011;31:7–15.
15. Nicolaides KH. The fetal medicine foundation. Available at: http://fetalmedicine.org. Accessed February 28, 2018.
16. D'Alton ME, Fuchs KM, Abuhammad A, et al. Implementation of a national nuchal translucency education and quality monitoring program. Nuchal Translucency Quality Review Program. Obstet Gynecol 2014;123:149–54.
17. Cuckle H, Platt LD, Thornburg LL, et al. Nuchal Translucency Quality Review (NTQR) program: first one and half million results. Ultrasound Obstet Gynecol 2015;45:199–204.
18. International Society of Ultrasound in Obstetrics and Gynecology. Official statement on safety. Ultrasound Obstet Gynecol 2003;21:100.
19. International Society of Ultrasound in Obstetrics and Gynecology. Official statement on the safe use of Doppler in the 11 to 13+6 week fetal ultrasound examination. Ultrasound Obstet Gynecol 2011,37.628.
20. Sheiner E, Hackmon R, Shoham-Vardi I, et al. A comparison between acoustic output indices in 2D and 3D/4D ultrasound in obstetrics. Ultrasound Obstet Gynecol 2007;29(3):326–8.
21. De Basio P, Prefumo E, Lantieri PB, et al. Reference values for fetal limb biometry at 10-14 weeks of gestation. Ultrasound Obstet Gynecol 2002;20:42–6.
22. Whitlow BJ, Economides DL. The optimal gestational age to examine fetal anatomy and measure nuchal translucency in the first trimester. Ultrasound Obstet Gynecol 1998;11:258–61.
23. Huggon IC, Ghi T, CookA C, et al. Fetal cardiac abnormalities identified prior to 14 weeks' gestation. Ultrasound Obstet Gynecol 2002;20:22–9.
24. Pitalis A, Basagiannis C, Eleftheriades M, et al. Evaluation of a two-step ultrasound examination protocol for the detection of major fetal structural defects. J Matern Fetal Neonatal Med 2012;25:1814–7.
25. Haak MC, van Vugt JM. Echocardiography in early pregnancy: review of literature. J Ultrasound Med 2003;22:271–80.
26. Gembruch U, Knöpfle G, Bald R, et al. Early diagnosis of fetal congenital heart disease by the echocardiography. Ultrasound Obstet Gynecol 1993;3:310–7.
27. Gembruch U, Shi C, Smrcek JM. Biometry of the fetal heart between 1 and 17 weeks of gestation. Fetal Diagn Ther 2000;15:20–31.
28. Johnson P, Sharland G, Maxwell D, et al. The role of transvaginal sonography in the early detection of congenital heart disease. Ultrasound Obstet Gynecol 1992; 2:248–51.
29. Vimpelli T, Huhtala H, Acharya G. Fetal echocardiography during routine first-trimester screening: a feasibility study in an unselected population. Prenat Diagn 2006;26:475–82.
30. Timor-Tritsch IE, Bashiri A, Monteagudo A, et al. Qualified and trained sonographers in the US can perform early fetal anatomy scans between 11 and 14weeks. Am J Obstet Gynecol 2004;191:1247–52.
31. Souka AP, Pilalis A, Kavalakis Y, et al. Assessment of fetal anatomy at the 11-14 week ultrasound examination. Ultrasound Obstet Gynecol 2004;24:730–4.
32. Sinkovskaya ES, Chaoui R, Karl K, et al. Fetal cardiac axis and congenital heart defects in early gestation. Obstet Gynecol 2015;125:453–60.

33. Timor-Tritsch IE, Fuchs KM, Monteagudo A, et al. Performing a fetal anatomy scan at the time of first-trimester screening. Obstet Gynecol 2009;113:402–7.
34. Luchi C, Schifano M, Sacchini C, et al. Detailed fetal anatomy assessment in the first trimester at 11, 12, and 13 weeks of gestation. J Matern Fetal Neonatal Med 2012;256:675–8.
35. Rossi CA, Prefumo F. Accuracy of ultrasonography at 11-14 weeks of gestation for detection of fetal structural anomalies. Obstet Gynecol 2013;122:1160–7.
36. Karim JN, Roberts NW, Salomon LJ, et al. Systematic review of first-trimester ultrasound screening for detection of fetal structural anomalies and factors that affect screening performance. Ultrasound Obstet Gynecol 2017;50:429–41.
37. Kenkhuis MJA, Bakker M, Bardi F, et al. Effectiveness of 12-13 week scan for early diagnosis of fetal congenital anomalies in the cell-free DNA era. Ultrasound Obstet Gynecol 2013;51:463–9.
38. Petousis S, Sotiriadis A, Margioula-Siarkou C, et al. Detection of structural abnormalities in fetuses with normal karyotype at 11-13 weeks using the anatomic examination protocol of the International Society of Ultrasound in Obstetrics and Gynecology (ISUOG). J Matern Fetal Neonatal Med 2019;1–7.
39. den Hollander, Wessels MW, Niermeijer MF, et al. Early fetal anomaly scanning in a population at increased risk of abnormalities. Ultrasound Obstet Gynecol 2002; 19(6):570–4.
40. Ebrashy A, El Kateb A, Momtaz M, et al. 13-14-week fetal anatomy scan: a 5-year prospective study. Ultrasound Obstet Gynecol 2010;35:292–6.
41. Hendler I, Blackwell SC, Bujold E, et al. The impact of maternal obesity on mid trimester sonographic visualization of fetal cardiac and craniospinal structures. Int J Obes Relat Metab Disord 2004;28:1607–11.
42. Tsai LJ, Ho M, Pressman EK, et al. Ultrasound screening for fetal aneuploidy using soft markers in the overweight and obese gravida. Perinat Diagn 2010;30: 821–6.
43. Grande M, Arigita M, Borobio V, et al. First-trimester detection of structural abnormalities and the role of aneuploidy markers. Ultrasound Obstet Gynecol 2012;39: 157–63.
44. Becker R, Schmitz L, Kilavuz S, et al. "Normal" nuchal translucency: a justification to refrain from detailed scan? Analysis of 6858 cases with special reference to ethical aspects. Prenat Diagn 2012;32:550–6.
45. Iliescu D, Tudorache S, Comanescu A, et al. Improved detection rate of structural abnormalities in the first trimester using an extended examination protocol. Ultrasound Obstet Gynecol 2013;42:300–9.
46. Rao R, Valderramos SG, Silverman NS, et al. The value of the first trimester ultrasound in the era of cell free DNA screening. Prenat Diagn 2016;36:1192–8.
47. Lawson HW, Frye A, Atrash HK, et al. Abortion mortality, United States,1972 through 1987. Am J Obstet Gynecol 1994;171:1365–72.
48. Dolkart LA, Reimers FT. Transvaginal fetal echocardiography in early pregnancy: normative data. Am J Obstet Gynecol 1991;165(3):688–91.
49. Gembruch U, Shi C, Smrcek JM. Biometry of the fetal heart between 10 and 17 weeks of gestation. Fetal Diagn Ther 2000;15(1):20–31.

# Coding and Legal Issues in Obstetric and Gynecologic Ultrasound

James M. Shwayder, MD, JD[a,*], Joshua A. Copel, MD[b], Hindi Stohl, MD, JD[c]

**KEYWORDS**

- Early pregnancy ultrasound • Obstetric ultrasound • Gynecologic ultrasound • Pelvic ultrasound • Ultrasound • Coding • Liability

**KEY POINTS**

- Current Procedural Terminology codes have specific requirements and parameters associated with each code.
- *International Classification of Diseases*, 10th edition, coding offers the ability to identify the reason for ultrasound performance, using the most specific codes available.
- Common errors leading to litigation include perception errors, interpretation errors, failure to suggest or properly counsel the next appropriate procedure or properly counsel patients about the implications of their findings, and failure to properly communicate critical findings to referring providers.

## INTRODUCTION

Areas not commonly addressed in ultrasound treatises are those of coding and liability related to ultrasound practice. The article discusses these important topics, initially addressing the proper Current Procedural Terminology (CPT) and *International Classification of Diseases*, 10th edition (ICD-10) coding in ultrasound practices while evaluating early pregnancy and gynecologic conditions. The second portion of the article discusses common errors leading to liability in obstetric and gynecologic ultrasound practice, using specific examples and cases to illustrate the concepts.

---

Disclosure Statement: J.M. Shwayder, Consultant: GE Ultrasound; J.A. Copel, Consultant: Jubel, LLC; H. Stohl, None.

[a] Shwayder Consulting, LLC, 13413 Orino Street, Venice, FL 34293, USA; [b] Yale School of Medicine, 333 Cedar Street, New Haven, CT 06510, USA; [c] Department of Obstetrics and Gynecology, Harbor-UCLA Medical Center, 1000 West Carson Street, Main Hospital, 7 West / Box 3, Torrance, CA 905509, USA
* Corresponding author.
*E-mail address:* jshwayder@hotmail.com

Obstet Gynecol Clin N Am 46 (2019) 853–862
https://doi.org/10.1016/j.ogc.2019.07.012
obgyn.theclinics.com

## GENERAL CONCEPTS FOR ULTRASOUND CODING

The rules for coding are established by the ICD-10 and the American Medical Association CPT books.[1,2] The ICD-10 book includes more than 141,000 codes that establish diagnoses that justify the performance of an ultrasound. The CPT code describes the ultrasound procedure(s) that was performed. When coding an encounter, one should use the ICD-10 code or codes that are confirmed or the definitive diagnosis documented in the ultrasound interpretation, using the greatest specificity available. If a definitive diagnosis is not available one then codes, in decreasing preference, the condition, problem, or symptom that led to the ultrasound examination.

There are 2 primary components of a CPT code: the professional component and the technical component. The professional component (denoted with the modifier -26) compensates the physician or provider for supervising the test, interpreting the test, and preparing a written report. The technical component (denoted with the modifier -TC) reimburses the costs associated with the sonographer's salary and benefits, the ultrasound equipment, and any necessary supplies. Each of the components has a relative value unit associated with it, adjusted for regional cost variants. The relative value unit for each CPT code is multiplied by a conversion factor established by the Centers for Medicare & Medicaid Services to determine the reimbursement for each CPT code. This factor often has a percentage adjustment to establish reimbursement for each procedural code, for example, Medicare plus 10%. CPT coding differs in provider-based (physician-owned) clinics and hospital-based clinics. An office owned by physicians bills a fully implemented nonfacility fee, without a modifier attached. The fee combines the professional component, the technical component, and includes any necessary supplies, including image storage. Thus, one cannot bill separately for supplies in a provider-based clinic. In contrast, in a hospital-based clinic the provider bills for the professional component by attaching the -26 modifier to the primary code, and the hospital bills separately for the technical component with the -TC modifier attached to the primary code. Hospital-based clinics can bill for supplies, such as catheters, needles, and medications, separately. If physicians perform scans themselves in the hospital, even with self-owned portable equipment, they must still attach the -26 modifier, unless they pay fair market value to the hospital for space or other supplies.

The Centers for Medicare & Medicaid Services also establishes the level of supervision required for various ultrasound procedures. Most obstetric and gynecologic ultrasound procedures only require general supervision. General supervision requires that the procedure is furnished under the physician's overall direction and control, with physician presence not required during the performance of the procedure. However, the training of the nonphysician personnel who perform the diagnostic procedure and equipment maintenance are the responsibility of the physician. Personal supervision is required for specific obstetric and gynecologic ultrasound procedures.[3] With personal supervision, the physician must be in attendance in the room during the performance of the procedure. The obstetric procedures requiring personal supervision include percutaneous umbilical cord blood sampling, chorionic villus sampling, and amniocentesis. The gynecologic ultrasound procedures requiring personal supervision include sonohysterography and sonosalpingography, also known as hysterocontrast-sonography.

## CODING FOR EARLY PREGNANCY ULTRASOUND EXAMINATIONS

Once pregnancy has been established, there are different codes for ultrasound scans. CPT (1) defines first trimester pregnancy as before 14 weeks + 0 days gestation. The code for first trimester sonography, 76801, includes evaluation of the fetus, uterus, and ovaries, so there are no additional codes to apply for examination of the uterus and adnexa. The location of the gestational sac should be described, and measurements of the fetus, if visible, are included. The optimal ultrasound tool for estimating gestational age is the crown-rump length (CRL). The mean diameter of the sac can also be used, but is subject to greater variance and should not be used if the CRL can be measured. Fetal cardiac activity should be documented either by real-time clips or m-mode. Owing to higher acoustic exposure of the fetus with pulsed Doppler ultrasound, this modality should be avoided. There are no additional applicable codes for including those.

Often it is necessary to scan vaginally for adequate visualization in the first trimester. When that is included, there should be image documentation and the 76817 code used. Both 76801 and 76817 can be used if both modalities are clinically indicated.

There is no maximum number of permissible 76801 scans, although there must be clinical indication for each encounter. Merely confirming fetal life at routine prenatal visits does not justify any ultrasound charge.

Suspected ectopic pregnancies can be handled either with obstetric or gynecologic codes. If a sac is established, even if it is ectopic, many use the obstetric codes, whereas if there is a suspected ectopic and no pregnancy can be identified, the gynecologic codes are more appropriate.

At present, there are no available codes for anatomy surveys performed before 14 weeks 0 days. The codes for fetal anatomic evaluation (76805 and 76811 for single or first gestations, 76810 or 76812 for additional fetuses in multiples), cannot be used in the first trimester. Short examinations in the first trimester can also be coded with 76815, for a limited examination, used when a single discrete clinical question is being evaluated.

When patients present for nuchal translucency evaluation the 76813 code is used (76814 for additional fetuses in multiples). The code includes CRL, fetal cardiac activity confirmation and measurement of the nuchal space. Further evaluation with 76801 should only be used if clinically indicated, and generally should not be included if a prior 76801 examination has occurred.

## CODING FOR GYNECOLOGIC ULTRASOUND EXAMINATIONS

The images required to bill for a gynecologic ultrasound are specified in the various CPT codes, which can be augmented by the practice guidelines developed by the American Institute of Ultrasound Medicine.[4,5] Transvaginal ultrasound, CPT 76830, specifies a complete evaluation of the female pelvic anatomy via the vaginal approach, including a description and measurement of the uterus and adnexal structures, including the cervix, measurement of the endometrium, and a description of the cul-de-sac and any fluid, the bladder (if applicable), and any pelvic pathology.[1] Similarly, the transabdominal approach, CPT 76856, specifies the same elements for evaluation, with the exception of the cervix. CPT 76857, gyn limited or follow-up, should be used if one performs an ultrasound, either vaginally or abdominally, that does not include all the required elements. This code is commonly used for follicular monitoring with ovulation induction or when an alternative approach is required to view a specific area, for example, an enlarged uterus, that cannot be adequately evaluated or visualized via a single approach. There is no specific code for Doppler assessment during a gynecology ultrasound, either for color flow Doppler or color power angiography. Thus, one must use a similar code, 93976, which is for a limited duplex scan of the arterial or venous flow in the abdomen and pelvis.

Sonohysterography or hysterosonography requires the application of 2 CPT codes. CPT 76831 is for the ultrasound component of the study. It includes the performance, interpretation, and documentation of the study. Of note, the code includes all elements of a vaginal ultrasound study, as well as color flow Doppler. Thus, one should not bill for a vaginal ultrasound or for a Doppler study in addition to hysterosonography. CPT 58340 is the code used for introducing a contrast agent or saline into the uterus. Thus, one typically submits CPT 76831 and CPT 58340 for sonohysterography. Sonosalpingography, also known as hystero-contrast-sonohysterography, is an office-based procedure to evaluate tubal patency. This examination is often performed in conjunction with sonohysterography. There is no specific or separate code for hystero-contrast-sonography. Thus, one should code this as one codes sonohysterography, that is, CPT 76831 and CPT 58340.

A specific code for gynecologic 3-dimensional (3D) studies does not exist. Thus, one should use the 3D codes 76376 (3D rendering by computed tomography scan, MRI, or ultrasound *not* requiring post processing on an independent workstation) or 76377 (3D rendering that requires post processing on an independent workstation).

Ultrasound guidance of various aspiration or injection techniques is not commonplace. CPT 76942 is used for ultrasound guidance for needle placement, for example, ilioinguinal nerve block, which includes the supervision and interpretation of the study. CPT 76998 is used for intraoperative ultrasound guidance for procedures such as follicular aspiration, embryo transfer, or insemination. This is also the appropriate code for ultrasound guidance of hysteroscopy and even intrauterine device insertion or retrieval.

Proper coding entails associating a diagnosis with the appropriate CPT code. One should strive for the greatest specificity for such diagnosis codes.[2] For example, the ICD-10 code for leiomyoma of the uterus is D25.9. Some payors will not acknowledge this general code for payment. More specificity is required, as illustrated below:

| | |
|---|---|
| D25.0 | Submucous leiomyoma of uterus |
| D25.1 | Intramural leiomyoma of uterus |
| D25.2 | Subserosal leiomyoma |

Providing such specificity enhances diagnostic coding accuracy, improves reimbursement, and may increase the case severity and case mix index, which can lead to improved compensation.

## GENERAL CONCEPTS IN ULTRASOUND-RELATED LIABILITY

Obstetrics and gynecology remains the specialty most affected by ultrasound-related liability issues.[6] As the specialty that has actively applied diagnostic ultrasound technology the longest, this finding is not surprising. Errors fall into 4 prime areas.[7] A perception error is when an abnormality is seen in retrospect, but was missed during the initial interpretation. The question is always, “Was it below the standard of care for the physician not to have seen the abnormality?” An example would be an obvious fetal anomaly missed on the initial evaluation. Clearly, such cases are difficult to defend, with 80% of cases lost that go to a jury trial. An interpretation error occurs when a finding is identified but improperly interpreted. The greatest liability of this type occurs when a malignant lesion is called benign. However, benign lesions called malignant can also result in liability actions, particularly if resultant surgery has significant complications. Consultant sonologists are expected to suggest the next appropriate study or procedure, or properly counsel patients based on the imaging findings and clinical information. This point is particularly important when findings are equivocal, or do not coincide with the clinical presentation. An example would include recommendations for additional imaging when a 4-chamber fetal heart view is not seen or when there is a suspected ectopic pregnancy with no specific or clear ultrasound findings. The fourth major area of liability occurs when the sonologist fails to properly communicate critical findings. Personal notification, with appropriate documentation of such notification, may be required with critical findings, such as a ruptured ectopic pregnancy or a fetal anomaly not relayed to the referring provider. This section separately reviews ultrasound-related liability for obstetric and gynecologic ultrasound practice.

## LIABILITY IN OBSTETRIC ULTRASOUND PRACTICE

Ultrasound examination is the primary imaging modality used in pregnancy. Although the number of prenatal ultrasound examinations varies significantly, most women in the United States have at least 2 ultrasound examinations performed during pregnancy. Typically, the first ultrasound examination evaluates the nuchal translucency and is performed at 10 to 13 gestational weeks. The second ultrasound examination occurs at 18 to 22 gestational weeks and involves an anatomic assessment of fetal structures. Obstetric ultrasound examinations are performed by a practitioner with specialized training in obstetric ultrasound examinations.

The American Institute of Ultrasound Medicine practice parameter on obstetric ultrasound examination is endorsed by the American College of Obstetricians and Gynecologists and Society for Maternal-Fetal Medicine and establishes guidelines for standard ultrasound examinations in the first, second, and third trimesters of pregnancy.[8] Specialty ultrasound examinations, such as detailed anatomic surveys, fetal echocardiograms, Doppler interrogation, cervical length assessments, biophysical profiles, or nuchal translucency assessments, may be required in a high-risk pregnancy or when a fetal abnormality is found or suspected.[9] Although failure to follow national guidelines does not automatically result in liability, the guidelines are often used in establishing the standard of care. A missed diagnosis by a practitioner who did not follow the American Institute of Ultrasound Medicine parameters will result in difficulty defending his or her actions.

Liability in obstetric ultrasound practice most commonly involves the lack of diagnosis, misdiagnosis or mismanagement of an abnormal fetal condition. Abnormalities may involve anatomic malformations (eg, congenital cardiac defects, intracranial lesions), genetic conditions (eg, Down syndrome, trisomy 18), infectious etiologies (eg, Parvovirus, Zika, and TORCH), fetal growth disturbances (eg, fetal growth restriction or acceleration), amniotic fluid imbalances (eg, oligohydramnios or polyhydramnios) or a host of other immune-mediated or non–immune-mediated conditions.

Congenital defects occur in an estimated 2% to 3% of fetuses.[10] However, not all conditions can be prenatally diagnosed or detected by ultrasound examination. Therefore, liability related to undiagnosed fetal anomalies does not occur per se when a fetal abnormality is missed, but rather when such a miss is below the standard of care for an obstetric ultrasound examination. Although the ultimate determination of standard of care is made by the jury, common obstetric practice is quite informative. Thus, there is likely to be greater liability for missing an anomaly that is routinely detected by ultrasound examination than for an anomaly that is difficult to detect prenatally.

Some malpractice cases result from a bona fide knowledge gap or skill deficit. A knowledge gap may occur when a physician does not have the requisite understanding of risks related to fetal anomalies and fails to perform or refer for an indicated ultrasound examination. Skills deficits occur when a physician's technical skills are subpar and result in uninterpretable images or inaccurate measurements. For example, a physician is likely to face liability for an undiagnosed cardiac anomaly in a patient with poorly controlled type I diabetes mellitus if a fetal echocardiogram was not obtained. This lapse would represent a gap in knowledge of risk factors for fetal cardiac abnormalities and that pregestational diabetes, particularly when poorly controlled, is an indication for a detailed evaluation of the fetal heart. Similarly, liability is likely when a deficiency in skills results in an otherwise preventable outcome. For example, liability is likely when calipers are inappropriately placed on a nuchal translucency resulting in a false estimation of aneuploidy risk, or when a shoulder dystocia occurs as a result of poor estimation of fetal weight owing to an abdominal circumference measurement that is obtained using the incorrect landmarks.

Many malpractice cases arise not from a knowledge gap or a skill deficit, but from inadequate counseling. In such cases, the practitioner may have performed a comprehensive and skilled ultrasound examination, but did not effectively communicate the findings to the patient, thus limiting her ability to exercise her full reproductive options, including termination of pregnancy. For example, the finding of a fetal atrioventricular canal defect in a woman with advanced maternal age significantly increases the fetus's risk for trisomy 21 (Down syndrome).[11] The cardiac defect in and of itself is a serious anomaly for which comprehensive counseling and multidisciplinary care is required. However, a practitioner would face liability if the counseling, even if fully comprehensive from a cardiac perspective, did not also include a comprehensive discussion about trisomy 21. Specifically, some issues that would need to be addressed would be the elevated risk of trisomy 21, the effects that aneuploidy may have on the pregnancy (eg, increased risk for fetal growth restriction, preeclampsia and other complications), delivery planning (including delivery mode, timing and location), and the diagnostic tests (eg, karyotype and microarray) that could be obtained prenatally.

Owing to the high costs associated with litigation, fetal abnormalities that result in death or significant physical or cognitive impairment have greater liability than those associated with only minor postnatal disability. This is because, in legal practice, it is not financially prudent to pursue a case with few compensatory damages. Of course, the financial calculus will vary by state depending on an individual state's tort laws, but, in general, misses that do not cause serious disability do not have significant liability. Thus, for example, failure to diagnose a minor renal pyelectasis is unlikely to result in liability, whereas failure to diagnose major anomalies, such as gastroschisis, agenesis of the corpus collosum, or transposition of the great vessels, would carry greater liability.

Careful and comprehensive documentation is typically one of the most helpful defenses against liability. Documentation of an obstetric ultrasound examination should include the ultrasound findings, technical limitations (eg, maternal habitus or fetal position), procedures performed (eg, amniocentesis, Doppler interrogation), and management plan, including additional work-up and testing that is recommended, as well as the counseling provided. Practitioners should be particularly mindful of problems associated with electronic medical records that may result in inaccurate or incomplete information. For example, electronic records allow for information to be cut and pasted from one document to another; practitioners using this function must always ensure that documentation for any given patient is accurate and complete for that specific patient. Furthermore, electronic records may have settings in an ultrasound report that default to "normal." Practitioners must be careful to change the documentation when anomalies are found or when visualization of a structure is inadequate such that it cannot be reported as being "normal."

## LIABILITY IN GYNECOLOGIC ULTRASOUND PRACTICE

Gynecologic ultrasound practice tends to have lower economic damages than obstetric ultrasound practice. However, liability cases related to gynecologic ultrasound practice have increased over the past several decades,[12] many related to errors in diagnosing intrauterine pregnancies as ectopic pregnancies and errors related to diagnosing adnexal masses. The following cases illustrate some of the errors that lead to litigation.

A 37-year-old Gravida 1, Para 0 transported to the emergency department by paramedics with complaints of abdominal pain and vaginal bleeding, with the history of a positive home pregnancy test. A quantitative human chorionic gonadotropin (hCG) was 6326 mIU/mL. An ultrasound examination was obtained that described a normal-sized uterus, with a small fluid collection with a decidual reaction within the uterine fundus. There was a large amount of fluid in the cul-de-sac and a left adnexal mass adjacent to the left ovary measuring approximately 3 cm in diameter. The diagnosis was a left adnexal ectopic pregnancy with a paraovarian mass measuring 3.6 × 2.3 × 3.0 cm. The patient was treated with methotrexate and she was given Rhogam, noting a negative blood type. An hCG 4 days later was 16,069 mIU/mL. The patient was seen by another physician with a definite yolk sac, fetal pole, and cardiac activity, with a CRL of 3.4 mm, consistent with 6 weeks 0 days of gestation. The patient subsequently miscarried. A suit was filed. In review of the images, the endometrium showed a definite sac-like structure (**Fig. 1**A), with 1 image showing a possible yolk sac. The left adnexal mass appears to be a left ovary with a corpus luteum present (**Fig. 1**B). This case demonstrates several errors:

1. Interpretation error. The intrauterine gestational sac was incorrectly interpreted to be a decidual reaction.
2. Perception error. The hemorrhagic corpus luteum was called an ectopic pregnancy.
3. Failing to suggest the next appropriate procedure.

Without the definitive diagnosis, for example, a gestational sac with a yolk sac or embryo in the adnexa,[13] the radiologist should have recommended serial hCG levels

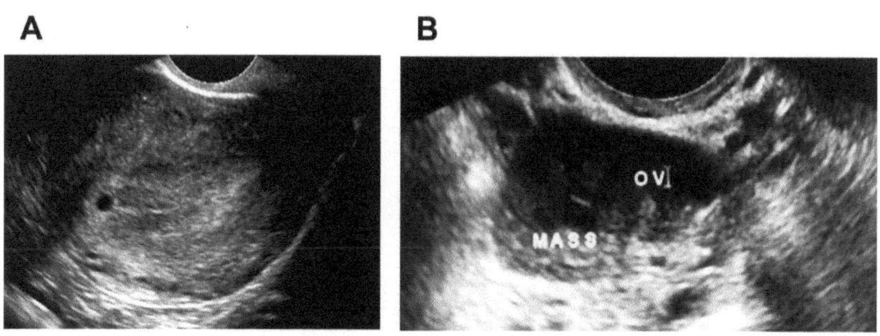


**Fig. 1.** (*A*) Sac-like structure within the endometrium. (*B*) Left ovary (mislabeled "mass") with a corpus luteum (mislabeled "ov").

and a repeat ultrasound examination. This case was settled for an amount approaching the cap in this particular state.

A 46-year-old Gravid 1, Para 1001 presents with a cul-de-sac mass. A sagittal view of the uterus revealed a cul-de-sac mass (**Fig. 2**A), with International Ovarian Tumor Analysis type 3 vascular flow (**Fig. 2**B).[14] The interpretation follows: "Cul-de-sac mass that appears to arise from the right ovary. It is primarily solid, with some cystic areas (**Fig. 2**C) and a papillation = 2.89 × 2.55 × 2.57 cm. The differential diagnosis includes a papillary serous carcinoma, an immature teratoma, tubal carcinoma, other solid ovarian tumors, a dermoid, a metastatic tumor (eg, from a gastrointestinal or breast primary), or an ovarian fibroma. My concern for malignancy is high: International Ovarian Tumor Analysis LR1 places the risk of malignancy at 94.5%."[15] The primary gynecologist was personally notified of the findings. A computed tomography scan was obtained the next day. It revealed a "15 cm complex cystic/solid multiloculated bilateral adnexal masses in the pelvis concerning for bilateral ovarian carcinoma inseparable from the uterus and distal ureters with extrinsic mass effect over the urinary bladder as detailed above. This mass extends up to encase the right ureter up to its midportion and there is mild bilateral ureteral prominence. Small amount of ascites along with hazy nodularity in the mesentery/omentum compatible with peritoneal carcinomatosis. Additionally, there is an enlarged right external iliac chain node and suspicious left para-aortic node concerning for nodal metastases. No evidence of metastatic disease in the chest." The patient underwent surgery that revealed bilateral ovarian adenocarcinoma, omental involvement, consistent with stage IIIC papillary ovarian adenocarcinoma. This case demonstrates the preferred method of management. The original ultrasound examination included the appropriate diagnosis, with an appropriate differential diagnosis. Communication to the ordering physician was

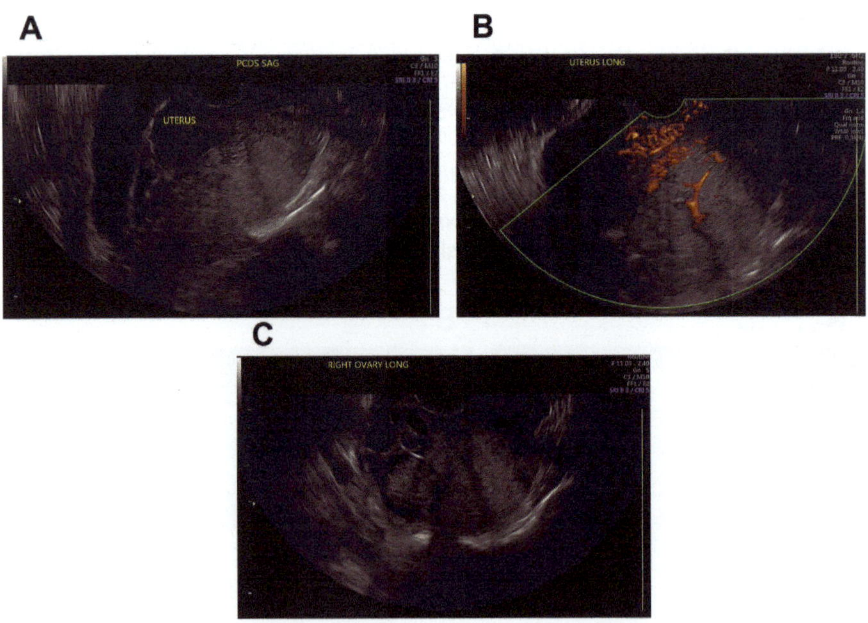


**Fig. 2.** (*A*) Cul-de-sac mass. (*B*) Cul-de-sac mass with central Doppler flow. (*C*) Cul-de-sac mass with multilocular, solid and cystic areas.

timely and direct, which prompted obtaining a computed tomography scan in a prompt fashion. As a result, the patient received optimal treatment.

A 46-year-old patient presents with abnormal uterine bleeding. A physician assistant saw the patient, performing an ultrasound examination interpreted as "negative" and a biopsy was not obtained. Images for this study could not be located. Eighteen months later, the patient presented with persistent bleeding. An ultrasound again was "negative," and a biopsy was not performed. These images were located (**Fig. 3**). The patient was seen 1 year after this visit by another physician, who performed an endometrial biopsy that revealed endometrial adenocarcinoma, subsequently found to be metastatic. The patient died shortly thereafter from her disease. A suit was filed against the original physician, who employed the physician assistant, because he was personally responsible for supervising the physician assistant. This case demonstrates the error of perception, because the thickened endometrium was not recognized. It also demonstrates a legal concept of respondeat superior, where an employer is liable for the wrong of an employee if it was committed within the scope of employment.[16] Whether the physician assistant was appropriately qualified to perform the ultrasound examination,[5] the physician was responsible to appropriately train and supervise the employee, which did not occur in this case. The case was settled for an amount just below the cap in this state ($800,000).

## SUMMARY FOR LIABILITY IN OBSTETRIC AND GYNECOLOGIC ULTRASOUND PRACTICE

These cases demonstrate the errors that are common in liability actions. One further note: many physicians routinely obtain both abdominal and vaginal images for gynecologic ultrasound examinations, regardless of the indication or necessity for appropriate imaging. The Department of Justice settled a claim for $10 million for routinely performing "unnecessary procedures," that is, adding a transabdominal ultrasound examination to all pelvic ultrasound examinations, many without a specific order for both studies. It is recommended that either the order include both studies, the caveat to perform both studies if necessary, or establish a protocol with referring physicians, or within a system, that allows the addition of an alternative approach, Doppler studies, or a 3D study when clinically indicated. Further, one should consider adding a comment in the interpretation, for example, "An abdominal ultrasound was required owing to the inability to adequately visualize both ovaries or the uterus on the vaginal study," to justify the additional studies. Such explanatory language can be helpful if there is an audit of one's practice.

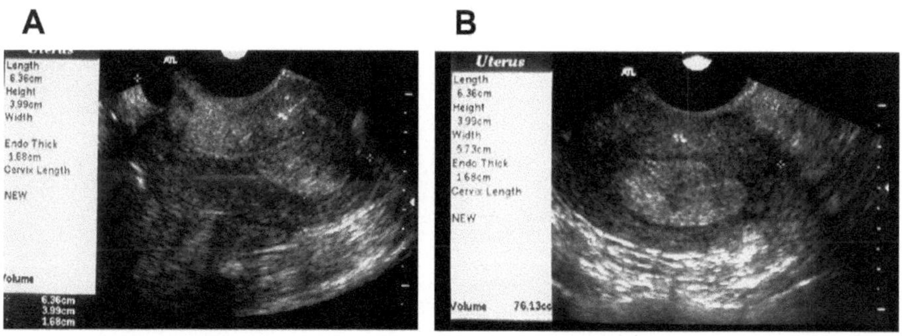


**Fig. 3.** (*A*) Sagittal view of the uterus with a thickened endometrium. (*B*) Transverse view of the uterus with a mass effect in the uterus.

## REFERENCES


1. AMA. CPT 2019 professional. Chicago: American Medical Association; 2019.
2. AMA. ICD 10-CM 2019. Chicago: American Medical Association; 2019.
3. Medicare requirements for physician supervision of sonographers. CMS; 2019. Available at: https://www.aium.org/resources/guidelines/sonohysterography.pdf. Accessed March 1, 2019.
4. AIUM practice guideline for the performance of saline infusion sonohysterography. Available at: https://www.aium.org/resources/guidelines/sonohysterography.pdf. Accessed May 16, 2011.
5. American Institute of Ultrasound in Medicine (AIUM), American College of Radiology (ACR), American College of Obstetricians and Gynecologists (ACOG), et al. AIUM practice guideline for the performance of ultrasound of the female pelvis. J Ultrasound Med 2014;33(6):1122–30.
6. Saunders RD, Shwayder JM, Nakajima ST. Current methods of tubal patency assessment. Fertil Steril 2011;95(7):2171–9.
7. Raskin MM. Liability of radiologists. Legal medicine. 6th edition. Philadelphia: Mosby; 2004. p. 456–60.
8. AIUM-ACR-ACOG-SMFM-SRU. AIUM-ACR-ACOG-SMFM-SRU Practice Parameter for the Performance of Standard Diagnostic Obstetric Ultrasound Examinations. J Ultrasound Med 2018;37(11):E13–24.
9. AIUM. AIUM practice parameter for the performance of limited obstetric ultrasound examinations by advanced clinical providers. J Ultrasound Med 2018; 37(7):1587–96.
10. Edwards L, Hui L. First and second trimester screening for fetal structural anomalies. Semin Fetal Neonatal Med 2018;23(2):102–11.
11. Morlando M, Bhide A, Familiari A, et al. The association between prenatal atrioventricular septal defects and chromosomal abnormalities. Eur J Obstet Gynecol Reprod Biol 2017;208(1):31–5.
12. Saunders R. Changing patterns of ultrasound-related litigation: a historical survey. J Ultrasound Med 2003;22(10):1009–15.
13. Barnhart K, van Mello NM, Bourne T, et al. Pregnancy of unknown location: a consensus statement of nomenclature, definitions, and outcome. Fertil Steril 2011;95(3):857–66.
14. Timmerman D, Ameye L, Fischerova D, et al. Simple ultrasound rules to distinguish between benign and malignant adnexal masses before surgery: prospective validation by IOTA group. BMJ 2010;341:c6839.
15. Kaijser J, Bourne T, Valentin L, et al. Improving strategies for diagnosing ovarian cancer: a summary of the International Ovarian Tumor Analysis (IOTA) studies. Ultrasound Obstet Gynecol 2013;41:9–20.
16. Garner B, editor. Black's law dictionary. 7th edition. St Paul (MN): West Group; 1999.

**UNITED STATES POSTAL SERVICE®**

# Statement of Ownership, Management, and Circulation (All Periodicals Publications Except Requester Publications)

| 1. Publication Title | 2. Publication Number | 3. Filing Date |
|---|---|---|
| OBSTETRICS AND GYNECOLOGY CLINICS OF NORTH AMERICA | 000 – 276 | 9/18/2019 |
| 4. Issue Frequency | 5. Number of Issues Published Annually | 6. Annual Subscription Price |
| MAR, JUN, SEP, DEC | 4 | $322.00 |

7. Complete Mailing Address of Known Office of Publication *(Not printer) (Street, city, county, state, and ZIP+4®)*
ELSEVIER INC.
230 Park Avenue, Suite 800
New York, NY 10169

Contact Person
STEPHEN R. BUSHING
Telephone *(Include area code)*
215-239-3688

8. Complete Mailing Address of Headquarters or General Business Office of Publisher *(Not printer)*
ELSEVIER INC.
230 Park Avenue, Suite 800
New York, NY 10169

9. Full Names and Complete Mailing Addresses of Publisher, Editor, and Managing Editor *(Do not leave blank)*

Publisher *(Name and complete mailing address)*
TAYLOR BALL, ELSEVIER INC.
1600 JOHN F KENNEDY BLVD. SUITE 1800
PHILADELPHIA, PA 19103-2899

Editor *(Name and complete mailing address)*
KERRY HOLLAND, ELSEVIER INC.
1600 JOHN F KENNEDY BLVD. SUITE 1800
PHILADELPHIA, PA 19103-2899

Managing Editor *(Name and complete mailing address)*
PATRICK MANLEY, ELSEVIER INC.
1600 JOHN F KENNEDY BLVD. SUITE 1800
PHILADELPHIA, PA 19103-2899

10. Owner *(Do not leave blank. If the publication is owned by a corporation, give the name and address of the corporation immediately followed by the names and addresses of all stockholders owning or holding 1 percent or more of the total amount of stock. If not owned by a corporation, give the names and addresses of the individual owners. If owned by a partnership or other unincorporated firm, give its name and address as well as those of each individual owner. If the publication is published by a nonprofit organization, give its name and address.)*

| Full Name | Complete Mailing Address |
|---|---|
| WHOLLY OWNED SUBSIDIARY OF REED/ELSEVIER, US HOLDINGS | 1600 JOHN F KENNEDY BLVD. SUITE 1800<br>PHILADELPHIA, PA 19103-2899 |

11. Known Bondholders, Mortgagees, and Other Security Holders Owning or Holding 1 Percent or More of Total Amount of Bonds, Mortgages, or Other Securities. If none, check box → ☐ None

| Full Name | Complete Mailing Address |
|---|---|
| N/A | |

12. Tax Status *(For completion by nonprofit organizations authorized to mail at nonprofit rates) (Check one)*
The purpose, function, and nonprofit status of this organization and the exempt status for federal income tax purposes:
☒ Has Not Changed During Preceding 12 Months
☐ Has Changed During Preceding 12 Months *(Publisher must submit explanation of change with this statement)*



| 13. Publication Title | 14. Issue Date for Circulation Data Below |
|---|---|
| OBSTETRICS AND GYNECOLOGY CLINICS OF NORTH AMERICA | JUNE 2019 |

| 15. Extent and Nature of Circulation | | | Average No. Copies Each Issue During Preceding 12 Months | No. Copies of Single Issue Published Nearest to Filing Date |
|---|---|---|---|---|
| a. Total Number of Copies *(Net press run)* | | | 216 | 207 |
| b. Paid Circulation *(By Mail and Outside the Mail)* | (1) | Mailed Outside-County Paid Subscriptions Stated on PS Form 3541 (Include paid distribution above nominal rate, advertiser's proof copies, and exchange copies) | 52 | 52 |
| | (2) | Mailed In-County Paid Subscriptions Stated on PS Form 3541 *(Include paid distribution above nominal rate, advertiser's proof copies, and exchange copies)* | 0 | 0 |
| | (3) | Paid Distribution Outside the Mails Including Sales Through Dealers and Carriers, Street Vendors, Counter Sales, and Other Paid Distribution Outside USPS® | 94 | 113 |
| | (4) | Paid Distribution by Other Classes of Mail Through the USPS (e.g., First-Class Mail®) | 0 | 0 |
| c. Total Paid Distribution *[Sum of 15b (1), (2), (3), and (4)]* ▶ | | | 146 | 165 |
| d. Free or Nominal Rate Distribution *(By Mail and Outside the Mail)* | (1) | Free or Nominal Rate Outside-County Copies included on PS Form 3541 | 58 | 26 |
| | (2) | Free or Nominal Rate In-County Copies Included on PS Form 3541 | 0 | 0 |
| | (3) | Free or Nominal Rate Copies Mailed at Other Classes Through the USPS (e.g., First-Class Mail) | 0 | 0 |
| | (4) | Free or Nominal Rate Distribution Outside the Mail *(Carriers or other means)* | 0 | 0 |
| e. Total Free or Nominal Rate Distribution *(Sum of 15d (1), (2), (3) and (4))* | | | 58 | 26 |
| f. Total Distribution *(Sum of 15c and 15e)* ▶ | | | 204 | 191 |
| g. Copies not Distributed *(See Instructions to Publishers #4 (page #3))* ▶ | | | 12 | 16 |
| h. Total *(Sum of 15f and g)* | | | 216 | 207 |
| i. Percent Paid *(15c divided by 15f times 100)* ▶ | | | 71.57% | 86.39% |

* If you are claiming electronic copies, go to line 16 on page 3. If you are not claiming electronic copies, skip to line 17 on page 3.

| 16. Electronic Copy Circulation | Average No. Copies Each Issue During Preceding 12 Months | No. Copies of Single Issue Published Nearest to Filing Date |
|---|---|---|
| a. Paid Electronic Copies ▶ | | |
| b. Total Paid Print Copies (Line 15c) + Paid Electronic Copies (Line 16a) ▶ | | |
| c. Total Print Distribution (Line 15f) + Paid Electronic Copies (Line 16a) ▶ | | |
| d. Percent Paid (Both Print & Electronic Copies) (16b divided by 16c × 100) ▶ | | |

☒ **I certify that 50% of all my distributed copies (electronic and print) are paid above a nominal price.**

17. Publication of Statement of Ownership
☒ If the publication is a general publication, publication of this statement is required. Will be printed in the DECEMBER 2019 issue of this publication. ☐ Publication not required.

18. Signature and Title of Editor, Publisher, Business Manager, or Owner
Stephen R. Bushing
STEPHEN R. BUSHING - INVENTORY DISTRIBUTION CONTROL MANAGER
Date
9/18/2019

I certify that all information furnished on this form is true and complete. I understand that anyone who furnishes false or misleading information on this form or who omits material or information requested on the form may be subject to criminal sanctions (including fines and imprisonment) and/or civil sanctions (including civil penalties).